<u>Understanding your automobile</u> and how to service and repair it is certainly useful.

<u>Understanding your body and</u> how to maintain and improve it is far more important.

<u>Understanding Healthcare</u> answers 100s of key questions and contains links to the best websites and other resources.

<u>Understanding Healthcare</u> is a visual encyclopedia—each spread making the complex clear.

<u>Understanding Healthcare</u> takes the powerful tools of information architecture to create a roadmap for each reader.

<u>Understanding Healthcare</u> empowers each of us to constructively navigate through our own patterns of health information as well as those for whom we care.

RSW

The book is **1** Understanding yourself
divided into three **2** **Understanding them**
color-coded sections: **3** **Making it happen**

Each spread
answers a **big question.**
Below are the subjects.
(⏱ = childcare related)

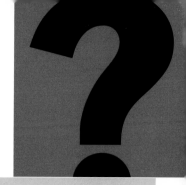

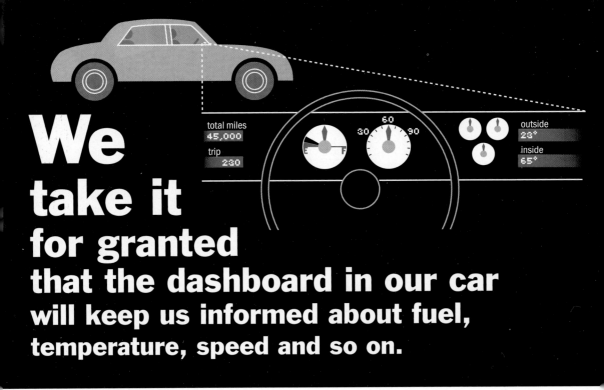

We
take it
for granted
that the dashboard in our car
will keep us informed about fuel,
temperature, speed and so on.

Most of us know more about our cars
than we do about the state of our bodies.

Why not

seek the same data from your body as from your car?

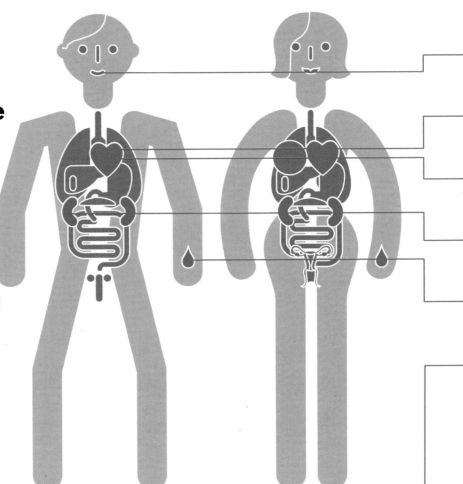

You should care more about your blood pressure than your tire pressure.

Knowing the state of your body is the first step in understanding how to live well.

Suppose there was a dashboard for the body.

What's my **temperature?**
What was it yesterday?

What's my **heart rate?**
And 6 months ago?

What are my
cholesterol levels?

What's my
blood sugar level?

What's my **blood pressure?**
Is that good or bad?
What was the last reading?

What's my **weight** now?
Compared to 3 years ago?

You may even carry it with you.

A handheld device could allow you to...

+ **Get data**
about your vital functions.

+ **Compare data**
with previous readings.

+ **Store information**

+ **Keep others informed**
by sending the data to doctors and
specialists in advance of consultations, or
to hospitals in case of emergency.

+ **Download your test results**
so everything is
in one place.

265

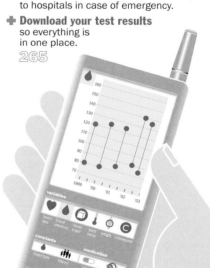

5

The **American Medical Association**, the **American College of Physicians** and the **US Preventive Services Task Force** no longer support the practice of annual physicals. Instead they suggest that patients would beneift more from periodic exams based on their health risks. And, the Task Force says that counseling patients remains one of the most underused, but important, parts of the health visit.

Because there is no definitive list of tests that all authorities or doctors agree should be performed routinely on asymptomatic persons, we have done our best to present those with the

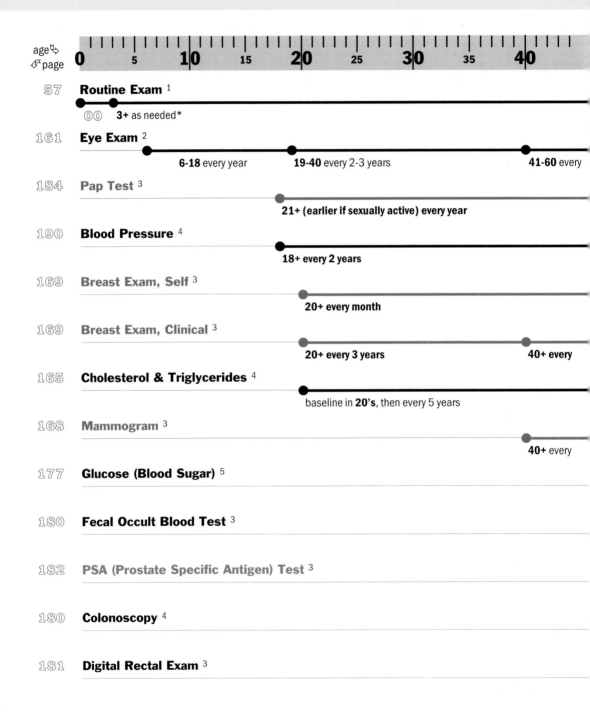

age ↘
↗ page

page		
57	**Routine Exam** [1]	00 **3+** as needed*
161	**Eye Exam** [2]	6-18 every year 19-40 every 2-3 years 41-60 every
184	**Pap Test** [3]	21+ (earlier if sexually active) every year
190	**Blood Pressure** [4]	18+ every 2 years
169	**Breast Exam, Self** [3]	20+ every month
169	**Breast Exam, Clinical** [3]	20+ every 3 years 40+ every
165	**Cholesterol & Triglycerides** [4]	baseline in **20's**, then every 5 years
168	**Mammogram** [3]	40+ every
177	**Glucose (Blood Sugar)** [5]	
180	**Fecal Occult Blood Test** [3]	
182	**PSA (Prostate Specific Antigen) Test** [3]	
180	**Colonoscopy** [4]	
181	**Digital Rectal Exam** [3]	

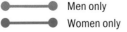

●———● Men only
●———● Women only
[1] US Preventive Services Task Force
[2] American Optometric Association
[3] American Cancer Society
[4] The Mayo Clinic
[5] The American Diabetes Association

Although the tests at right are not widely recommended for purely preventive purposes, ask your doctor if some of these tests might make sense for you as part of a thorough maintenance program based on your risk factors (age, family history, lifestyle, etc.). ↘

best substantiation in our estimation. All are recommended by a major health organization or the **Mayo Clinic**.

These screening recommendations are for otherwise healthy people with no complaints or symptoms, and no risk factors for a particular disease. If a disease or condition runs in your family, or if you have some high-risk history or habits, then you and your doctor should discuss more frequent testing for those specific problems.

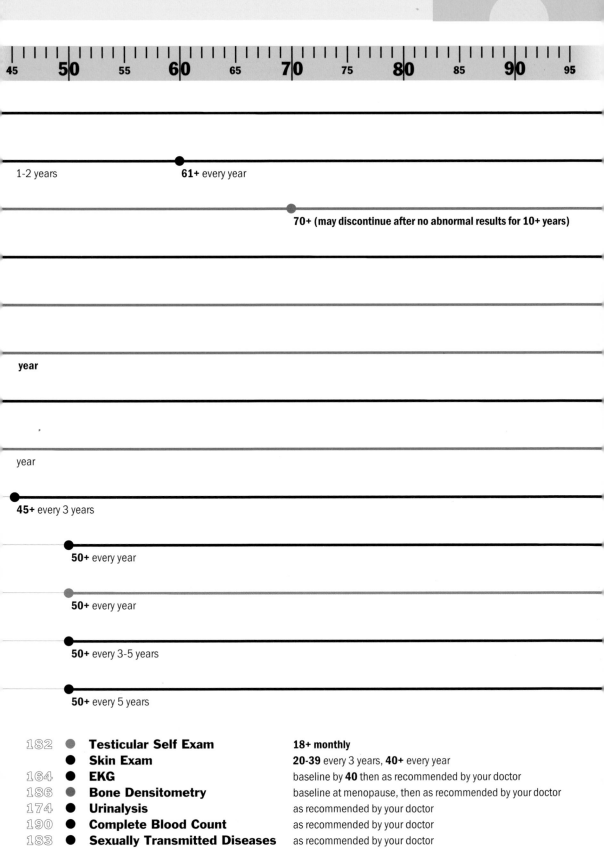

45 50 55 60 65 70 75 80 85 90 95

1-2 years | 61+ every year

70+ (may discontinue after no abnormal results for 10+ years)

year

year

45+ every 3 years

50+ every year

50+ every year

50+ every 3-5 years

50+ every 5 years

182	●	**Testicular Self Exam**	18+ monthly
	●	**Skin Exam**	20-39 every 3 years, **40+** every year
164	●	**EKG**	baseline by **40** then as recommended by your doctor
186	●	**Bone Densitometry**	baseline at menopause, then as recommended by your doctor
174	●	**Urinalysis**	as recommended by your doctor
190	●	**Complete Blood Count**	as recommended by your doctor
183	●	**Sexually Transmitted Diseases**	as recommended by your doctor

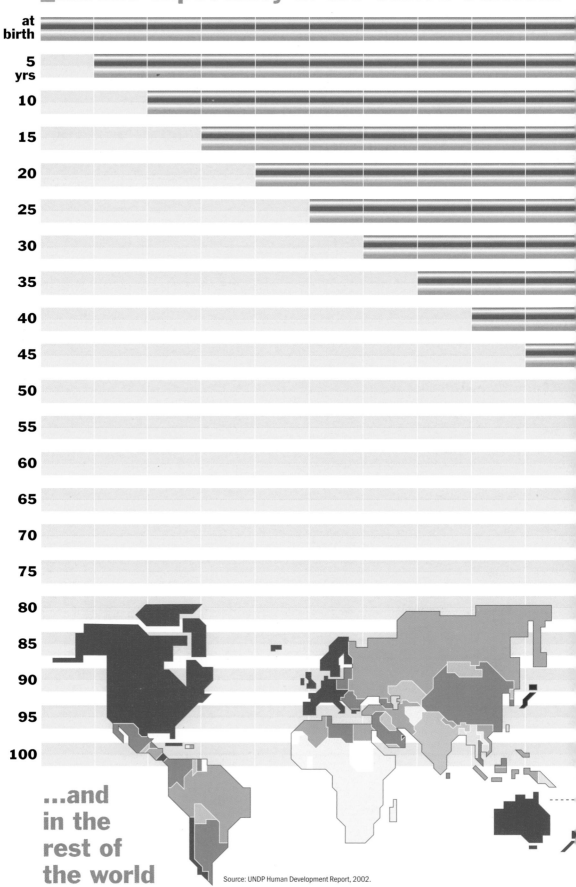

Source: UNDP Human Development Report, 2002.

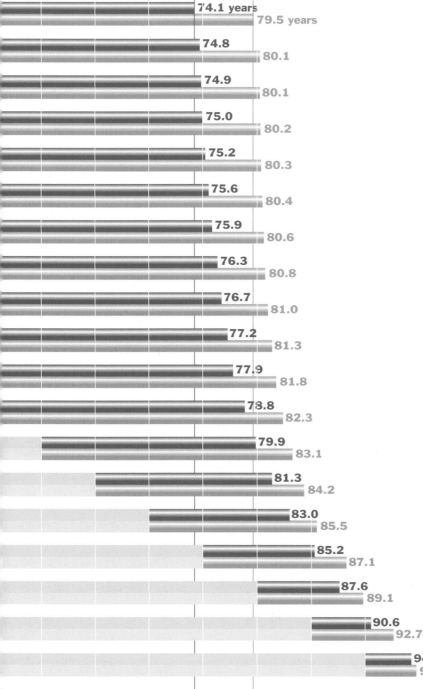

Men	Women
74.1 years	79.5 years
74.8	80.1
74.9	80.1
75.0	80.2
75.2	80.3
75.6	80.4
75.9	80.6
76.3	80.8
76.7	81.0
77.2	81.3
77.9	81.8
78.8	82.3
79.9	83.1
81.3	84.2
83.0	85.5
85.2	87.1
87.6	89.1
90.6	92.7
94.2	94.8
98.1	98.5
102.4	102.7

Horace Deets, former Executive Director of the AARP, was often asked how long we can live.
His answer was:
121 years.
When asked how he knew this, he replied that a Frenchwoman, Jeanne Calment, had lived to that age.

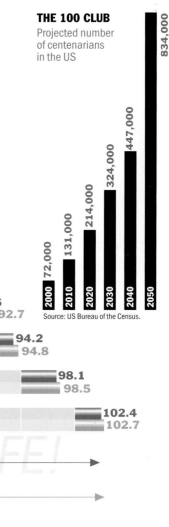

THE 100 CLUB
Projected number of centenarians in the US

2000	2010	2020	2030	2040	2050
72,000	131,000	214,000	324,000	447,000	834,000

Source: US Bureau of the Census.

Men, at birth: 74.1 years

Women, at birth: 79.5 years

KEY Years of life expectancy, at birth

Representative countries:

80–85	Japan
75–80	N. America, W.Europe
70–75	China
65–70	Russia
60–65	India
55–60	
under 55	Most of Africa
n/a	

Source: National Vital Statistics Report, 2002.
Numbers are for 2000, all races, both sexes.

EXTRA LIFE!

❶ Aging 133

If science cured every known disease of the elderly, it would add only 15 years to the current life expectancy of 75 years.

❷ Allergy 125

Allergies tend to improve with age, possibly because the immune system becomes less responsive with age.

❸ Alzheimer's 109

Alzheimer's is the ninth leading cause of death in adults over 65 years of age.

❻ Breast Cancer 93

75% of breast cancers occur in women 50 years and older.

❼ Cancer 87

Nearly 80% of all cancers are diagnosed at age 55 and older.

❽ Carpal Tunnel 117

Carpal tunnel syndrome occurs most often in people 30 to 60 years old.

⓫ Depression 129

The elderly are at higher risk for depression because they are more likely than younger people to have experienced illness, death of loved ones, impaired function and loss of independence.

⓬ Diabetes 121

Your risk of developing diabetes increases after the age of 45, with significant increased risk in persons 65 years of age or older.

❹ Arthritis 107

Arthritis may first appear without symptoms between the ages of 30 and 40. Before age 55, it occurs equally in both sexes. After age 55, the incidence is higher in women. It is present in almost everyone by age 70.

❺ Asthma 97

50% of the people with asthma develop it before age 10 and most develop it before age 30.

❾ Colds 99

On average, adults have 2 to 4 colds per year. The elderly average less than 1 per year.

❿ Colon Cancer 89

Colon cancer occurs most often in older adults. Incidences of cancer begin to rise around age 40 and peak at age 70.

⓭ Disability 135

80% of all Americans will have at least one backache a year. Backaches are most common between the ages of 25-45.

⓮ Dying 137

Two million people die in the US annually, and 80% of these deaths occur in hospitals, nursing homes or hospice centers.

15 GERD 123

GERD occurs monthly in 50% of American adults and weekly in 20%. People of all ages are susceptible to GERD, but the elderly tend to have more serious symptoms than younger people.

18 High Blood Pressure 111

In men, the risk of developing hypertension begins to rise sharply at age 45; in women, the risk increases at age 55.

19 HIV/AIDS 103

More than 10% of new AIDS cases in the US occur in people over the age of 50.

22 Prostate Cancer 95

The risk of prostate cancer increases with age; usually men are between the ages of 60 and 70 when diagnosed.

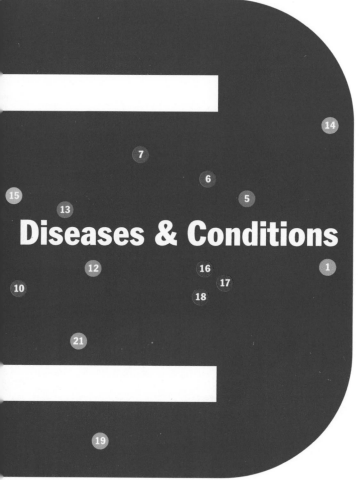

Diseases & Conditions

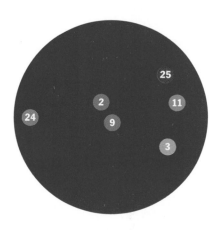

23 STD/ Chlamydia 105

25% of all chlamydia cases occur in people over age 25.

24 Strep Throat 101

8,800 cases of severe Group A streptococcal disease were reported in 2000.

16 Heart Attack 77

80% of people who die from heart attacks are 65 years or older.

17 Heart Disease 75

Congestive heart failure is the single most frequent cause of hospitalization for people aged 65 years and older.

20 Menopause 131

The average woman reaches menopause around age 51.

21 Obesity 127

Nearly 170 million Americans are overweight or obese.

25 Stroke 115

72% of stroke victims are 65 years or older.

Top 10 causes of death in the US, by age

More people die as a result of **medical errors** than from motor vehicle accidents, breast cancer or AIDS. Reports of the numbers vary widely, but some are as high as **180,000 deaths a year.** It is also possible that some deaths due to hospital errors are never reported as such. **Medication errors** alone, occurring either in or out of the hospital, are estimated to account for over **7,000 deaths** in the US annually.

Source: *To Err is Human: Building a Safer Health System,* National Academy Press, 1999.

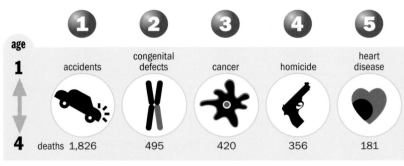

age	1 accidents	2 congenital defects	3 cancer	4 homicide	5 heart disease
1–4	deaths 1,826	495	420	356	181

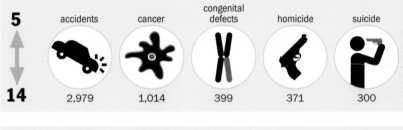

age	1 accidents	2 cancer	3 congenital defects	4 homicide	5 suicide
5–14	2,979	1,014	399	371	300

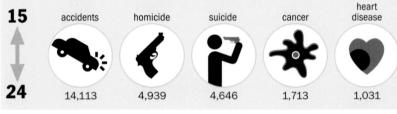

age	1 accidents	2 homicide	3 suicide	4 cancer	5 heart disease
15–24	14,113	4,939	4,646	1,713	1,031

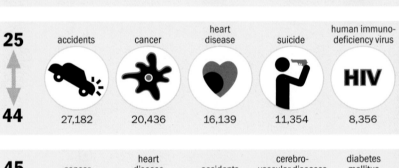

age	1 accidents	2 cancer	3 heart disease	4 suicide	5 human immuno-deficiency virus
25–44	27,182	20,436	16,139	11,354	8,356

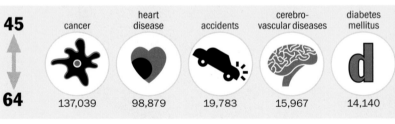

age	1 cancer	2 heart disease	3 accidents	4 cerebro-vascular diseases	5 diabetes mellitus
45–64	137,039	98,879	19,783	15,967	14,140

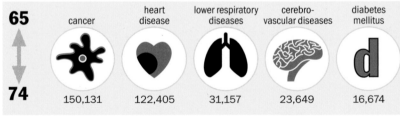

age	1 cancer	2 heart disease	3 lower respiratory diseases	4 cerebro-vascular diseases	5 diabetes mellitus
65–74	150,131	122,405	31,157	23,649	16,674

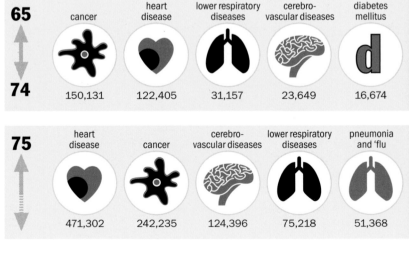

age	1 heart disease	2 cancer	3 cerebro-vascular diseases	4 lower respiratory diseases	5 pneumonia and 'flu
75+	471,302	242,235	124,396	75,218	51,368

12

Source: National Vital Statistics Report, 2002.
Numbers are for 2000, all races, both sexes.

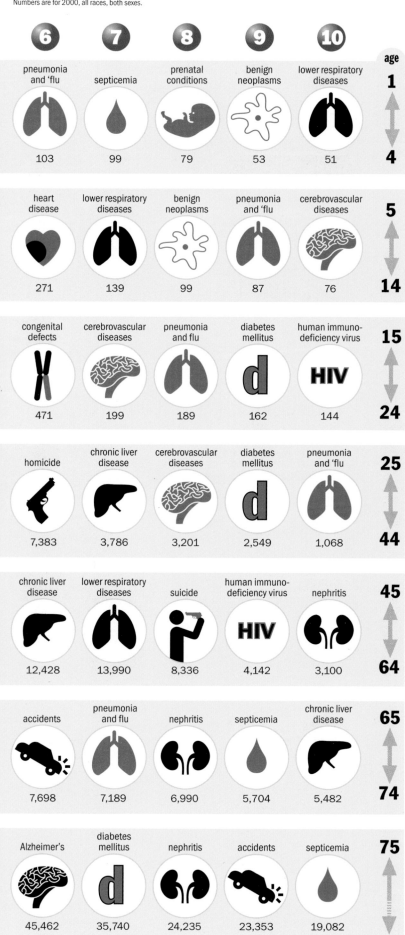

6	7	8	9	10	age
pneumonia and 'flu	septicemia	prenatal conditions	benign neoplasms	lower respiratory diseases	**1**
103	99	79	53	51	**4**
heart disease	lower respiratory diseases	benign neoplasms	pneumonia and 'flu	cerebrovascular diseases	**5**
271	139	99	87	76	**14**
congenital defects	cerebrovascular diseases	pneumonia and flu	diabetes mellitus	human immuno-deficiency virus	**15**
471	199	189	162	144	**24**
homicide	chronic liver disease	cerebrovascular diseases	diabetes mellitus	pneumonia and 'flu	**25**
7,383	3,786	3,201	2,549	1,068	**44**
chronic liver disease	lower respiratory diseases	suicide	human immuno-deficiency virus	nephritis	**45**
12,428	13,990	8,336	4,142	3,100	**64**
accidents	pneumonia and flu	nephritis	septicemia	chronic liver disease	**65**
7,698	7,189	6,990	5,704	5,482	**74**
Alzheimer's	diabetes mellitus	nephritis	accidents	septicemia	**75**
45,462	35,740	24,235	23,353	19,082	

What are the leading causes of death?

Overall, they are:

1 heart disease
710,760 deaths; 29.6% of total deaths

2 cancer
553,091; 23.0%

3 cerebro-vascular diseases
167,661; 7.0%

4 lower respiratory diseases
122,009; 5.1%

5 accidents
97,900; 4.1%

6 diabetes mellitus
69,301; 2.9%

7 pneumonia and 'flu
65,313; 2.7%

8 Alzheimer's
49,558; 2.1%

9 nephritis
37,251; 1.3%

10 septicemia
31,224; 1.3%

The diseases people fear most are not necessarily the ones most likely to kill them. For instance, in a survey of women aged 25 or older, these were what they perceived to be their greatest health problems:

BREAST CANCER	34%
STROKE	1%
HEART DISEASE	7%

…but, at the time of the survey, the actual number of deaths from these causes were:

BREAST CANCER	43,000
STROKE	97,500
HEART DISEASE	234,000

Source: *Archives of Family Medicine.*

13

Internal Medicine
Internist

Family Practice
Family Practitioner

Infants & Children
Pediatrician

Senior Care
Geriatric Specialist

Anesthesia
Anesthesiologist

Surgery
Surgeon

Emergency Medicine
Emergency Physician

Allergies
Allergist

Diseases in General
Pathologist

Cancer
Oncologist

Medical Genetics
Clinical Geneticist

Physical Medicine & Rehabilitation
Physiatrist

Nuclear Medicine
Nuclear Medicine Specialist

Preventive Medicine
Occupational Specialist

Brain & Nervous System
Neurologist

Neurological Surgery
Neurosurgeon

Psychiatric Medicine
Psychiatrist

Head & Neck Surgery
Otolaryngologist

Surgery of the Chest
Thoracic Surgeon

Heart
Cardiologist

Kidneys
Nephrologist

Glands & Metabolism
Endocrinologist

Stomach & Intestines
Gastroenterologist

Colon & Rectal Surgery
Colon & Rectal Surgeon

Urinary Tract & Prostate
Urolologist

Blood
Hematologist

Skin
Dermatologist

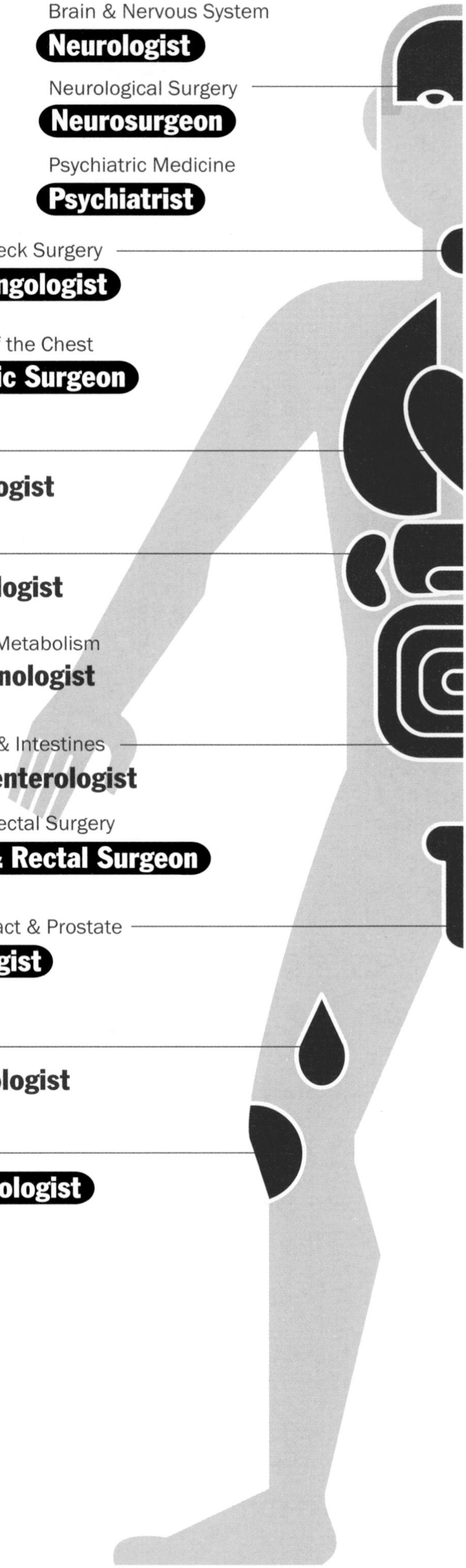

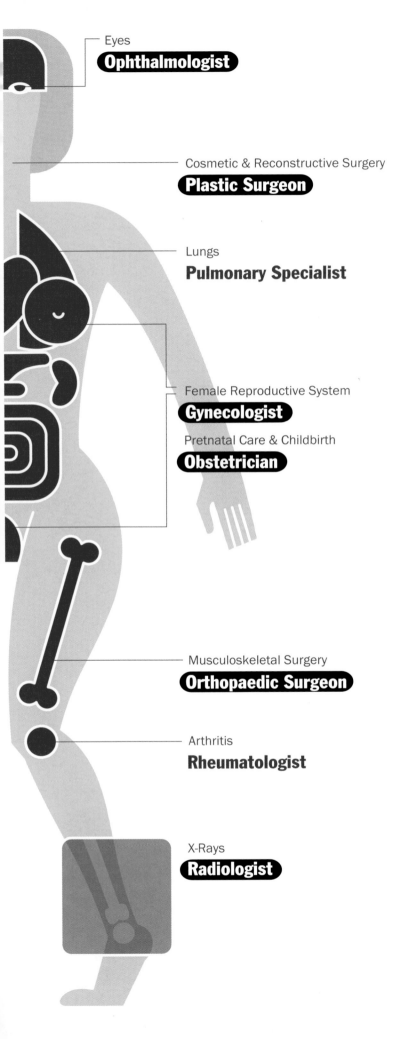

Eyes
Ophthalmologist

Cosmetic & Reconstructive Surgery
Plastic Surgeon

Lungs
Pulmonary Specialist

Female Reproductive System
Gynecologist

Pretnatal Care & Childbirth
Obstetrician

Musculoskeletal Surgery
Orthopaedic Surgeon

Arthritis
Rheumatologist

X-Rays
Radiologist

What types of medical doctors are there?

Twenty-four medical specialty boards are approved by the American Board of Medical Specialites.

At least one specialty from each is shown here along with some popular subspecialties of internal medicine. To find out if your doctor is certified by one of these boards, call 866.ASK.ABMS.

Source: abms.org.

Specialists
Subspecialists

Health facilities in the US

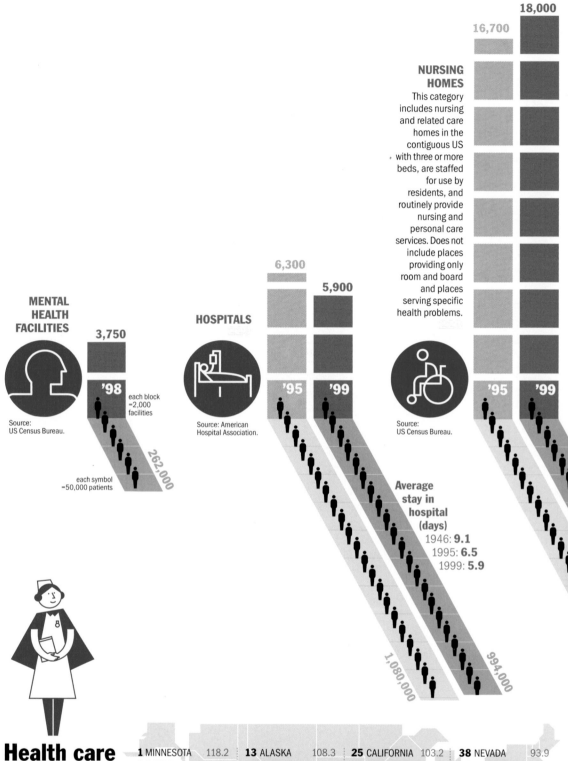

MENTAL HEALTH FACILITIES

3,750

'98

each block =2,000 facilities

Source: US Census Bureau.

each symbol =50,000 patients

262,000

HOSPITALS

6,300

5,900

'95   '99

Source: American Hospital Association.

1,080,000

NURSING HOMES

18,000

16,700

This category includes nursing and related care homes in the contiguous US with three or more beds, are staffed for use by residents, and routinely provide nursing and personal care services. Does not include places providing only room and board and places serving specific health problems.

'95   '99

Source: US Census Bureau.

994,000

Average stay in hospital (days)
1946: **9.1**
1995: **6.5**
1999: **5.9**

Health care quality by state

This ranking was created from data on 46 individual measures relating to health, based on information from medical associations and US government agencies. The average score is 100.

Source: Health Risk Management, Inc.

1 MINNESOTA	118.2	**13** ALASKA	108.3	**25** CALIFORNIA	103.2	**38** NEVADA	93.9
2 HAWAII	115.7	**14** NEBRASKA	108.1	**25** MONTANA	103.2	**39** ARIZONA	93.6
3 WISCONSIN	114.6	**15** N. DAKOTA	107.7	**27** ILLINOIS	102.8	**40** W. VIRGINIA	93.2
4 N. HAMPSHIRE	113.9	**16** RHODE IS.	107.2	**28** MICHIGAN	101.9	**41** KENTUCKY	92.5
5 VERMONT	113.1	**17** NEW JERSEY	107.0	**29** MARYLAND	101.6	**42** TEXAS	92.1
6 MASS.	112.8	**17** KANSAS	107.0	**30** NEW YORK	100.6	**43** ALABAMA	91.0
7 CONNECTICUT	111.9	**19** VIRGINIA	106.7	**31** INDIANA	99.8	**44** NEW MEXICO	90.4
8 WASHINGTON	110.2	**20** WYOMING	106.6	**32** DELAWARE	98.8	**45** S. CAROLINA	90.0
9 MAINE	110.0	**21** S. DAKOTA	105.3	**33** IDAHO	98.1	**46** OKLAHOMA	88.9
10 IOWA	109.3	**22** OREGON	105.0	**34** MISSOURI	98.0	**47** TENNESSEE	87.1
11 UTAH	108.8	**23** OHIO	103.7	**35** FLORIDA	96.6	**48** ARKANSAS	86.6
12 COLORADO	108.4	**24** PENN.	104.5	**36** GEORGIA	95.8	**49** MISSISSIPPI	83.1
				37 N. CAROLINA	95.7	**49** LOUISIANA	83.1

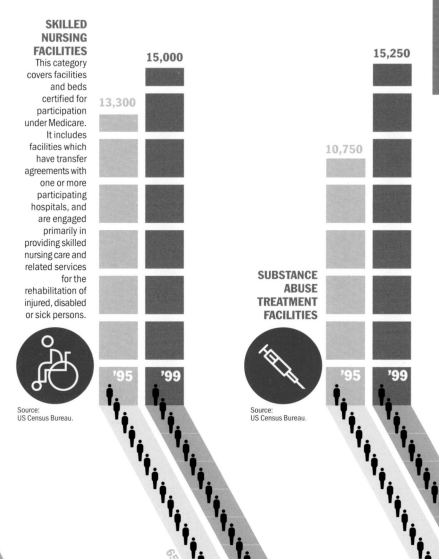

SKILLED NURSING FACILITIES

This category covers facilities and beds certified for participation under Medicare. It includes facilities which have transfer agreements with one or more participating hospitals, and are engaged primarily in providing skilled nursing care and related services for the rehabilitation of injured, disabled or sick persons.

15,000

13,300

'95 '99

657,000

1,038,250

Source:
US Census Bureau.

SUBSTANCE ABUSE TREATMENT FACILITIES

15,250

10,750

'95 '99

833,700

1,009,127

1,038,250

Source:
US Census Bureau.

1,009,127

1,038,250

How we compare

Total investment in medical facilities per capita, 1998. Figures for ten selected countries where data was available.

Source: Hospital Management.net.

	Country	$
1	AUSTRIA	$136
2	NETH.	97
3	UK	79
4	DENMARK	78
5	ICELAND	69
6	US	57
7	FRANCE	56
8	FINLAND	48
9	CANADA	47
10	CZECH REP.	35

Top 10

Research areas funded by drug companies, US
1999-2000
Source: Pharmaceutical Research and Manufacturers of America, Annual Membership Survey, 2002.

1	2	3	4	5
Central nervous system diseases *Psych. conditions; pain relief*	Cancer; diabetes; hormonal conditions	Infections *(viral, bacterial); parasitic diseases*	Cardiovascular diseases	Gastrointestinal & genito-urinary condtions
$ 4 bil	$ 3.9 bil	$ 2.7 bil	$ 2.3 bil	$ 846 mil

Prescription drugs sold, by disease category, Global
2002
Source: MedAd News, May 2003.

1	2	3	4	5
High cholesterol	Cardiovascular diseases	Psychological conditions *Depression, anxiety, schizophrenia*	Gastrointestinal conditions *Ulcers, reflux disease (heartburn)*	Respiratory conditions *Asthma, nasal inflammation (allergy)*
$ 21.4 bil	$ 20.7 bil	$ 19.8 bil	$ 16.8 bil	$ 16 bil

Causes of death and disability, Global
1990
Source: The Global Burden of Disease: Executive Summary, Vol. 1.

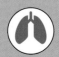

1	2	3	4	5
Pneumonia and flu	Diarrheal diseases	Newborn health problems *Effects of prematurity, poor pregnancy care, birthing injury, et al.*	Major depression	Heart disease

Causes of death, US
1999-2000
Source: National Vital Statistics Report, Vol. 50, No. 16, September 16, 2002.

  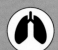

	1	2	3	4	5
	Heart disease	Cancer	Stroke	Lung disease *Emphysema, chronic bronchitis*	Accidents
Number:	710,760	553,091	167,661	122,009	97,900
% of total deaths:	29.6%	23.0%	7.0%	5.1%	4.1%

How we died then: Causes of death, US, 1900
Source: 1900-1940 tables ranked in National Office of Vital Statistics, December, 1947.

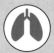 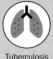

	1	2	3	4	5
	Pneumonia and flu	Tuberculosis	Diarrhea, intestinal ulcers	Heart disease	Stroke
Number:	40,362	38,820	28,491	27,427	21,353
% of total deaths:	11.7%	11.3%	8.3%	7.9%	6.2%

What about your tax dollars?

Whereas drug companies focus on developing new medicines, government-funded research generally addresses "basic science" issues, helping to advance knowledge of human biology and diseases. However, the NIH (**National Institutes of Health**) does occasionally collaborate with drug companies on the product-development side of the process, spending government funds on new compounds and some clinical trials. In these collaborative arrangements, drug companies still fund the majority of R&D costs.

Top 10 drug companies by sales
Global pharmaceutical sales, 2002 *Source: Pharmaceutical Executive, May 2003.*

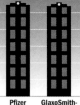

Pfizer	GlaxoSmith-Kline	Merck	Astra-Zeneca	Aventis	Johnson & Johnson	Novartis	Bristol-Myers Squibb	Pharmacia*	Wyeth
$ 28.3 bil	$ 28.2 bil	$ 21.6 bil	$ 17.8 bil	$ 17.3 bil	$ 17.2 bil	$ 15.4 bil	$ 14.7 bil	$ 12 bil	$ 11.7 bil

Acquired by Pfizer in 2003.

Top 10 drug companies by R&D expenditures
Research and Development, 2002 *Source: Pharmaceutical Executive, May 2003.*

Pfizer	GlaxoSmith-Kline	Aventis	Astra-Zeneca	Johnson & Johnson	Merck	Novartis	Roche	Pharmacia*	Bristol-Myers Squibb
$ 5.2 bil	$ 4.3 bil	$ 3.7 bil	$ 3.1 bil	$ 2.7 bil	$ 2.67 bil	$ 2.6 bil	$ 2.4 bil	$ 2.3 bil	$ 2.2 bil

Acquired by Pfizer in 2003.

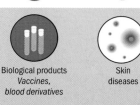

What are the top areas of drug research?

6	7	8	9	10
Respiratory diseases	Biological products *Vaccines, blood derivatives*	Skin diseases	Diagnostic agents	Vitamins and nutrients
$696 mil	$664 mil	$182 mil	$107 mil	$0.2 mil
Cancer	Infections (*viral, bacterial, fungal*)	Blood disorders *Anemia, hemophilia*	Arthritis	Diabetes
$14.1 bil	$13.6 bil	$12.7 bil	$9.6 bil	$6.1 bil
Stroke	Tuberculosis	Measles	Road traffic accidents	Birth defects
Diabetes	Pneumonia and flu	Alzheimer's disease	Kidney disease	Blood infection
69,301 2.9%	65,313 2.7%	49,558 2.1%	37,251 1.5%	31,224 1.3%
Kidney disease	Accidents	Cancer	Senility	Diphtheria
17,699 5.1%	14,429 4.2%	12,769 3.7%	10,015 2.9%	8,056 2.3%

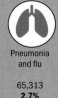

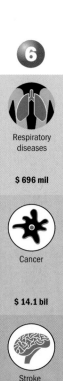

Pharmaceutical companies, which develop more than 90% of new drugs, spent over $30 billion* in research and development (R&D) in 2001. Factors driving increased R&D costs include: the need to treat degenerative diseases (which requires longer-term testing), more stringent drug-approval regulations and economics research required to show that new drugs will be cost-effective to consumers.

*Estimated

Where are the top drug companies located?

(Top 50 worldwide by healthcare revenue)

Denmark: 1
Netherlands: 1
United Kingdom: 3
Belgium: 1
Ireland: 1
Germany: 5
United States: 17
France: 2
Switzerland: 4
Japan: 13
Israel: 1
Bermuda: 1

Orphan Drug Act

In 1982, the FDA (Food and Drug Administration) passed the Orphan Drug Act, which gives drug companies financial incentives to develop medicines for rare diseases like muscular dystrophy, Tourette syndrome, ALS (Lou Gehrig's disease) and Huntington's disease.

US Department of Health & Human Services

United States government's principal agency for protecting the health of all Americans and providing essential human services, especially for those who are least able to help themselves. The Department includes more than 300 programs, covering a wide spectrum of activities. HHS is the largest grant-making agency in the federal government, providing some 60,000 grants per year. HHS' Medicare program is the nation's largest health insurer.

$502 billion (FY2003)

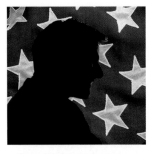

Office of the Secretary

The Secretary of Health and Human Services advises the president on health, welfare and income security plans, policies and programs of the federal government. He administers these functions through the Office of the Secretary and the Department's 11 operating systems. The department operates with a budget of $502 billion and a workforce of 65,000 employees.

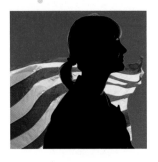

Inspector General

The office of the Inspector General protects the integrity of Department of Health and Human Services programs and its beneficiaries. The Inspector General has a responsibility to report both to the Secretary and to the Congress, management problems and make recommendations to correct them. The Inspector General's duties are carried out through a nationwide network of audits, investigations, inspections and other mission-related functions.

CMS
Centers for Medicare & Medicaid Services

Formerly the Health Care Financing Administration, this agency oversees our Medicare and Medicaid 303 programs.

www.medicare.gov

410.786.3000

$378 billion

ACF
Administration for Children & Familes

ACF is responsible for some 60 programs that provide assistance to needy children and families including family assistance and Head Start.

www.acf.dhhs.gov

800.424.2246

$44.5 billion

NIH
National Institutes for Health

NIH is the world's premier medical research organization.

www.nih.gov

301.496.4000

$23.7 billion

HRSA
Health Resources & Services Administration

HRSA helps provide health resources for medically underserved populations by supporting a nationwide network of community and migrant health centers,

www.hrsa.gov

301.443.3376

$7.1 billion

CDC
Centers for Disease Control and Prevention

The CDC provides a system of health surveillance to monitor and prevent outbreak of diseases. This agency also maintains national health statistics, guards against international disease transmission, provides for immunization services and supports research on disease and injury prevention.

www.cdc.gov

800.311.3435

$6.8 billion

 National Cancer Institute

 National Eye Institute

 National Heart, Lung, and Blood Institute

 National Human Genome Research Institute

 National Institute on Aging

 National Institute on Alcohol Abuse and Alcoholism

 National Institute of Allergy and Infectious Diseases

 National Institute of Arthritis and Musculoskeletal and Skin Diseases

 National Institute of Biomedical Imaging and Bioengineering

 National Institute of Child Health and Human Development

 National Institute on Drug Abuse

SAMHSA
**Substance Abuse &
Mental Health Services
Administration**

This agency works to improve
the quality and availability of
substance abuse prevention,
addiction treatment and
mental health services.

www.samhsa.gov

301.443.5700

$3.2 billion

IHS
**Indian Health
Services**

The IHS supports a network of
hospitals and health stations
that provide services to
American Indians and Alaskan
natives.

www.ihs.gov

301.443.1083

$3.5 billion

FDA
**Food & Drug
Administration**

The FDA assures the safety of
foods and cosmetics and the
safety and efficacy of pharma-
ceuticals, biological products
and medical devices.

www.fda.gov

888.INFO.FDA

$1.7 billion

AoA
**Administration
on Aging**

AOA supports programs like
Meals on Wheels that provide
services to the elderly.

www.aoa.gov

800.677.1116

$1.4 billion

AHRQ
**Agency for Healthcare
Research & Quality**

This agency supports research
designed to improve the outcomes and quality of healthcare, reduce its costs, address
patient safety and medical
errors and broaden access to
effective services.

www.ahrq.gov

301.594.1364

$309 million

ATSDR
**Agency for Toxic Substances
& Disease Registry**

ATSDR works with states and
other federal agencies to prevent exposure to hazardous
substances from waste sites by
conducting public health
assessments and health education training around waste sites
on the Environmental
Protection Agencies National
Priorities List.

www.atsdr.cdc.gov

888.42.ATSDR

$81 million

PSC
**Program Support
Center**

This service-for-fee organization provides support services
to HHS and other departments
and federal agencies.

$452 million

U.S. Public Health Service

In 1798, Congress established
the U. S. Marine Hospital
Service—predecessor of today's
U.S. Public Health Service—to
provide health care to sick and
injured merchant seamen.
Today, as one of the seven
Uniformed Services of the
United States, the mission of
the Public Health Service
Commissioned Corps is to provide highly trained and mobile
health professionals who carry
out programs to promote the
health of the Nation, understand and prevent disease and
injury, assure safe and effective
drugs and medical devices,
deliver health services to
Federal beneficiaries, and furnish health expertise in time of
war or other national or international emergencies.

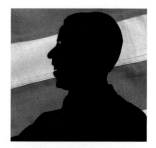

The Surgeon General

The **Surgeon General** is
appointed by the President of
the United States with the
advice and consent of the
United States Senate for a four-
year term of office. In carrying
out all responsibilities, the
Surgeon General reports to the
Assistant Secretary for Health,
who is the principal advisor to
the Secretary on public health
and scientific issues.

 **National Institute
on Deafness
and Other
Communication
Disorders**

 **National Institute of
Dental and
Craniofacial
Research**

 **National Institute of
Diabetes and
Digestive and
Kidney Diseases**

 **National Institute of
Mental Health**

 **National Institute of
Environmental
Health Sciences**

 **National Institute of
General Medical
Sciences**

 **National Institute of
Neurological
Disorders and Stroke**

 **National Institute of
Nursing Research**

 **National Library of
Medicine**

Total budget in 2000: $1,300,000,000,000

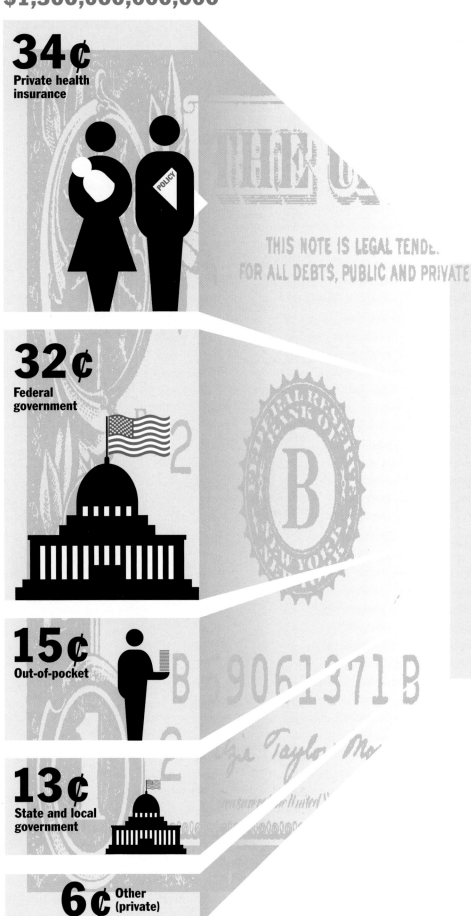

34¢
Private health insurance

32¢
Federal government

15¢
Out-of-pocket

13¢
State and local government

6¢ Other (private)

33¢
Hospital care

23¢
Physician and clinical services

10¢
Prescription drugs

7¢
Nursing home care

27¢
Other spending

Source: US Census Bureau

Something is wrong with the
US healthcare system when people
say things like this...........

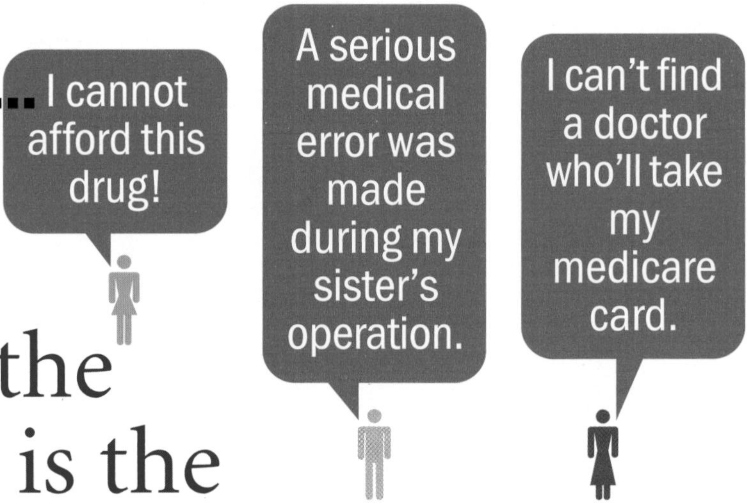

I cannot afford this drug!

A serious medical error was made during my sister's operation.

I can't find a doctor who'll take my medicare card.

"The heart of the problem is the basic nature of the system— the way insurance is paid and the way doctors are paid. The system is fragmented and there is no overall accountability."

—Arnold Relman, M.D., former editor of the *New England Journal of Medicine*, quoted in *Bruised and Broken: US Health System*, in the *AARP Bulletin*, March, 2003

---

41 million people in the US have no health insurance. That's... 20% of Americans uninsured

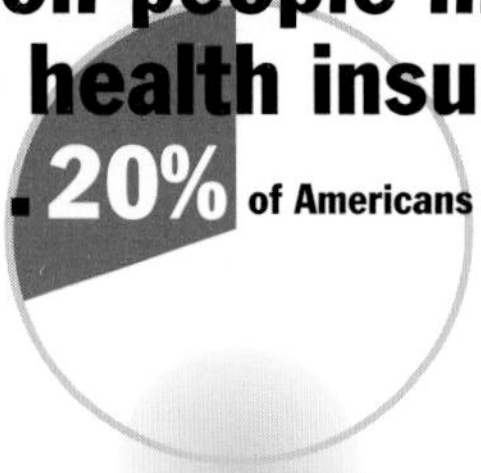

In **1993, 46%** of large firms offered health insurance to early retirees.

By **2001, 29%** of large firms offered retiree health benefits.

Source: *AARP Bulletin*, March 2003.

Amount spent on healthcare as a % of GDP

US **14.1%**

The US spends more of its GDP on health care than any other country.

Germany **11%**

Canada **9%**

Both Germany and Canada insure all their citizens, and have lower prices for prescription drugs.

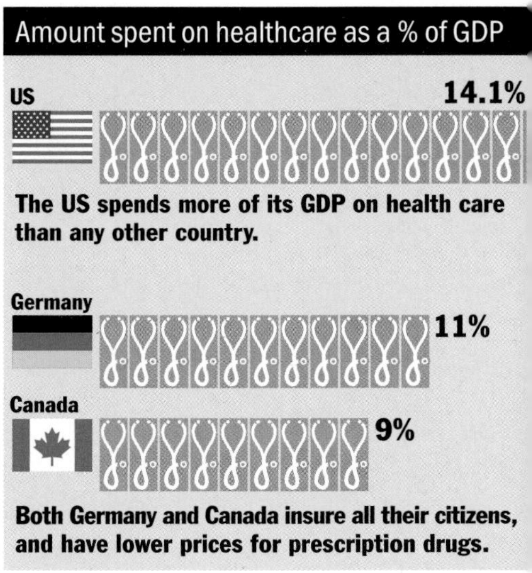

Doctors are paid the same whether they give good or bad care. You have to be on top of all healthcare decisions.

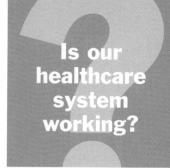

Tips for 3 crucial areas

① Costs

Investigate **state programs** that help pay for drugs.

Fast answer: NO. But there are steps to help you cope.

Ask your doctor about **pharmaceutical assistance programs** offered by drug companies. These are based on income.

Use **generic drugs** when appropriate. Ask your doctor about all your medication options. (Don't be taken in by TV and magazine advertisements.)

If you can't make Medicare Part B payments, you may be eligible for **Medicaid programs** that will help pay these costs. Your **state insurance counselling program** will tell you how to apply.

If you are eligible for health care through **Veterans Affairs or Medicaid**, you may be able to get coverage for prescription drugs.

② Access to coverage

If you leave your job, you must elect **COBRA** health coverage to keep your eligibility for an individual policy.

If you have used up the COBRA benefits and try to get new individual coverage within 63 days, you are eligible for a policy regardless of any health problems you have.

When considering **early retirement,** don't leave your job unless you've planned for continued coverage until you are eligible for Medicare.

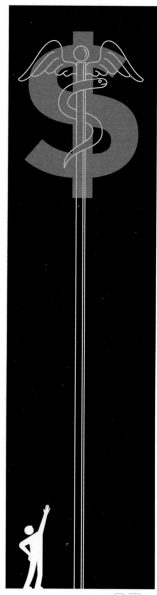

③ Quality of care

Keep a list of all medications you are taking. That includes everything: non-prescription and vitamin and herbal supplements as well as prescription drugs. Make sure your doctor knows what you are taking. If you go to the hospital give your list to hospital administration. If you are transferred to another hospital, make sure the list is given to the new facility.

After a hospital stay, ask for a copy of your **medical records,** and check it for accuracy.

Source: *Bruised and Broken: US Health System* by Trudy Lieberman, *AARP Bulletin*, March 2003.

Keeping track is up to you

Your doctor relies heavily on your medical history and records to make an accurate diagnosis. Often, these vital records are incomplete. **Why?** Even if you ask your doctor to forward your records when you switch to a new doctor, she may only pass along information gathered while under her care. **Doctors are not required to forward records from specialists or previous physicians.**

Source: The Savard Health Record.

? What can I do?

Keep a health file and share it with your doctor. Working together from the same current information helps avoid unnecessary tests and solves health problems earlier. And it's complete because you keep and update your personal health file on a regular basis. It's not easy, but gathering your records is worth the effort.

Ask your doctor if you can get your info via the Web! More doctors are computerizing your health information and some health systems are providing their patients with electronic access to their medical records over the Internet.

Source: Irene Maher's Medical Report.

> **Everyone should have a "health buddy" or advocate to go with them to the doctor's office.**
> Source: The Savard Health Record.

? How should I keep my health records?

The two most commons methods of keeping your records are on paper in a file you keep in your home or on a personal computer. If you have a potentially life-threatening allergy or illness, you may want to wear a medical identification bracelet and keep an **emergency medical card** in your purse or wallet. ·········

The Savard Health Record is a six-step paper-based system for managing your health care and includes detailed information on record-keeping. Check it out. www.drsavard.com.

Your employer and health plan may offer personal health records that you can fill in with your personal information. We have provided some basic forms at the back of this book . 326 — 333 Or, you can find electronic systems online at WebMD www.webmd.com or Protocol Driven Healthcare, Inc. www.pdhi.com . Some organizations offer these free and others charge a fee. If you do decide to go online, check out the privacy and security policies to ensure your information is secure.

Online programs can record medical conditions, allergies, medications, tests and treatments. Some can even store laboratory reports and digital images of x-rays, CT and MRI scans and EKGs. You can then print out and mail or e-mail your records to physicians, specialists or health care facilities.

Consumers are ahead of doctors in this technology. **Fewer than 10% of doctors keep medical records electronically.**

Source: CapMed® Corporation.

Many pharmacies allow you to review your entire medication history on their secure web site.

Source: Merck-Medco.com.

> **Many doctors and their office staff don't even realize that people are entitled to copies of their records.**
> Source: The Savard Health Record.

EMERGENCY MEDICAL CARD

Name ....
Address ....
Phone ....

In an emergency, contact
Name ....
Address ....
Day phone ....
Night phone ....

Medical conditions ....

Allergies ....

Medications taken ....

Living will? ☐ Yes ☐ No

A typical format for medical cards. Others include names and numbers of your doctor and the pharmacy you generally use.

Emergency medical/ID wallet cards can be downloaded from the Internet, to be printed and laminated by yourself. Try www.medids.com/free-id , or www.medcardalert.com.

ACTION ITEMS Medical records checklist

Gather the following materials for a comprehensive personal health record

- ☐ Immunization records
- ☐ Primary care doctor name and phone number
- ☐ Chronic conditions: arthritis, diabetes, hypertension, asthma, etc.

- ☐ Allergies to food, medications, insects, material (latex)
- ☐ Side effects of your experience with medications and anesthesia
- ☐ Names, amounts and frequency of medications
- ☐ Dates of major illnesses, surgeries and injuries (pneumonia, cancer, broken bones)

❓ Why is it important to keep personal health records?

Incomplete medical information can lead to a misdiagnosis, delay in proper treatment and, in some situations, death. More than 98,000 people are killed every year in America due to medical mistakes. Keeping your own records helps ensure that your doctor has all the information necessary to give you the best care without medical mistakes due to a lack of information.

Another reason to keep a personal health file is that it makes your life easier. If you have a personal health record, every time you see a new doctor or a specialist, you have all the information they need to give you the best care. And it may save you from some paperwork. Take your records with you to every visit.

Sources: Institute of Medicine; Wall Street Journal.

Make a list of medications and allergic reactions

include drug names and dosages:

- **prescription medications**
- **over-the-counter medications** (aspirin, ibuprofen, etc.)
- **vitamins**
- **supplements**
- **herbal remedies** (echinachea, St. John's wort, etc.)

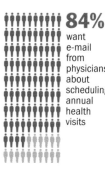

❓ What should my family know about my health?

Does your family know what to do in an **emergency** situation? Do they know the **name of your doctor, your medications and your allergies?** Important medical details are hard to remember and even more difficult in an emergency. Keeping your records and letting your family know where they are can ease anxiety and help you get the care you need quickly.

Source: Irene Maher's Medical Report.

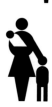

❓ What is the future for medical records?

A Harris Interactive poll of consumers across all age, geographic and income groups shows that **consumers want Internet-based tools** to manage their healthcare:

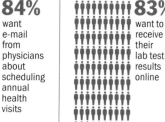

84% want e-mail from physicians about scheduling annual health visits

83% want to receive their lab test results online

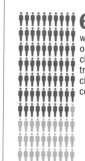

80% want personalized medical information online from their physician

69% want online charts for tracking chronic conditions

Source: Harris Interactive.

What should I know about keeping my health records?

Everything

Know the dates of your immunizations, and health screening results, like blood pressure, cholesterol and vision. Keep records of major illnesses and injuries, and a list of all your medications.

CONSUMER ALERT

Americans change doctors frequently and often see a variety of specialists and other health care providers. Unfortunately, there is no centralized system that allows your providers to share health records or knowledge about you. The responsibility of making sure your doctors have complete and up-to-date information is yours.

Source: Markle Foundation

- ❑ Important factors: deaf, blind, hearing aid, pacemaker
- ❑ Health screening results: blood pressure, cholesterol
- ❑ Health habits: exercise, smoking, alcohol consumption
- ❑ Family medical history tree: major illnesses and causes of death of parents, grandparents and siblings

- ❑ Laboratory reports: blood work, pap smears, biopsies, cultures, urinalysis
- ❑ Body scans: x-rays, mammogram, CT scan, MRI, PET scan, ultrasound

Sources: Healthwise Handbook: A Self-care Guide for You. The Savard Health Record.

Genetics studies how characteristics are passed from one generation to the next. It tries to answer questions like: Do I have blue eyes because one of my parents did? Am I likely to get a certain disease because it is "in the family?"

? What health problems are most likely to pass fom generation to generation?

These diseases are known to have a strong genetic component:

Alcoholism	Cancer:	Diabetes	Lupus
Allergies	colon	Epilepsy	Multiple sclerosis
Alzheimer's	colorectal	Hearing loss	Obesity (in children)
Asthma	prostate	Heart disease	Parkinson's
Cholesterol	breast	Huntington's	Sickle cell anemia

In the last 30 years, research has shown that the genes we inherit from our parents are implicated in almost every disease. But not all diseases are purely genetic in origin: environmental influences play a role, too.

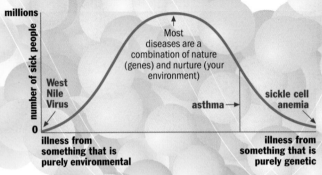

millions — number of sick people

Most diseases are a combination of nature (genes) and nurture (your environment)

West Nile Virus

asthma →

sickle cell anemia

illness from something that is purely environmental

illness from something that is purely genetic

The science of genetics is just beginning to understand how diseases arise in humans. Most diseases arise from mutations of a single gene or, more likely, from mutations in several genes combined with a variety of environmental influences. Scientists are learning that those genes that give rise to a disease may be different from those influencing the progression of the disease.

? Can genetic testing tell me what diseases I am likely to get?

If a disease is caused by a mutation in a single gene, then testing will show that. Some 4,000 genetic diseases we know about arise from a mutation in a single gene. **Sickle cell anemia** is an example of a single-gene disease: if you have inherited these defective genes, you have sickle cell anemia. Other diseases are not as clear cut. For instance, **breast cancer** is a complex genetic disease, and certain mutations of the BRCA1 gene will increase a woman's chance of having cancer to about 80%. But unlike sickle cell anemia, this gene mutation does not always lead to cancer, so some women with mutations of the BRCA1 gene will never develop the disease. In the future, many more tests will be available for gene mutations such as the BRCA1 that show increased risk of getting a disease.

A timeline of **genetic milestones**

1859 Charles Darwin publishes *The Origin of Species,* by means of natural selection.

1866 Gregor Mendel, in experiments with peas, shows that some traits are passed on to the next generation and some disappear.

1953 James Watson and Francis Crick discover the double helix structure of DNA.

1973 Stanley Cohen and Herbert Boyer perfect the technique of cutting and pasting DNA to reproduce new genes.

1976 Genentech is the first company to use recombinant DNA technology.

1982 Genentech produces the first drug to be made from genetically modified bacteria that gains FDA approval.

ACTION ITEMS   Putting together a family health history

One of the easiest ways to create a health history is to simply list all of the people in your family, starting with yourself, and include the following information about each person:

- Full legal name, date of birth, location of birth
- How they are related to you (i.e., brother, sister, maternal aunt, paternal uncle, etc.)
- Ethnic background (ancestry or country of origin)
- Type of health problem or disease for which the person has taken medication or been in the hospital for treatment
- Dates of illnesses

- How old the person was when the illness developed
- For cancers, include:
  - The site where the tumor began
  - Whether it was bilateral (both sides of the body)
  - How the diagnosis was made
  - The stage of cancer at diagnosis

Write down all of the above information for:

- Yourself and your spouse
- Your children and your children's children

❓ How accurate is genetic testing?

Genetic tests can be quite accurate. However, in all but simple, single-gene diseases, **accuracy can be deceiving.** The results do not give clear cut, positive or negative answers. They are percentages that indicate the risk of contracting a disease.

The results of a genetic test have many implications. If a person carries an inherited gene mutation, then **family members** probably do as well. They should therefore have the test themselves.

This raises all sorts of ethical problems: if a person is likely to develop a disease in the future, **should an employer or insurance company know** about it?

The average family doctor today is not equipped to answer the kind of question brought up by genetic testing. They may refer you to trained **genetic counselors.**

In the future, predictive genetic testing for complex problems such as heart disease will be available, and doctors will be able to recommend great care with diet and exercise.

❓ What do genetic counselors do?

They work with doctors, offering information on the consequences of genetic disorders, the probability of developing the disorder and passing it on to children. They are certified with masters degrees in genetic counseling. They take **family histories** and show how diseases are inherited.

Genetic counselors help with:
● family histories of late-onset disorders that have a genetic component, such as Huntington's, schizophrenia, breast cancer, prostate cancer.
● the birth of a child with spina bifida, dwarfism or cystic fibrosis
● family history of a relative with a birth defect or genetic disorder
● A stillborn infant
● recurring miscarriage
● exposure to chemicals known to cause birth defects
● an older mother

Source: WebMD Health.

How do genetics affect my health?

Genetics play a significant role in your health. With the advances made in the study of genetics, we are able to understand more exactly how many diseases or the susceptibility to them are passed on.

Even when heredity is a large factor, however, the environment usually plays a significant role.

1983 Kary Mullis invents chain-reaction technique to make unlimited copies of genes.	**1980** US Supreme Court approves patenting of recombinant life forms.	**1986** Chiron develops the first genetically engineered vaccine (hepatitis B) for humans.	**1995** Craig Venter sequences the first living organism, an influenza bacterium.	**1997** Dolly is cloned from an adult sheep cell at Roslin Institute, Scotland.	**1998** Researchers at the University of Wisconsin-Madison grow the first embryonic stem cells.	**2001** The Human Genome Project publishes the human genome. Source: US News & World Report.

● Your siblings and your siblings' children (your nieces and nephews)

● Your parents and your parents' siblings (your aunts and uncles), their children (your first cousins)

● Your grandparents and their siblings (your great aunts and uncles)

Go back as many generations as possible—at least to your grandparents' generation.

When all of this information is gathered and put into a diagram format, it is referred to as a family pedigree. (A genetic counselor can work with you to put the information into a pedigree format.)

Share this information with your family. Since genetics is a family affair, passing on the family health history could prove vital to the health of anyone in your family or your extended family. Providing copies to everyone in your family is a helpful gesture.

After you record all of the above information about family health history, you can expand your research to include more relatives. Everyone in your family and extended family can choose whether or not to share the family health history with other family members and/or the family physician.

Source: cancercare.org.

? What health problems am I more likely to have if I am male?

Compared to women, men...

...die

7 years younger

...die
twice as often
from heart disease

...have a suicide rate
four times
higher

...are the victim in
4 of 5 every
homicides

...die
twice as often
from accidents

...die more often from cancer, and don't survive as long once diagnosed.

Source: Health Care Directions.

There appear to be **two reasons** for these differences between men and women:

1 men are more likely to engage in high-risk activities

2 men don't use the health care system to prevent problems or catch them before it's too late

Men are at higher risk for certain kinds of
cancer:
new cancer cases, 2001

	MEN	WOMEN
mouth	20,200	9,900
esophagus	9,900	3,300
lung/respiratory	102,400	82,200
liver	92,000	59,000
urinary (bladder, kidney)	59,400	28,100
prostate	198,100	–

Source: American Cancer Society, *Cancer Facts & Figures 2001.*

MALE HEALTH MYTHS

Breast cancer does not affect men
Wrong. Male breast cancer affects less than 1% of men, but that means there are about 1,400 cases each year. So if you have unexplained lumps in your breasts, you should get medical attention as soon as possible.
Source: *Truly Yours*, United Heathcare.

Hair loss is a "man's disease"
Wrong. Female hair loss can be caused by medication, hormonal changes and stress.
Source: American Hair Loss Council.

ACTION ITEMS
Find out more

Men

- **American Medical Association Complete Guide to Men's Health**
  American Medical Association

- **The Harvard Medical School Guide to Men's Health**
  Harvey B. Simon

- **Dr. Timothy Johnson's On Call Guide to Men's Health**
  Timothy Johnson

- **The Complete Book of Men's Health**
  edited by Men's Health

- **The Men's Health Network**
  www.menshealthnetwork.org

Women

- **Women's Heart Foundation**
  www.womensheartfoundation.org

- **National Women's Health Information Center**
  www.4women.org

❓ What health problems am I more likely to have if I am female?

Headaches occur more frequently in women than men. The prevalence in women is

15–17%

versus 3–6% in men.

Drugs are metabolized differently in women. Sometimes the affect is slower than in men, meaning that women may need smaller doses.

Osteoporosis affects more women than men, and after menopause the loss the bone mass in the hip is # 33%

more rapid in women than men.

A woman's immune system is different than a man's. For this reason, women are far more likely to suffer from lupus erythematosus, Sjogren's syndrome, rheumatoid arthritis and multiple sclerosis.

Source: Health Alliance, *Healthy Living.*

Previously thought primarily to affect men, coronary heart disease 75 also affects women in substantial numbers.

In addition, statistics show big differences between men and women in the survival rate following a heart attack:

42%

of women who have a heart attack **die within 1 year,** compared with **24%** of men.

A reason for this may be that women get heart disease later in life than men, and are more likely to have coexisting chronic conditions. Also, women are not diagnosed and treated as agressively as men, and some drugs that work successfully in treating heart disease in men have serious adverse effects in women.

FEMALE HEALTH MYTHS

Breast cancer 93 is the #1 killer of women.
Wrong. Cardiovascular diseases are the #1 cause of death. However, since women often exhibit less common symptoms of heart disease (such as fatigue and dull chest pain) doctors may not notice. Women are protected by estrogen until they are 45 or 50, but then there's a 400% increase in their chance of heart attack.
Source: American Heart Association; *Heart Sense for Women*, Stephen T. Sinatra, MD.

Arthritis 107 affects men and women equally
Wrong. Nearly two-thirds of arthritis sufferers are women. The most common conditions (osteoarthritis, rheumatoid arthritis and fibromyalgia) are more likely to affect women.
Source: *Truly Yours*, United Heathcare.

There are certain and sometimes obvious health advantages and risks to being a man or a woman.

There are many myths, however, about gender differences that are not true.

- **Society for Women's Health Research**
  www.womens-health.org
- **US Department of Health and Human Services Health Resources and Services Administration**
  www.hrsa.gov/WomensHealth
- **Estronaut: A Forum for Women's Health**
  www.womanshealth.org

The growing gap

Both men and women are living longer today than in the early years of the 20th century. But women live longer, and the gap has been growing—from just 2 years in 1920 to 5.4 years today—mainly because men don't take the necessary health-protective steps. If men and women equally took those steps, it's likely that the gap would virtually disappear, and both sexes could expect to live nearly 100 years.

Source: Consumer Reports on Health.

t was hard for me to ask for help," said Carla, a 27-year-old veterinarian. "When I did, I was really surprised about the response I received from my school's counselor."

Like many adolescents, Carla had concerns about her appearance. "I first realized that 'thin is in' when I started junior high. The popular girls were thin and I wanted to be popular. I learned from other kids about binging and purging," Carla said.

"I've always been pretty healthy so I hardly ever went to a doctor," Carla said. "It was easy for my parents to miss what was going on, especially since I would stop periodically."

During her first year at college, Carla realized her eating disorder was serious."

"I went to the school infirmary and talked to a counselor. 215 At first, she told me that I didn't have an eating disorder—that minorities and men

Eating disorders lead to death in 1 out of every 10 cases from starvation, suicide or heart failure.
Source: Eating Disorders, Kid Source Online.

One-third to one-forth of people with binge eating disorders are men.
Source: Eating Disorders, Kid Source Online.

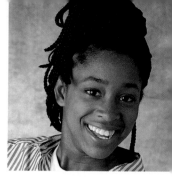

are rarely diagnosed with anorexia or bulimia."

Carla returned to her dorm and thought about her options. "I decided to make an appointment with a doctor. I know the counselor meant well, but I was ready to take action."

Carla called her parents and talked to them for the first time about her situation. "It took some convincing. They didn't want to believe that their straight-A daughter could have this problem."

Together, they saw an eating disorder specialist who outlined treatment options. "My doctor helped me understand that eating disorders aren't limited to affluent white women, though some profession-als still believe that myth."

"I still take it one day at a time," Carla said. "I know recovery will take work on my part. I'm working on it and the support I'm getting from my doctor and my family is making the difference."

Carla persisted and got help when her condition was overlooked because of her race.

Psychotherapy is recommended for people with eating disorders as well as treatment for the illness.
Source: Eating Disorders, Kid Source Online.

Recurrent binge eating, a common feature of bulimia, is shown in some studies as more common among black women than white women.
Source: Recurrent Binge Eating in Black American Women, Archives of Family Medicine, January 2000.

What constitutes a race might seem obvious to most people, but it doesn't mean much to biologists.

Of course, genetic differences exist between chimps and humans.

And, some **small differences** can have **big effects:** chimps and humans share 99.4% of their genetic code. 0,06% makes a big difference!

But in humans, genetic differences are not found along racial lines.

Even the most obvious differences—skin color—can vary widely within a race, and then be similar *across* races—the dark color of a sub-Saharan African is not unlike the dark skin of a Caucasoid in India.

Most scientists see race as a social construct, not a biological one. This means that social rules determine what a race is, not science.

For instance you are considered black if you have one black and one white parent (or even just one black grandparent). Biologically speaking, such labelling makes no sense.

Source: Pittsburgh *Post-Gazette.*

❓ What are some health-related differences between ethnic groups or "races"?

Long-term **alcohol dependence** [49] appears to have a more damaging effect on the immune system of blacks than whites, putting them at increased risk for infection and death from a number of infectious diseases (tuberculosis, hepatitis C, HIV).

A national **breast cancer** [98] screening program showed that white women have a higher incidence of the disease than women of other races.

breast cancer per 1,000 women:

WHITE	7.7
AFRICAN-AMERICAN	6.4
ASIAN/PACIFIC ISLANDER	6.2
AM. INDIAN/ALASKAN/HISPANIC	4.9

A recent study indicates that **menopause** [131] symptoms vary depending on ethnicity.

Japanese and Chinese women reported fewer overall symptoms. African women seemed to experience more hot flashes or night sweats. Hispanic women reported more urine leakage, vaginal dryness, heart pounding and forgetfulness.

In the past, endocrinologists have considered all women to be the same, but this study said that hormonal levels may differ by ethnicity.

Black and hispanic adults are more likely to suffer from **arthritis** [107] than are whites, according to a national survey of 7,500 adults aged 70 or more. Lower levels of education and lower income were associated with the disease. The reasons certain ethnic groups have more severe atrthritis is not clear, but this survey supports previous ones showing higher rates among some minorities.

% of adults seeing a doctor for **arthritis** the previous year:

WHITE	25%
AFRICAN-AMERICAN	40%
HISPANIC	44%

African Americans aged 65+ living in the US are more likely to develop **Alzheimer's disease** [109] than are those living in Nigeria. A 5-year study found that environmental and cultural factors play a role.

new cases of **alzheimer's** in those...

...LIVING IN THE US	2.52%
...LIVING IN NIGERIA	1.15%

Source for all items: The Queen's Medical Center.

ACTION ITEMS
Learn more

● **Office of Minority Health**
www.omhrc.gov

A national resource and referral service for minority health issues, the Office of Minority Health Resource Center collects and distributes information on topics including substance abuse, cancer, heart disease, violence, diabetes, HIV/AIDS and infant mortality in minority populations.

● **Race, Gender and Health**
Edited by Marcia Bayne-Smith

● **Racial and Ethnic Differences in the Health of Older Americans**
Edited by Linda G. Martin and Beth J. Soldo

● **Health Care Divided: Race and Healing a Nation**
David Barton Smith

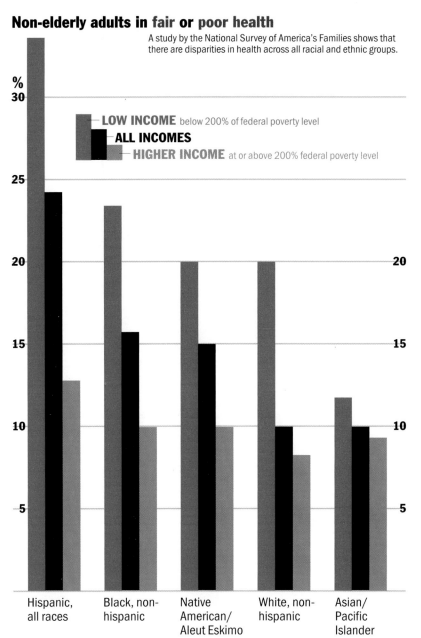

Non-elderly adults in fair or poor health

A study by the National Survey of America's Families shows that there are disparities in health across all racial and ethnic groups.

%
30

— LOW INCOME below 200% of federal poverty level
— ALL INCOMES
— HIGHER INCOME at or above 200% federal poverty level

25

20 — 20

15 — 15

10 — 10

5 — 5

Hispanic, all races | Black, non-hispanic | Native American/ Aleut Eskimo | White, non-hispanic | Asian/ Pacific Islander

Source: Urban Institute, *New Federalism: National Survey of America's Families, 1997.*

As far as genetics are concerned, nothing differentiates one race from another. All humans share the same set of genes.

If race has a bearing on health, it may simply be as a marker for the geographic origins of certain populations.

Source: *Genetics and race: Researchers explore why rates of diseases vary from one population to another,* Byron Spice, Science Editor, Post-Gazette.

● An American Health Dilemma, Volume One: A Medical History of African Americans and the Problem of Race: Beginnings to 1900
W. Michael Byrd and Linda A. Clayton

● Health and the American Indian
Edited by *Pricilla A. Day* and *Hilary N. Weaver*

● Dying in the City of the Blues:

● Sickle Cell Anemia and the Politics of Race and Health
Keith Wailoo

Recent studies show that money matters when it comes to fitness and health. The more money you have, the better your odds of being physically fit. **But,** discussion about the relationship between health and money misses a point that researchers have recently discovered: just because you can afford good medical care does not necessarily mean that you will be healthy.

? How does education affect income levels?

This chart shows the mean annual income for all persons 18 years and older in the US, according to their highest educational level.
Source: US Bureau of the Census.

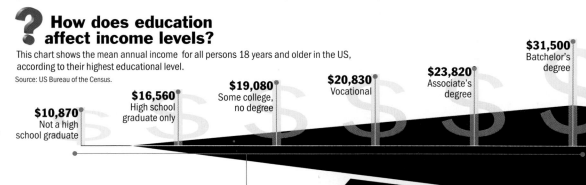

$10,870
Not a high
school graduate

$16,560
High school
graduate only

$19,080
Some college,
no degree

$20,830
Vocational

$23,820
Associate's
degree

$31,500
Batchelor's
degree

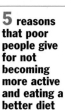

People with lower incomes are more likely to be obese and to smoke, and less likely to wear seat belts and to exercise.

47 million households in the US have annual incomes below $35,000.

In the event of a layoff or medical crisis in the household, **40% of American families would run out of cash within 3 days.**
Source: *New York Times.*

The CDC* says that some unemployed people report feeling sick 20 days a month. (People without a high school diploma are sick on average 7.2 days a month compared to high school graduates at 5.3 days a month and college graduates at 4 days.)
Source: *Centers for Disease Control.

5 reasons that poor people give for not becoming more active and eating a better diet

- No one to watch the children
- Lack of access to parks
- Inability to afford gym or health club
- High cost of healthier foods such as fruit and vegetables
- Neighborhood safety factors

The result is that low-income parents (and their children) sit at home in front of the TV.

Of those people watching the most TV, 62% have incomes below $25,000 a year.
Source: Shape Up America.

ACTION ITEMS Work to overcome obstacles

1 Talk to your doctor.
Take it upon yourself to make the most of your doctor's visits.

Get clear instructions. Make sure you understand how and when to monitor your health status and take medications. Ask questions, and try to get specifics in writing. If you have questions later, call the office for clarification.

Ask questions. Make sure your physician knows you're interested in your own welfare. Ask what you can do to improve your health status.

2 Find a way to fit in exercise.
Don't let obstacles to getting exercise keep you from getting fit.

Make time. If you work too many jobs, try to switch one to a position with built-in physical activity like lawn care or cleaning homes. If you have trouble getting time away from the kids, get them involved with active play like hide-and-seek or bike riding.

Look for low-cost fitness opportunities. An exercise video is more affordable than a gym membership. Activities like walking and jumping rope require only modest equipment. Look, too, for opportunities

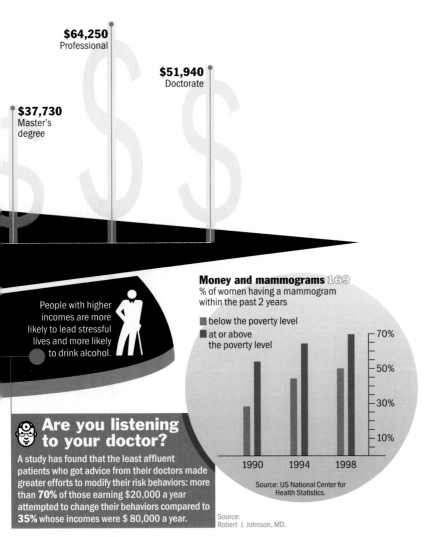

$64,250
Professional

$51,940
Doctorate

$37,730
Master's degree

Education and income levels have an impact on your health, but often in ways that might surprise you.

People with higher incomes are more likely to lead stressful lives and more likely to drink alcohol.

Money and mammograms 169
% of women having a mammogram within the past 2 years

■ below the poverty level
■ at or above the poverty level

70%
50%
30%
10%

1990   1994   1998

Source: US National Center for Health Statistics.

Are you listening to your doctor?

A study has found that the least affluent patients who got advice from their doctors made greater efforts to modify their risk behaviors: more than **70%** of those earning $20,000 a year attempted to change their behaviors compared to **35%** whose incomes were $80,000 a year.

Source: Robert J. Johnson, MD.

How does income affect health insurance?

Household income	people covered by Medicaid		people covered by private insurance		people with no insurance	
less than $25,000	17,600,000	(27.2%)	26,500,000	(41.0%)	15,600,000	(24.1%)
$25,000–$49,999	6,700,000	(8.6%)	54,200,000	(70.2%)	14,000,000	(18.2%)
$50,000–$74,999	2,000,000	(3.6%)	47,300,000	(83.1%)	6,700,000	(11.8%)
$75,000 or more	1,600,000	(2.1%)	62,700,000	(88.4%)	6,300,000	(8.3%)

Source: US Bureau of the Census.

that will get you active. Sign your whole family up for a charity walk or exercise dogs at the local animal shelter. You'll feel good!

Find a safe and enjoyable place to exercise. If your neighborhood is unsafe, see if there is a nearby park or school with facilities that you can use. Otherwise, check the library for information on exercises you can do at home.

3 Get help to quit smoking.
It can be tough to quit smoking. 51 Ask your doctor if he knows of free or low-cost programs or check with your local hospital and community centers for free

support groups. If you need the assistance of a nicotine medication, remember how much you'll save by not buying cigarettes.

4 Upgrade your diet. 43
Try to overcome the "healthy food is too expensive" excuse by checking out some cookbooks on low-cost, healthy meal preparation from your local library. Look, too, for free recipe demonstrations at supermarkets and health fairs. Ask for suggestions on substituting lower-cost ingredients without sacrificing nutrition.

Sources: The Physician and Sportsmedicine, AOL Health News, WebMD.

After my mother died, my mentally handicapped sister came to live with us," said Jim, a 45-year-old father of three. "Jenny has multiple health problems and her care was overwhelming at first."

Jim's mother had died suddenly leaving little information about the care Jenny needed. "We sorted through Mom's things looking for medical records that would give us a clue about what to do. We even looked on her computer."

After finding doctors' names on prescription bottles, Jim began piecing together his sister's medical history. "It taught me a lesson," he said. "I realized that we didn't even have our kids' immunization records. If something were to happen to me and my wife, someone else would be just as confused. I realized we had to get organized."

But the task was easier said than done. Jim called all the doctors' offices and tried to get copies

A Harris Interactive survey showed that 47 percent of people would likely use computerized medical records if access were available.
Source: Computer Health Benefits Survey, Harris Interactive, 2002.

Vaccination records of children who've switched doctors often have incomplete or unavailable immunizations records, which could lead to these children receiving more than the recommended dosage of vaccines.
Source: American Academy of Family Physicians.

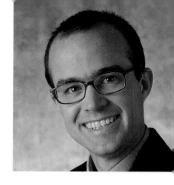

You are legally entitled to copies of your medical records.
Source: The Savard Health Record.

Jim found out that piecing together someone's medical history is hard work when good records haven't been kept.

of Jenny's medical records. In all cases, he had to prove he was Jenny's legal guardian and there the similarities ended. "A couple offices told me that they didn't give records to patients and some charged me a photocopying fee. One doctor kept his records on the computer and was able to email me the information. One large medical practice had destroyed some of the records."

Persistence paid off and Jim eventually gathered his sister's medical records. "At first I organized everything in folders and made handwritten lists. Then I searched the Internet and found several web sites that allow you to store your medical records online at no cost—available to access and print out whenever you need them."

"I learned the hard way that we need to share the responsibility of coordinating records with our healthcare providers and insurance companies."

Some physician practices destroy medical records after keeping them on file for several years. Each state has laws and regulations on how long these files must be kept. Contact your state health department or medical society for the laws in your state.
Source: When Can a Doctor Destroy Your Records?, WebMD.

Websites that provide free online storage of health records:

WebMD
www.webmd.com

Dr.I-Net
www.drinet.com

My Online Medical Record
www.myonlinemedicalrecord.com

? What is the HIPAA privacy rule?

The Health Insurance Portability and Accountability Rule (HIPAA) creates national standards to protect individuals' medical records and other personal health information.

It gives patients more control over their health information.

It **sets boundaries** on the use and release of health records.

It establishes appropriate **safeguards** that health care providers and others must achieve to protect the privacy of health information.

It holds violators accountable, with civil and criminal penalties that can be imposed if they violate patients'privacy rights.

It strikes a balance when public responsibility supports disclosure of some forms of data—for example, to protect public health.

For patients, it means being able to make informed choices when seeking care and reimbursement for care based on how personal health information may be used.

It enables patients to find out how their information may be used, and about certain disclosures of their information that have been made.

It generally gives patients the right to examine and obtain a copy of their own health records and request corrections.

It empowers individuals to control certain uses and disclosures of their health information.

Source: US Department of Health and Human Services.

? Who has access to my medical records?

By signing a **"blanket waiver,"** or **"general consent form"** when you obtain medical care, you are allowing the health care provider to release your medical information to government agencies, insurance companies, employers and the Medical Information Bureau:

Government agencies[21]
may need your medical records to verify claims made through Medicare, etc.

Insurance companies
require you to release your records before they will issue a policy, or make a payment under an existing policy. Medical information that is obtained by one insurance company may be shared with other insurance companies.

Employers
often ask their employees to authorize disclosure of records. This happens when the employer is paying for the medical insurance. Some large corporations are self-insured, and set up a fund to cover the claims of employees.

The Medical Information Bureau
is a central database. About 15 million Americans and Canadians are on file. Over 750 insurance companies use the service to get information about life insurance and health insurance policy applicants. A decision on whether to insurance you is NOT supposed to be based solely on this report.

If your medical information is on file, be sure it's correct. You can get a copy (there is a fee) by writing to: Medical Information Bureau, PO Box 105, Essex Station, Boston, MA 02112

ACTION ITEMS Protect your medical information

Here are some tips for limiting others' access to your medical records:

 Be wary of waivers.
When you sign a waiver for the release of your medical records, try to limit the information being shared. Instead of signing a blanket waiver, edit the text to allow only the release of certain information. For example, "I authorize my records to be released from [facility/doctor name] for the [date of treatment] as relates to [the condition being treated]."

 Be specific.
If you want a specific condition kept private, bring a written request the revokes your consent to release that information to your insurance company/employer. To keep information from your insurance company you will probably have to pay for treatment of the condition you want kept private.

3 Be careful filling out forms.
Be very careful filling out medical questionnaires. Your information could also be passed on from informal health screenings, web sites and online discussion groups. Be sure to find out if a questionnaire is required and who will have access to it.

40

? How can my health information be misused?

Direct marketers can buy your medical information from informal health screenings, such as the free tests for cholesterol levels, blood pressure, weight and fitness that are held at pharmacies, health fairs and shopping malls. **Your information may end up in a data bank that will be used to sell products related to the tests.**

The Internet 325 has many chat rooms that people use to discuss their specific health problems with people who have similar conditions. There is seldom any guarantee that the information you give out is confidential. Use a pseudonym. Don't register your name on these websites.

? How are my doctors and others required to protect my health information?

By sticking to the age-old tradition of doctor-patient privilege. While many states have laws that make it difficult for others to gain access to your medical records, the laws have exemptions; often you lose the right to confidentiality in return for insurance coverage.

When you seek treatment from a health care provider they must give you a notice of information practices that states your privacy rights and explains how the provider intends to use or disclose your information. While they are required to make an effort to get you to acknowledge that you have read it, your signature is not required.

How do I keep my medical information private?

Know your rights and exercise them.

New privacy rules help you to protect your privacy.

? What if my privacy is violated?

Contact a privacy officer. Every health care provider and plan must have one.

File a federal complaint with the Department of Health and Human Services, Office for Civil Rights. This office has the the authority to impose penalties if they find a violation of the law. The process is outlined at www.healthprivacy.org.

Seek state-level recourse. Among officials in your state who may be willing to help are your state attorney general, your state insurance commissioner and your state medical board.

You do not have the right to sue a healthcare provider or health plan for a violation of the federal privacy law but a documented violation of the law may strengthen a privacy case you bring in state court.

Source: Health Privacy Project.

? What do my records contain?

Medical records are created whenever you receive treatment from a doctor, nurse, dentist, chiropractor or psychiatrist. They may include:

- **your medical history**
- **details about your lifestyle** (such as smoking or participation in high-risk sports)
- **family medical history**
- **laboratory test results**
- **medications prescribed**
- **reports showing the results of operations or medical procedures**

Source: Health Privacy Project.

You have the right to see, copy and supplement your own records.

Copies must be supplied to you within 30 days of your request. (The holder can charge you a reasonable fee for copying .)

4 **Watch the copies.**
Ask your healthcare providers to use discretion when copying your records for others. Sometimes more information than required is distributed.

5 **Ask for discretion in legal matters.**
In the event your medical records are subpoenaed for a legal matter, some of your private information will become public record. Ask the court to allow only what is absolutely necessary to be open. And, ask the judge to seal the records after the case is decided.

6 **Protect against eavesdroppers.**
Ask your healthcare providers if they have a policy on the use of cell phones and fax machines. Phone conversations on cell and cordless phones can be overheard and fax machines are often available to multiple people.

7 **Get help if you need it.**
The Health Privacy Project of Georgetown University has a helpful web site on medical records confidentiality that will help you find out about federal and state privacy regulations.

Source: privacyrights.org.

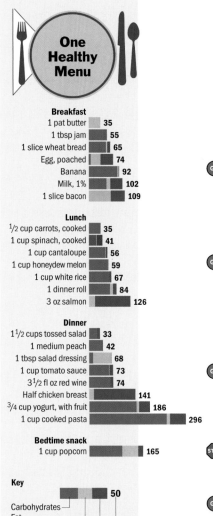

One Healthy Menu

Breakfast

	Calories
1 pat butter	35
1 tbsp jam	55
1 slice wheat bread	65
Egg, poached	74
Banana	92
Milk, 1%	102
1 slice bacon	109

Lunch

	Calories
1/2 cup carrots, cooked	35
1 cup spinach, cooked	41
1 cup cantaloupe	56
1 cup honeydew melon	59
1 cup white rice	67
1 dinner roll	84
3 oz salmon	126

Dinner

	Calories
1 1/2 cups tossed salad	33
1 medium peach	42
1 tbsp salad dressing	68
1 cup tomato sauce	73
3 1/2 fl oz red wine	74
Half chicken breast	141
3/4 cup yogurt, with fruit	186
1 cup cooked pasta	296

Bedtime snack

	Calories
1 cup popcorn	165

Key

50

Carbohydrates
Fat
Protein
Calories

The above sample menu reflects the USDA food pyramid guidelines for good nutrition.

Source: usda.gov.

What nutrients and vitamins support the systems of my body?

Below is a partial list of body systems and the nutrients and vitamins that support them, plus the foods that contain these nutrients and vitamins.

Vision

GO Foods rich in vitamins A and C: citrus fruit, cantaloupe, strawberries, almonds, peanuts and sunflower seeds

Lungs

GO Foods rich in beta-carotene: mangoes, sweet potatoes, carrots, pumpkin, spinach, butternut squash and red peppers

Liver

GO Sulfur-rich foods: garlic, legumes, onions and eggs
Broccoli, cabbage, brussels sprouts, beets and carrots
Licorice, cinnamon, turmeric

STOP Alcohol

Bones

GO Dairy products and foods enriched with calcium
Dark green leafy vegetables
Nuts and seeds

STOP Carbonated beverages
Alcohol

ACTION ITEMS

Eat more fruits and vegetables

1 Aim for variety.
Try different kinds of fruit and vegetables: fresh, frozen, canned, dried, juices. All provide vitamins and minerals.

2 Keep it clean.
Don't forget to wash fresh fruits and vegetables before using.

3 Try something new.
Serve fruits and vegetables in ways you haven't tried. For example, add shredded vegetables to your next meatloaf.

4 Buy wisely.
Frozen or canned fruits and vegetables are sometimes better buys, and they are rich in nutrients. If fresh fruit is very ripe, buy only enough to use right away.

5 Store properly.
Refrigerate most fresh fruit (not bananas) and vegetables (not potatoes or tomatoes) for longer storage, and arrange them so you'll use the ripest ones first. If you cut them up or open a can, cover and refrigerate afterward.

Brain

GO Carrots, broccoli and fish
Fruits and vegetables rich in antioxidants

STOP Too much meat
Too much fat or salt

Heart/Cardiovascular

GO A variety of fruits and vegetables
A variety of grain products
Fat-free and low-fat products, fish, legumes, skinless poultry and lean meats

STOP Too much fat or salt

Digestion

GO Fiber-rich foods: fruits, vegetables and whole-grain foods
Plenty of non-caffeinated and non-alcoholic beverages
Yogurt

Kidneys

GO Low-potassium foods: apples, cherries, strawberries, grapes, watermelon, green beans, onions, corn, carrots, rice, noodles, breads and cereals

STOP Foods that are high in potassium

Colon

GO High-fiber foods: oats, fruits and vegetables

STOP Alcohol

Skin

GO Foods with vitamin A: carrots, apricots, sweet potatoes, spinach, collard greens and broccoli
Plenty of non-caffeinated and non-alcoholic beverages

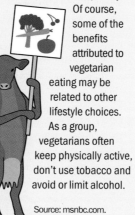

THINK PLANT FOOD, NOT ANIMAL FOOD!
Studies generally show that vegetarians face about a 30% lower risk of death from heart disease than those who eat meat, fish or poultry. Of course, some of the benefits attributed to vegetarian eating may be related to other lifestyle choices. As a group, vegetarians often keep physically active, don't use tobacco and avoid or limit alcohol.

Source: msnbc.com.

We are what we eat.

As Americans gain more and more weight, it's time to take a hard look at the link between our diet and our health. Diet-related diseases are on the rise, and include heart disease, cancer and stroke. Beginning in 2006, the FDA will require that trans-fats be listed on food labels.

Source: Business Week.

CONSUMER ALERT

The nutrition pyramid was created to give the public a clear understanding of what people need to eat and in what quantity to stay healthy. New research, however, shows that the familiar diagram is too simplistic. The USDA is reassessing the pyramid to reflect the new understanding of the complex relationship between diet and health. While nutritionists still encourage consumption of healthy fats and grains, they recommend avoiding refined carbohydrates, butter and red meat.

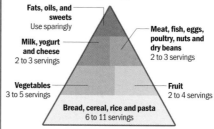

Fats, oils, and sweets — Use sparingly
Milk, yogurt and cheese — 2 to 3 servings
Meat, fish, eggs, poultry, nuts and dry beans — 2 to 3 servings
Vegetables — 3 to 5 servings
Fruit — 2 to 4 servings
Bread, cereal, rice and pasta — 6 to 11 servings

Source: Scientific American.

TIP
Foods that cling to your teeth promote tooth decay. So when you snack, try to avoid soft, sweet, sticky foods.

6 Prompt yourself.
Keep ready-to-eat raw vegetables handy in a clear container in the front of your refrigerator for snacks or meals on the go. Keep a day's supply of fresh or dried fruit handy on the table or counter.

7 Pay attention at restaurants.
When eating out, choose a variety of vegetables at a salad bar.

8 Have a happy ending.
Enjoy fruits as a naturally sweet finish to a meal.

Source: Dietary Guidelines for Americans.

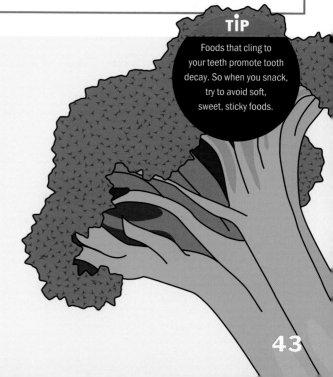

Manage your expectations

Weight loss is a $30-billion industry with skimpy results. Hope usually outruns common sense and willpower. Of 50 million Americans who'll diet this year, only 5% will manage to stay thinner in the long run.

Ideally speaking

Gender, age and other factors influence the ideal weight for your height. A few guidelines:

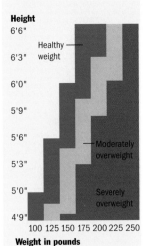

Source: US Food & Drug Administration.

Feature	Pros
THE ZONE	
Food is consumed in exact proportions of carbohydrates, protein and fat—40/30/30. The average number of calories consumed per day is about 1,400.	Fairly easy to follow since the average American diet is already about 40/30/30. Saturated fat consumption is lowered.
ATKINS DIET	
Eat all the protein you want as long as you eliminate sugar and carbohydrates. Plan allows between 1,200 and 1,800 calories per day.	Simple and easy to follow. Significant calories are eliminated through the restriction of carbs and sugar.
PRITIKIN/ORNISH DIETS	
This diet restricts fat intake to 10–15% of total calories. Consumption of complex, fibrous CHO's such as fruits and vegetables is encouraged.	Low fat reduces calories and the risk of heart disease.
BLOOD TYPE DIET	
Foods to eat or avoid are chosen based on your blood type (A, B, AB, or O.) Calorie restriction is not severe.	All blood types are encouraged to eat fruits and vegetables along with lean sources of protein.
GRAPEFRUIT DIET	
Requires you to eat one grapefruit at every meal, with small amounts of protein, black coffee, and salad. Average calorie consumption: 800 per day.	You will get high amounts of vitamin C and fiber.
CAVEMAN DIET	
Processed foods are replaced with lean meats, nuts, berries, fresh fruits and salads.	Whole foods are more nutritious than processed foods. Calories are not severely restricted.
CABBAGE SOUP DIET	
This is a seven-day diet with severe calorie restrictions. It consists of eating a vegetable-based soup (cabbage, onions, peppers, tomatoes and celery.)	Rapid weight loss.

ACTION ITEMS Get the skinny on these diets

The Zone

The Zone
Barry Sears, with Bill Lawren

A Revolutionary Life Plan to Put Your Body in Total Balance for Permanent Weight Loss

www.drsears.com

Atkins Diet

Dr. Atkins' New Diet Revolution
Robert C. Atkins

www.atkins.com

Pritikin Diet

The Pritikin Weight Loss Breakthrough
Robert Pritikin

5 Easy Steps to Outsmart Your Fat Instinct

www.pritikin.com

Ornish Diet

Eat More, Weigh Less
Dean Ornish

Dr. Dean Ornish's Life Choice Program for Losing Weight Safely While Eating Abundantly

www.ornish.com

Cons	Daily calorie count (not to exceed)

Plan is difficult to maintain since the number of calories is so low.

1400

All pose some risk; few offer permanent results.

High protein intake can increase saturated fats, leading to risk of heart disease. Low in whole grains, fruit and fiber necessary for good health.

1800

Sudden, radical changes in your eating habits are almost impossible to sustain. Better solution: Set goals with your doctor's advice, eat less of a balanced selection of food.

A diet low in fat is difficult to maintain over time. Users don't always distinguish between good fats found in fish and vegetables, and bad fats, like butter.

1500

Food suggestions are unusual and can be hard to find. Difficult for families with differing blood types. Not supported by scientific research.

Varies according to blood type and ancestry

NO FAST FIXES FOR FAT!
Quick and easy solutions just don't work but exercise and calorie control do. Be sure to consult your doctor to set sensible goals for weight loss based on your height, build and age.

Source: fda.gov.

This diet is nutritionally deficient and since the caloric intake is so restricted it is difficult to maintain for very long.

800

Does nothing to counter the carbohydrate craving, and weight gain will occur as carbohydrates are added back.

3000

Weight lost—mostly water— is temporary and is practically impossible to maintain.

1000

TIP
Don't even try to lose more than two pounds per week. You'll stress yourself mentally and physically, and you'll never keep it off.

Blood Type Diet

Eat Right 4 Your Type
Peter J. D'Adamo, with Catherine Whitney

The Individualized Diet Solution to Staying Healthy, Living Longer and Achieving Your Ideal Weight

www.dadamo.com

The Caveman Diet

Neanderthin
Ray V. Audette, Troy Gilchrist, Michael Eades and Tony Gilchrist

Eat Like a Caveman to Achieve a Lean, Strong, Healthy Body

www.neanderthin.com

Cabbage Soup Diet

The New Cabbage Soup Diet
Margaret Danbrot

Can you afford to take it easy?

A study in the October issue of *The Physician and Sportsmedicine* found that physically active individuals had lower direct annual medical costs than inactive people. The cost difference was

$865 per person.

The potential savings if all inactive American adults became physically active could be as much as

$76.6 billion.

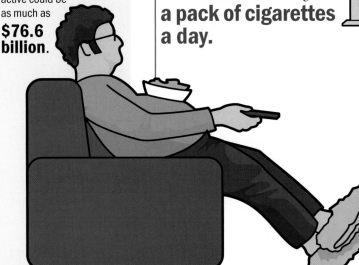

Estimates are that **250,000 deaths** per year in the US—about 12 percent of total deaths—are due to a lack of regular physical activity.

COUCH POTATO

No exercise

3 times as many adults with incomes below the poverty level are as likely to be physically inactive as adults in the highest income group.

28% of Americans age 18 or older aren't active at all.

An inactive lifestyle increases your risk of heart disease as much as smoking **a pack of cigarettes a day.**

OFFICE WORKER

Occasional exercise

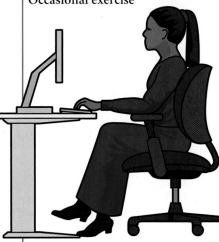

44% of adults get some exercise but don't do it regularly or intensely enough to protect their hearts.

34 million (33%) Americans are obese (20% overweight).

RISKS

 High blood pressure 111 and progressive heart disease 75

 Buildup of excess fat, possibly leading to obesity 127

 Clinical depression, lethargy and anxiety 129

ACTION ITEMS

Find the time to exercise

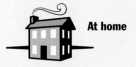 At home

- Work in the garden or mow the grass. Using a riding mower doesn't count! Rake leaves, prune, dig and pick up trash.
- Go out for a short walk before breakfast, after dinner or both! Start with 5–10 minutes and work up to 30 minutes.
- Walk or bike to the corner store instead of driving.
- When walking, pick up the pace from leisurely to brisk. Choose a hilly route.
- Stand up while talking on the phone.
- Walk the dog.

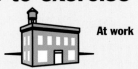 At work

- Brainstorm project ideas with a coworker while taking a walk.
- Walk down the hall to speak with someone rather than using the phone.
- Take the stairs instead of the elevator.
- Stay at hotels with fitness centers or swimming pools–and use them–while on business trips.
- Join a fitness center near your job. Exercise before or after work to avoid rush-hour traffic.
- Get off the bus a few blocks early and walk the rest of the way to work or home.
- Walk around your building for a break during the day or during lunch.

OUTDOOR PERSON

Frequent exercise

27% of American adults get enough leisure-time exercise to achieve cardiovascular fitness.

30 minutes a day is the minimum adults should spend doing aerobic and strength-building activities.

Light or moderate activity is defined as exercise lasting at least 10 minutes. The activity should cause light sweating or a slight to moderate rise in breathing and heart rate.

ATHLETE

Faithful exercise

21.3% of men and **16.9%** of women engage in a high level of overall physical activity.

1 in 4 adults with an advanced degree engages in a high level of overall physical activity.

1 in 7 adults without a high school diploma engages in a high level of physical activity.

31% of American adults engage in regular leisure-time physical activity.

Vigorous activity is defined as exercise that causes profuse sweating, heavy breathing and a pounding heart rate.

How does exercise affect my health?

Exercise keeps your body running efficiently.

Although most people know that exercise is good for them, many do not realize the dangers of not exercising. Our bodies are designed for exercise. Without it, we break down.

Source: med.umich.edu.

WHAT'S AN EFFECTIVE EXERCISE SESSION?

Warm-up:	5 minutes
Aerobic activity:	5 to 10 minutes at first, then gradually increasing to 45 minutes
Cool-down:	5 minutes
Stretching:	5 to 10 minutes

BENEFITS

 Blood pressure control and cardio-vascular health

 Healthier bones, limber muscles and joints

 Reduced risk of colon cancer 89 and Type 2 diabetes 121

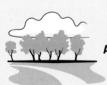 **At play**

- Plan outings and vacations that include physical activity (hiking, backpacking, swimming, etc.)
- See the sights in new cities by walking, jogging or bicycling.
- Dance with someone or by yourself. Take dancing lessons. Hit the dance floor on fast numbers instead of slow ones.
- Join a recreational club that emphasizes physical activity.
- At the beach, sit and watch the waves instead of lying flat. Better yet, get up and walk, run or fly a kite.
- When golfing, walk instead of using a cart.

- Play singles tennis or racquetball instead of doubles.
- At a picnic, join in a game of volleyball or badminton.
- At the lake, rent a rowboat or canoe instead of a powerboat.

Source: American Heart Association.

58,960

LIGHT DRINKING

Research shows that moderate amounts of alcohol can reduce the risk of cardiovascular disease.
75

MODERATE DRINKING

People who drink regularly can develop a tolerance to alcohol. They then need to drink more to experience the same effect.

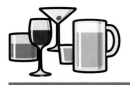

BINGE DRINKING

Drinking heavily over a short period can cause hangovers, headaches, nausea, shakiness and vomiting.

LONG-TERM EFFECTS

If you drink heavily over a long period of time, alcohol can have a negative effect on the body's systems.

Brain and Nervous System
- Loss of memory
- Confusion
- Hallucinations
- Tingling
- Loss of sensation in hands and feet

Lungs
- Greater chance of infections

Heart
- High blood pressure
  111
- Irregular pulse
- Enlarged heart

Liver
- Severe swelling and pain
- Hepatitis
- Cirrhosis
- Liver cancer

Pancreas
- Inflammation

Skin
- Flushing
- Sweating
- Bruising

Digestive Tract
- Cancer of airway and digestive tract, including mouth, pharynx, larynx, esophagus
- Bleeding stomach, ulcers

Reproductive System
- Impotence
- Shrunken testicles
- Damaged and/or fewer sperm
- Greater risk of gynecological problems
- Damage to fetus if pregnant

ACTION ITEMS

Learn how to spot problem drinking

Alcoholics Anonymous® is a fellowship of men and women who share their experience, strength and hope to solve their common problem and help others recover from alcoholism.

AA uses the following quiz to help people face alcoholism. Answer yes or no to each question. If you answer yes four or more times, you may be in trouble with alcohol.

1. Have you ever decided to stop drinking for a week or so, but only lasted for a couple of days?

2. Do you wish people would mind their own business about your drinking and stop telling you what to do?

3. Have you ever switched from one kind of drink to another in the hope that this would keep you from getting drunk?

4. Have you had to have a morning eye-opener during the past year?

alcohol-induced deaths

occurred in the United States in 2000. Here's the breakdown: **26,552** deaths from cirrhosis and chronic liver disease; **13,050** deaths from auto accidents; and **19,358** deaths from other alcohol-induced afflictions.

Source: cdc.gov.nchs.

Alcohol is a depressant drug, not a stimulant as many people think.

It slows down the activity of the central nervous system, including the brain, affecting concentration and coordination and slowing down response times in unexpected situations.

In small quantities, alcohol can make people more relaxed, confident and extroverted. In larger quantities, alcohol has been blamed for many chronic illnesses and diseases.

Source: adf.org.au.

? Can a glass of wine a day be good for me?

Yes. One drink per day has been shown to be the amount of alcohol for balancing the cardiovascular benefit with the increase in risk for other health problems.

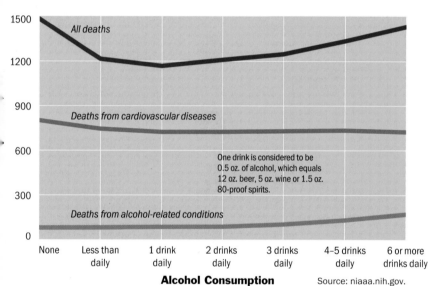

All deaths

Deaths from cardiovascular diseases

One drink is considered to be 0.5 oz. of alcohol, which equals 12 oz. beer, 5 oz. wine or 1.5 oz. 80-proof spirits.

Deaths from alcohol-related conditions

| None | Less than daily | 1 drink daily | 2 drinks daily | 3 drinks daily | 4–5 drinks daily | 6 or more drinks daily |

Alcohol Consumption

Source: niaaa.nih.gov.

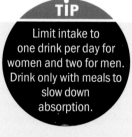

TIP

Limit intake to one drink per day for women and two for men. Drink only with meals to slow down absorption.

5 Do you envy people who can drink without getting into trouble?

6 Have you had problems connected with drinking during the past year?

7 Has your drinking caused trouble at home?

8 Do you ever try to get extra drinks at a party because you do not get enough?

9 Do you tell yourself you can stop drinking any time you want to, even though you keep getting drunk when you don't mean to?

10 Have you missed days of work or school because of drinking?

11 Do you have blackouts?

12 Have you ever felt that your life would be better if you did not drink?

Source: aa.org.

There are over **4,000** chemicals in tobacco smoke, many of which are poisonous, and 43 alone have been proven to be carcinogenic. They include:

Nicotine The drug that causes addiction. Nicotine addiction is said to be as strong or stronger than heroin addiction.

Tar The main cause of lung and throat cancer in smokers.

Carbon monoxide A colorless, odorless and very toxic gas which the lungs take up more readily than oxygen.

Smoking-Related Deaths

Source: kickbutt.org.

For every 1,000 smokers, 6 will die by homicide, 12 from auto accidents, and 500 from smoking-related causes. **Each icon represents 2 people.**

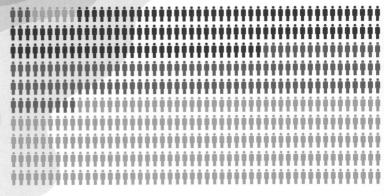

- Homicide
- Auto accident
- Smoking-related death in middle age
- Smoking-related death in old age
- Smokers who will die a non-smoking related death

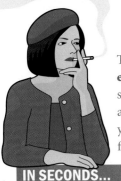

The **negative effects** of smoking begin as soon as you take that first puff.

DAYS...

You may experience nausea, dizziness, watery eyes and acid in the stomach.

Appetite, taste and smell are weakened.

The flow of blood to extremities like fingers and toes is decreased.

MONTHS...

Smoking may cause as many as one quarter of all psoriasis cases. The risk of the disease increases the longer you continue to smoke. Psoriasis from smoking is more prevalent in women than in men.

Although smokers tend to be thinner than non-smokers, body fat can be stored in an abnormal distribution. Smokers are more likely to store fat around the waist and upper torso, increasing the risk of diabetes 121, heart disease 75 and high blood pressure 111.

IN SECONDS...

Smoking one cigarette immediately raises your blood pressure and heart rate.

Brain and nervous system activity is stimulated for a short time, then reduced.

ACTION ITEMS

You can quit

There are many programs to help you quit smoking. Their cost may vary from almost nothing to hundreds of dollars. But a higher cost does not guarantee success. Many health plans and workplaces provide free quit-smoking programs, and some health plans cover the cost of medications to help you quit. Check with your insurance carrier or employer for more information.

Some steps you can take to kick the habit:

1 Make it personal.
Identify your own reasons for quitting.

2 Set a quit date.
If you smoke mostly at work, try quitting on the weekend. If you smoke mostly when socializing, try quitting during the week.

3 Identify your barriers to quitting.
What makes it hard to quit? Does your spouse smoke? Did you gain weight the last time you tried to quit?

4 Make specific plans ahead of time for dealing with temptation.
Have a friend you can call to talk you through a weak moment. Or take a walk to refocus.

A LIFETIME

Smoking increases your risk of cancer (lung, throat, mouth and bladder), stomach ulcers and emphysema.

Smoking increases risk of amputation if blood vessels in your legs deteriorate.

A long-term smoker has

20–30

times higher risk of mouth and throat cancers.

A long-term smoker has

10–20

times the risk of lung cancer.

A long-term smoker is twice as likely to die from a heart attack.

Loss of bone density associated with smoking increases the risk of hip fractures.

Breathing secondhand smoke can cause lung cancer and heart disease.

YEARS...

Smokers typically experience shortness of breath, persistent coughs and reduced fitness.

Smokers get yellow stains on fingers and teeth and a diminished sense of taste and smell.

Smokers have more colds than non-smokers and find it harder to recover from minor illnesses.

Smoking can cause impotence in men and reduced fertility in women.

People who smoke acquire facial wrinkles much earlier, and in general, look older than non-smokers of the same age.

How will smoking affect my health?

Dramatically, and starting with your first pack.

The degree of the effects depends upon you and several other factors: your susceptibility to chemicals found in tobacco, the number of cigarettes you smoke daily, your age when you began smoking and the number of years you've been smoking.

Source: National Institute of Occupational Safety and Health (NIOSH).

www.cdc.gov/niosh/jobstres.html

Smoking costs the United States approximately **$97.2 billion** each year in healthcare costs and lost productivity.

If you gave up a $4 a day cigarette habit, you would save an extra $1,460 per year. After 15 years, you would save $21,900.

Source: kickbutt.org.

TIP

Low tar or nicotine cigarettes are not safer than other cigarettes, nor do they reduce the risk of smoking-related diseases.

---

5 **Get cooperation from family and friends.**
They can't quit for you, but they can help by not smoking around you, providing encouragement when you need it and leaving you alone when you need space.

6 **Consider using medications.**
Unlike cigarettes, which contain thousands of harmful chemicals, nicotine medications contain small doses of nicotine alone to combat cravings. Medications can optimize your chances of success, but not everyone will want or need to use them. Some medications may require a prescription. If you are pregnant, consult your physician; if you are taking other medications, consult your doctor or your pharmacist.

7 **Work to stay smoke-free.**
The average person makes two to four attempts at quitting before becoming smoke-free. If you return to smoking, it doesn't mean you can't quit. It just means you need to try again by figuring out what caused you to slip and improving your plan for next time.

Source: American Lung Association.

It all adds up

Public and private funds are depleted by drug-related social ills: crime, AIDS, poverty, homelessness, teen pregnancy, family violence and illness.

Students who have experimented with an illegal drug

Marijuana
8th Graders	22%
10th Graders	40.9%
12th Graders	49.7%

Cocaine
8th Graders	4.7%
10th Graders	7.7%
12th Graders	9.8%

Ecstasy
8th Graders	4.3%
10th Graders	7.3%
12th Graders	11%

Heroin
8th Graders	2.3%
10th Graders	2.3%
12th Graders	2%

Marijuana

remains the most commonly used illicit drug in the US

33%

of all Americans have tried marijuana at least once.

Source: drugabuse.gov.

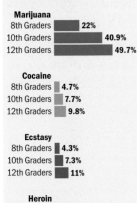

Drug abuse cost $110 billion in the

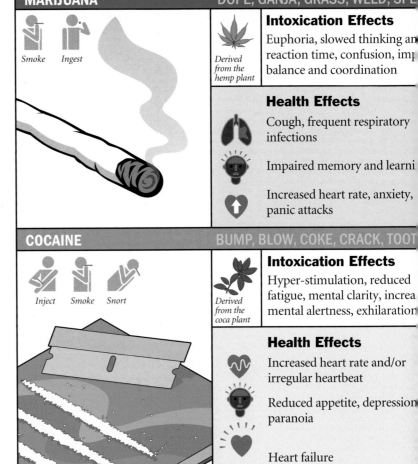

MARIJUANA — DOPE, GANJA, GRASS, WEED, SPL

Smoke   Ingest

Derived from the hemp plant

Intoxication Effects
Euphoria, slowed thinking an reaction time, confusion, imp balance and coordination

Health Effects
Cough, frequent respiratory infections

Impaired memory and learni

Increased heart rate, anxiety, panic attacks

COCAINE — BUMP, BLOW, COKE, CRACK, TOOT

Inject   Smoke   Snort

Derived from the coca plant

Intoxication Effects
Hyper-stimulation, reduced fatigue, mental clarity, increa mental alertness, exhilaration

Health Effects
Increased heart rate and/or irregular heartbeat

Reduced appetite, depression paranoia

Heart failure

ACTION ITEMS

Learn the signs of drug abuse

It may be possible to recognize drug abuse by observing a person's physical appearance or behavior. Keep in mind that these are guidelines. We all have days when we're not at our best, but a drug abuser is likely to exhibit more than one of these symptoms for a prolonged period.

1 **Tired appearance**
Drug-induced depletion of B-complex vitamins can make users look chronically run-down.

2 **Aimless walk or gestures**
A drug user may show one set of mannerisms when high and another when coming down. Causes can be B-complex vitamin depletion, especially vitamin B1.

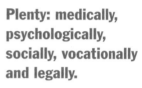

PREGNANCY AND POT JUST DON'T MIX

Research shows more anger and more regressive behavior (thumb sucking, temper tantrums) in toddlers whose parents use marijuana than in toddlers of non-using parents.

Source: drugabuse.gov.

What harm can illegal drugs do?

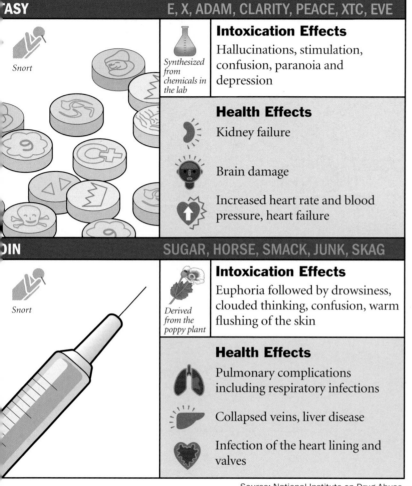

'ASY	E, X, ADAM, CLARITY, PEACE, XTC, EVE	
Snort	*Synthesized from chemicals in the lab*	**Intoxication Effects** Hallucinations, stimulation, confusion, paranoia and depression
		Health Effects Kidney failure · Brain damage · Increased heart rate and blood pressure, heart failure
DIN	SUGAR, HORSE, SMACK, JUNK, SKAG	
Snort	*Derived from the poppy plant*	**Intoxication Effects** Euphoria followed by drowsiness, clouded thinking, confusion, warm flushing of the skin
		Health Effects Pulmonary complications including respiratory infections · Collapsed veins, liver disease · Infection of the heart lining and valves

Source: National Institute on Drug Abuse.

Plenty: medically, psychologically, socially, vocationally and legally.

At left are just four of the dozens of commonly abused substances. Available drugs and drug-related problems have multiplied in recent decades.

Drug abuse can do more than harm your health. It can increase your likelihood of other risky behaviors and associated personality disorders.

No easy answers have emerged, although some directions show promise: consider addiction a disease, not a crime; improve education; raise economic prospects.

Source: Drug Foundation, adf.org.au.

3 Undependable behavior
A drug user may begin to arrive late for, or miss, important commitments like school or work.

4 Sudden energy shifts
Variations in alertness can signal drug abuse. An unexplained spurt of energy in a person who has been dragging may indicate a lift from drugs.

5 Sadness or lack of interest
Melancholy in someone who is generally happy may suggest drug abuse.

6 Odors
Cigarette smoke, incense or room deodorizers may cover the telltale scent of drugs such as marijuana.

7 Sudden change in friends
It's common for a drug user to suddenly acquire a new social circle almost overnight.

Source: Friends of Narcanon.

Do you know who you'r[e

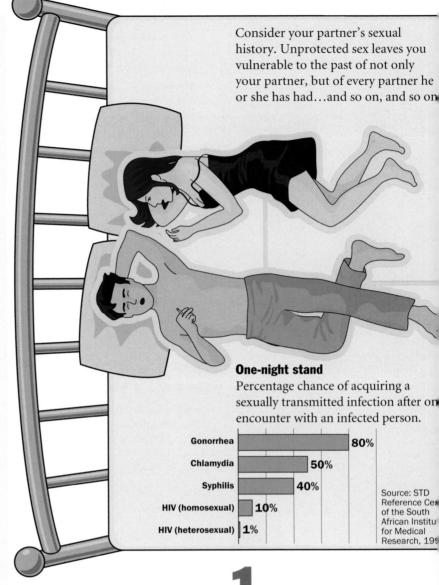

At your own risk

EXTREMELY HIGH RISK
- Unprotected anal intercourse (receptive partner)

HIGH RISK
- Unprotected vaginal intercourse (receptive partner)
- Unprotected vaginal intercourse (insertive partner)
- Protected anal intercourse (receptive partner)
- Unprotected anal intercourse (insertive partner)

LESS RISK
- Unprotected oral intercourse (fellatio) (receptive partner)
- Unprotected oral intercourse (cunnilingus) (receptive partner)

LOW RISK
- Receptive oral intercourse with a barrier (condom or dental dam)
- Insertive oral intercourse
- Anilingus ("rimming")
- Brachioproctal/brachio-vaginal manipulation ("fisting")

SAFE ACTIVITIES
- Masturbation
- Kissing (dry or wet)
- Intimate but non-sexual contact
- Use of sex toys (single-person use)
- Prolonged casual contact

The risks listed above are only for HIV 103 transmission. (For example, anilingus is extremely dangerous for the transmission of parasites and viruses like hepatitis.)

Source: University of Michigan.

Consider your partner's sexual history. Unprotected sex leaves you vulnerable to the past of not only your partner, but of every partner he or she has had…and so on, and so on

One-night stand
Percentage chance of acquiring a sexually transmitted infection after on encounter with an infected person.

Gonorrhea	80%
Chlamydia	50%
Syphilis	40%
HIV (homosexual)	10%
HIV (heterosexual)	1%

Source: STD Reference Ce of the South African Institu for Medical Research, 199

1 partner

ACTION ITEMS

Negotiate safe sex with your partner

There's more talk about "negotiated safety" lately. It's a way of deciding to practice unprotected sex with your permanent partner without condoms.

You have to ask yourself some tough questions. How sure are you that your partner is not doing anything else unsafe? If you're thinking about not using condoms with your main squeeze, or if you are already having unprotected sex, then read the following guidelines:

1 **Decide whether having unprotected sex is important to you.**
If you're perfectly happy using condoms all the time, keep it up. If not, read on.

2 **Both of you should get tested for HIV and other STDs.**
If you both test negative, wait! There's still the window period to be concerned about.

3 **Wait six months, then get tested again.**

4 **If you both still test negative, now it's time to make some tough agreements.**
Have a long, honest conversation about fidelity, trust, love and your mutual health. If one of you feels uncomfortable with the agreement at any point, agree to go back to condoms, no questions asked.

...leeping with?

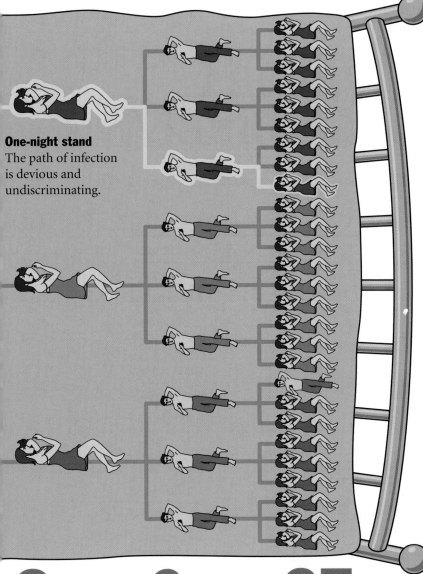

One-night stand
The path of infection is devious and undiscriminating.

3 partners 9 partners 27...

Each year in the US, 15,000,000 men and women are infected by STDs 105.

Sexually transmitted diseases (STDs), once called venereal diseases, are among the most common infectious diseases in the United States today. More than 25 STDs have now been identified. The annual cost of STDs in the US is estimated to be well in excess of $10 billion.

Source: National Institute of Allergy and Infectious Diseases.

? Is oral sex "sex"?

Any activity that involves the exchange of body fluids (blood, semen and vaginal secretions) is considered sex and can be unsafe.

TIP
When stored in a cool, dry place, condoms are good for about two years from the date they were made.

5 Agree to be monogamous, or if you agree to some sort of open relationship, define exactly what is acceptable outside.
If you are both completely safe outside the relationship, this could still work. But are you comfortable with the possible risk that your partner is experimenting when you're not around? Set up clear guidelines.

6 If one of you slips and does something unsafe outside the relationship, agree that you both will be honest about it so the two of you can go back to safe sex until you can get tested again.
Also, agree that this honesty will be rewarded with understanding. If the revelation automatically means the end of the relationship,

then why would your partner tell you? This is the tough one. If you don't feel there's enough trust or honest communication in your relationship, you're better off using condoms every time.

7 Periodically bring up the subject again.
Check to make sure your partner still feels this is the right thing to do.

If any of these steps seem unrealistic for your situation, you should use condoms every time.

Source: aris.org.

Why have a periodic health exam?

Evaluate new symptoms you may be experiencing.

Monitor and manage chronic medical problems.

Prevent new problems through early diagnosis.

Immunizations aren't just for kids

Hepatitis B is a virus that can cause serious damage to the liver. A series of three shots is given to provide immunity.

Influenza is caused by several viruses that the flu shot protects against. An annual flu shot is important for people over 50 and those with chronic illnesses.

Mumps, Measles and Rubella re-vaccination may be necessary for people born between 1956 and 1975. The vaccines used during those years have been found not to provide lifelong immunity.

Pneumonia can be caused by several different bacteria and viruses. Vaccination protects against 23 of the most common types. One shot typically provides lasting immunity.

Tetanus is caused by bacteria that enter the skin through open wounds. Vaccination should be given once every 10 years.

Source: hopkinsmedicine.org.

Periodic health exams based on individual health risks are the rule of the day.

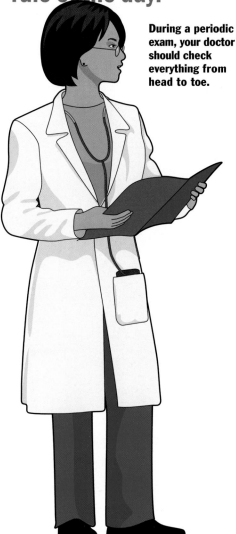

During a periodic exam, your doctor should check everything from head to toe.

"First, I'll look in your ears."

"Now, watch my finger."

"Say aahhh."

"Swallow."

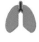
"Breathe normally."

"Take a deep breath."

"Do you feel pain or just pressure?"

"Push back against my hand."

ACTION ITEMS
How to make the most of your exam

1 Be prepared.
Take along any information that the doctor may need, including insurance cards, names of your other doctors, prescriptions you're taking and medical records.

2 Make a list.
Before arriving for your appointment, make a list of the items you want to discuss. For example, are you having any new problems? Are you experiencing any new symptoms from an existing condition?

3 Consider bringing support.
It can be helpful to bring a family member or close friend with you. Tell the person what you want from the visit in advance.

4 Update the doctor.
Be specific about any changes in your appetite, weight, sleep patterns, energy level or medications. Share any life events that might affect your well-being, such as a death in the family or a new living situation.

5 Be honest.
It's tempting to say what you think the doctor wants to hear—that you've quit smoking, that you've improved your diet and exercise, etc.

6 Stick to the point.
The doctor has a limited amount of time to spend with each patient. Coming prepared with a list of questions or problems will help you stay focused.

- Visual inspection checks for excessive wax build-up and ear drum ruptures
- Blowing air into the ear checks for ear infections and excess pressure

- Following finger movement from side to side and top to bottom checks three different nerves in the eye
- Following finger movement toward and away from your nose checks your pupils
- Shining a bright light in your eyes enables a check of your retinas

- Saying "aahhh" lifts the soft pallet, checking an important nerve function
- Visual inspection checks for ulcers, infections and cancerous areas

- Checking your neck looks for swollen lymph nodes, a possible sign of infection or cancer

- Listening with a stethoscope on your chest checks heart rate, rhythm, and listens for murmurs

- Listening with a stethoscope on your back checks the symmetry between left and right lungs and can indicate wheezing or cracking, possible signs of asthma, pneumonia or bronchitis
- Tapping the back lightly can indicate whether fluid is present in the lungs

- Pressing on areas of the belly can indicate an enlarged liver, infected gall bladder or enlarged spleen
- Listening with a stethoscope on your belly checks for normal bowel sounds

- Using push/pull tests checks the strength in your arms and legs
- Touching your palms and feet verifies normal sensation between left and right, as do hot/cold and pin-prick sensation tests
- Tapping your knee with a reflex hammer checks for normal reflex action

Each year, Americans make 59,300,000 visits to the doctor for periodic health exams.

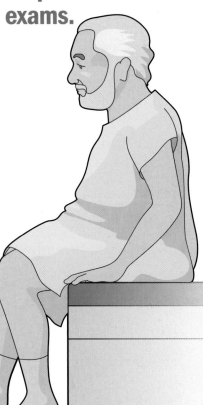

Do I need to see my doctor if I'm not sick?

The American Medical Association, the American College of Physicians, and the US Preventive Services Task Force no longer support the practice of annual physicals.

Instead, they suggest that patients would benefit more from periodic exams based on their health risks.

To determine how frequently to schedule a periodic exam and what tests are right for you, discuss your family history and personal health priorities with your doctor. Your age, gender and other individual risks will factor into your care.

Source: nsc.org.

TIP

Know your family history to help identify your at-risk factors. Then, schedule a health exam. Finally, follow your doctor's advice about future care.

7 Ask questions.
Don't be shy. Asking questions is key to getting what you want from the visit. If you don't ask questions, your doctor may think you understand all that's being said or that you don't want any more information.

8 Share your point of view.
Your doctor can't read your mind. It is important to let him or her know what's working for you and what's not. During the visit, if you're feeling rushed or uncomfortable, try to voice your feelings in a positive way. If necessary, schedule a follow-up visit to continue the discussion.

9 Take notes.
Medical terminology can be difficult to remember. Take along a note pad and pencil to write down the main points of what the doctor says, or ask your doctor to write them down for you.

10 Get more information.
Ask your doctor for brochures, video tapes or web site recommendations to help you learn more about your condition. Often, it's helpful to review detailed information on your own and ask follow-up questions later.

Source: National Institute on Aging.

*I*t wasn't just one thing; it was everything. I had pressure from school, pressure from friends, my grandmother was sick and Mom and I were fighting a lot," Angela said of her depression. "I was angry and sad."

At 17, Angela was well into her adolescent years. Her parents and teachers put her symptoms down to typical teenage behavior. "I felt like I had no one to talk to, even though we have school counselors, I just didn't want the kids at school talking about me."

Angela coped with her feelings by withdrawing from her friends and family. Sleeping and eating seemed to help a little so she did both excessively. It was a classmate's suicide that shocked her into action. "I saw how sad everybody was and I was sad too. I'd been collecting pills. I thought I'd just go to sleep and not wake up. John's death made me realized I needed help."

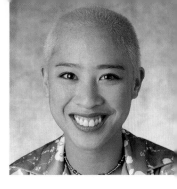

Angela learned to control her depression with a combination of therapy and medication.

"I asked my mom if I could see our family doctor," Angela said. "He suggested I talk to a mental health nurse practitioner. We were concerned about the money, but the doctor said there are programs that can help. He really gave me hope."

Angela's mental health nurse practitioner started her on Prozac with positive results. After nine months the dosage was lowered. "Our therapy sessions helped me too. I learned that rather than yell and slam doors when my mom's driving me nuts I can choose an alternative like breathing deeply until I calm down or going for a walk."

Angela's mother occasionally sits in on therapy sessions. She says she's learned how to better communicate with her daughter. Angela reports their relationship has improved. "We still have our moments," she says. "And I still get down once in awhile, but I work through it and I know it will always get better."

How vulnerable are you to mental illness?

Genetics 29
There is an increased risk of developing mental illness when there is a family history of it.

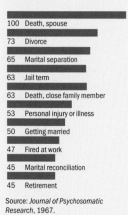

Brain chemistry
Research has proven that many mental health problems are biological in origin. For example, chemical imbalances in the brain's neurotransmitters can result in clinical depression.

Life
Experiencing life-altering events, then returning to normal, subjects all of us to stress. Here are the **top 10** stressful human experiences. (On this scale, death of a spouse rates 100 points; a traffic ticket rates 11.)

100	Death, spouse
73	Divorce
65	Marital separation
63	Jail term
63	Death, close family member
53	Personal injury or illness
50	Getting married
47	Fired at work
45	Marital reconciliation
45	Retirement

Source: *Journal of Psychosomatic Research*, 1967.

Am I crazy?

What's crazy for one person could be considered normal for another. We're all unique human beings.

But there are times when changes in our thoughts and moods indicate a clinical psychological condition. Here's a list of identifiable mental health problems and some of their warning signs.

Depression 129
Persistent sadness, weight loss or gain, fatigue, irritability, sleeplessness

Bipolar disorder
Periods of depression alternating with periods of elation

Anxiety
Long-term unrealistic fears, extreme worry, panic

Post-traumatic stress
Reliving traumatic experience, unresponsiveness, detachment

Substance abuse 53
Low concentration, nervousness, low self-esteem, sadness

Eating disorders
Sudden weight loss, irritability, obsessiveness

Sexual dysfunction
Loss of interest and pleasure in sex

Get help.

No need to suffer
If you're consistently experiencing any of the symptoms at left, talk to your doctor. Psychotherapy 215 and/or various medications can effectively treat symptoms.

 Cultural healing arts
Acupuncture (Chinese), yoga (Indian) and chanting (Native American) can help promote the balance between our spiritual, physical and mental selves, relieving depression, stress and anxiety.

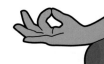

Relax!
But it takes a little work. Biofeedback, or retraining your breathing habits during stress, can induce relaxation and lower your heart rate. Equally effective is visualizatio in which you create a mental image of recovery and wellness

---

ACTION ITEMS

Learn how to cope with loss

The loss of a loved one is one of life's most stressful events and can cause a emotional crisis. Some emotions you may experience include denial, disbelief, confusion, shock, sadness, yearning, anger, humiliation, despair and guilt. The best thing you can do is allow yourself to grieve.

1 Seek out caring people.
Find relatives and friends who can understand your feelings of loss. Join support groups with others who are experiencing similar losses.

2 Express your feelings.
It will help you work through the grieving process.

3 Take care of your health.
Maintain regular contact with your family physician and be sure to eat well and get plenty of rest.

4 Accept that life is for the living.
Postpone major life changes.
Try to hold off on making any major changes, such as moving, remarrying, changing jobs or having another child. You should give yourself time to adjust to your loss.

5 Be patient.
It can take months or even years to absorb a major loss and accept your changed life.

6 Seek outside help if necessary.

Diet and nutrition 43

Improving your diet can help manage symptoms of mental illness and promote recovery.

Expressive therapies

Art, dance and music help foster self-awareness as well as personal growth. They stimulate the body's "feel-good" chemicals, improving blood pressure, pulse rate, breathing and posture.

Support groups

Sharing your problems with people who have similar needs can be very helpful. It's good to know you're not the only one. Groups tend to be confidential and free.

Exercise

Beat depression and lift your mood by becoming active. Start small, but start.

Technology 323

The boom in electronic tools in the home and office makes access to mental health information just a phone call or mouse click away. Before you jump into any therapy, however, learn as much as you can about it.

Pastoral counseling

For many, a good dialogue with a pastor, rabbi or priest can be effective in managing mental illness.

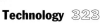

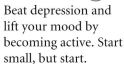

body, mind & spirit

How can I avoid mental health problems?

Understand the warning signs, and don't let the stigma of mental illness prevent you from seeking help if you need it.

Emotional health is just as important as physical health. But many Americans don't recognize the warning signs of mental illness or know where to go if they need help.

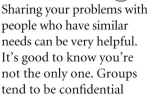

A **psychiatrist** is an MD. A **psychologist** is a professional with a PhD. Though both treat disorders involving behavior, feelings, motives and thinking, only a psychiatrist can write prescriptions.

Sources: KEN Publications/Catalog, mentalhealth.org.

If someone you care about has lost a loved one, here are some things you can do to help him or her through the grieving process.

1 Share the sorrow.
Allow them—even encourage them—to talk about their feelings of loss and share memories of the deceased.

2 Don't offer false comfort.
It doesn't help the grieving person when you say "it was for the best" or "you'll get over it in time."Instead, offer a simple expression of sorrow and take time to listen.

3 Offer practical help.
Babysitting, cooking and running errands are all ways to help someone who's in the midst of grieving.

4 Be patient.

5 Encourage professional help when necessary.
Don't hesitate to recommend professional help when you feel someone is experiencing too much pain to cope alone.

Source: National Mental Health Association.

Healthy States

1

New Hampshire
Minnesota
Massachusetts
Utah
Connecticut
Vermont
Iowa
Colorado
North Dakota
Maine
Washington
Wisconsin
Rhode Island
Hawaii
Nebraska
South Dakota
Oregon
Virginia
New Jersey
Idaho
Kansas
Indiana
Pennsylvania
Montana
California
Wyoming
Ohio
Maryland
Michigan
Alaska
Illinois
New York
Missouri
Arizona
Delaware
North Carolina
Texas
Nevada
Kentucky
Georgia
West Virginia
New Mexico
Florida
Tennessee
Alabama
Oklahoma
Arkansas
South Carolina
Mississippi
Louisiana

50

Farm Living is the Life for Me

South Dakotans are fairly healthy and are likely to call in sick the least. They reported feeling sick only 4 days a month. Residents of Kentucky and Nevada reported feeling sick most often—6.3 days a month.

A City Slicker is Sicker

A study from the Centers for Disease Control and Prevention found that city dwellers are sick more often than people who live in the country.

Air Pollution

Children are more sensitive to pollution than adults. They also experience more illness in areas of high pollution.

Sunburn Hurts

Excessive sun exposure is the main cause of skin cancer—about 90% of skin cancers occur on exposed areas of the body.

Radon

This radioactive gas comes from soil and rock beneath and around building foundations, groundwater wells and some construction materials.

Pesticides

In 1990, the American Association of Poison Control reported 79,000 children involved in pesticide poisonings or exposures.

Cell Phones

There is no conclusive proof that cell phones pose a health risk. Ongoing studies focus on the association of certain brain cancers and cell phone use.

Carbon Monoxide

Sources include unvented fossil-fuel space heaters, gas stoves and ovens, and backdrafting furnaces and water heaters.

Formaldehyde

Carpeting, pressed wood products and some types of insulation give off formaldehyde, a potential carcinogen.

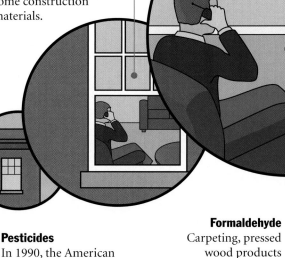

Source: unitedhealthfoundation.org.

ACTION ITEMS

Avoid secondhand smoke

At home:

- Don't smoke in your house or permit others to do so.
- If a family member insists on smoking indoors, increase ventilation.
- Do not smoke if children are present.
- Don't allow babysitters or others who work in your home to smoke while on duty.

In restaurants and bars:

- Know the law concerning smoking in your community. Some communities have banned smoking in places such as restaurants entirely; others require separate smoking areas.
- If smoking is permitted, smoking areas should be located where the ventilation minimizes nonsmoker exposure.
- Ask to be seated in nonsmoking areas as far from smokers as possible.

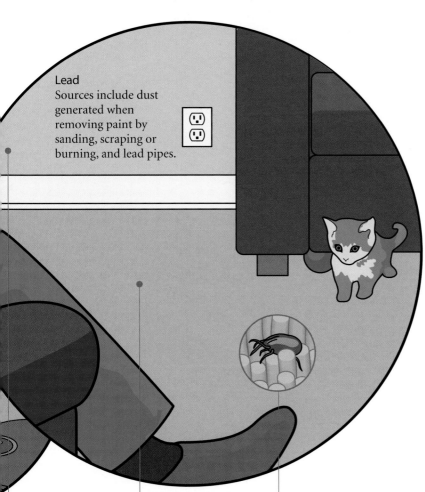

Lead
Sources include dust generated when removing paint by sanding, scraping or burning, and lead pipes.

We live with countless potential hazards.

We are surrounded by potential allergens and dangerous substances, but the good news is that with a little research and some work, we can make our homes safe.

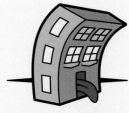

Sick Building Syndrome
Building occupants may experience acute health and comfort effects that appear to be linked to time spent in a building, even if no specific illness or cause can be identified.

Household Pollutants
Beware of volatile compounds from paints, solvents, air fresheners, adhesives and additives in carpeting and furniture. Avoid asbestos, including pipe insulation, fireproofing and floor tiles.

Moisture, Mold and Mildew
Mold and mildew can cause severe allergic reactions. Keep your home clean and dry. Use a disinfectant to clean moldy surfaces.

Dust Mites
These tiny creatures eat dead skin that collects in bedding and upholstered furniture. Dust mites are a normal part of life, but many people with asthma are allergic to their droppings.

Source: healthatoz.com.

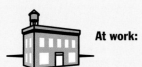

At work:

- If your company does not have a smoking policy that effectively controls secondhand smoke, work with management and labor organizations to establish one.

- Simply separating smokers and nonsmokers within the same area, such as a cafeteria, may reduce exposure, but nonsmokers will still be exposed to recirculated or drifting smoke.

- Prohibiting smoking indoors or limiting smoking to rooms that have been designed to prevent smoke from escaping are options that will effectively protect nonsmokers.

- Designated outdoor smoking areas should be as far away from doors and ventilation system air intakes as possible. Nonsmokers should be able to enter and exit without passing through the smoke of smokers congregating near doorways.

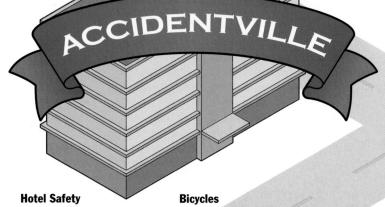

Accidents Waiting to Happen

Below are the five top causes of accidental death in the US each year. **Each icon represents roughly 1,000 people.**

Motor vehicles—41,200

Falls—16,600

Poisonings—8,400

Drownings—4,100

Fires and burns—3,700

Source: National Safety Council Report on Injuries in America.

In the US, cooking is the leading cause of home fires—101,000 fires per year.

Smoking materials are the leading cause of home fire deaths—840 per year.

Source: cdc.gov.

Hotel Safety
After checking into a hotel, review the safety information in your room. Find the closest exits and fire alarms.

Bicycles
Wear a bike helmet. One out of seven children under age 15 suffers a head injury in a bike crash. Helmets can prevent head injuries.

Sun Exposure
There's no such thing as a healthy suntan. Wear appropriate sun-screens.

Drowning
Fence all home pools and keep the gate closed and locked. Never dive into water unless you know beforehand how deep it is. Supervise young children in the tub, the swimming pool or any other body of water.

Learn CPR for potentially life-threatening emergencies.

Poisoning
In 1998, more than 2.2 million people called pois control centers in the US in r to poisoning incidents.

ACTION ITEMS
Check for home safety

Here are some things you can do to make your home safer.

- ❑ Install smoke detectors and check the batteries regularly.
- ❑ Keep dangerous materials (medicine, cleaning supplies, alcohol, etc.) out of the reach of children.
- ❑ Never leave a burning candle or fireplace fire unattended.
- ❑ Establish an emergency escape plan for your home and review it periodically.

- ❑ Keep at least one fully charged fire extinguisher on each level of your home and know how to use it.
- ❑ Store flammable materials away from heat sources.
- ❑ Install sturdy handrails in all stairways.
- ❑ Provide proper lighting in all entryways.
- ❑ Use nonslip floor and bath mats in the bathroom.

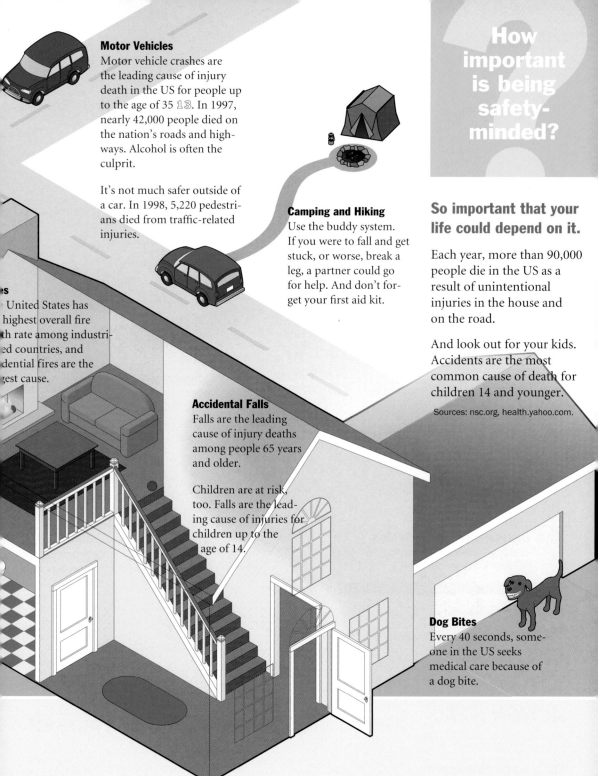

Motor Vehicles
Motor vehicle crashes are the leading cause of injury death in the US for people up to the age of 35 13. In 1997, nearly 42,000 people died on the nation's roads and highways. Alcohol is often the culprit.

It's not much safer outside of a car. In 1998, 5,220 pedestrians died from traffic-related injuries.

Camping and Hiking
Use the buddy system. If you were to fall and get stuck, or worse, break a leg, a partner could go for help. And don't forget your first aid kit.

...es
United States has ...highest overall fire ...th rate among industri-...ed countries, and ...dential fires are the ...gest cause.

Accidental Falls
Falls are the leading cause of injury deaths among people 65 years and older.

Children are at risk, too. Falls are the leading cause of injuries for children up to the age of 14.

Dog Bites
Every 40 seconds, someone in the US seeks medical care because of a dog bite.

So important that your life could depend on it.

Each year, more than 90,000 people die in the US as a result of unintentional injuries in the house and on the road.

And look out for your kids. Accidents are the most common cause of death for children 14 and younger.

Sources: nsc.org, health.yahoo.com.

- ❏ Immediately mop up spills that may cause someone to slip and fall.
- ❏ Turn pot handles toward the back when cooking on the stove.
- ❏ Don't use electrical appliances when you are wet or near water.
- ❏ Wear protective eyewear when working with tools.
- ❏ Keep unused electrical outlets covered.
- ❏ Replace frayed electrical cords or throw the item away.
- ❏ Install a carbon monoxide detector in your home, and have your furnace checked regularly for leaks.
- ❏ Keep your hot water heater set to no higher than 120°F.

? What are the early warning signs of job stress?

- *Headache*
- *Sleep disturbances*
- *Difficulty concentrating*
- *Short temper*
- *Upset stomach*
- *Job dissatisfaction*
- *Low morale*

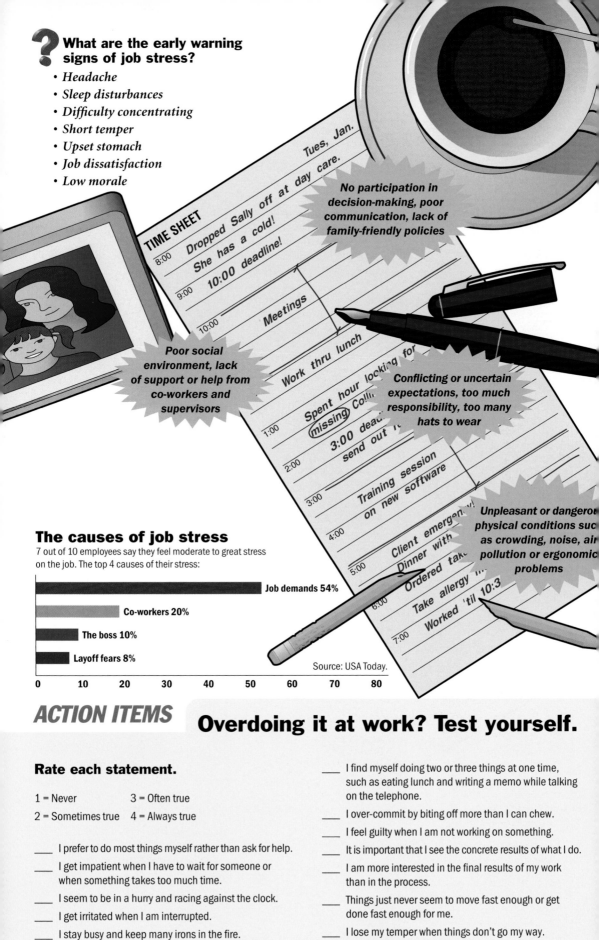

No participation in decision-making, poor communication, lack of family-friendly policies

Poor social environment, lack of support or help from co-workers and supervisors

Conflicting or uncertain expectations, too much responsibility, too many hats to wear

Unpleasant or dangerous physical conditions such as crowding, noise, air pollution or ergonomic problems

TIME SHEET

Tues, Jan.

8:00 — Dropped Sally off at day care. She has a cold!

9:00 — 10:00 deadline!

10:00 — Meetings

Work thru lunch

1:00 — Spent hour looking for missing Coll..

2:00

3:00 — 3:00 dea.. send out ..

Training session on new software

4:00

5:00 — Client emergen.. Dinner with Ordered tak..

6:00 — Take allergy ...

7:00 — Worked 'til 10:3..

The causes of job stress

7 out of 10 employees say they feel moderate to great stress on the job. The top 4 causes of their stress:

Cause	Percentage
Job demands	54%
Co-workers	20%
The boss	10%
Layoff fears	8%

0 10 20 30 40 50 60 70 80

Source: USA Today.

ACTION ITEMS

Overdoing it at work? Test yourself.

Rate each statement.

1 = Never   3 = Often true
2 = Sometimes true   4 = Always true

____ I prefer to do most things myself rather than ask for help.

____ I get impatient when I have to wait for someone or when something takes too much time.

____ I seem to be in a hurry and racing against the clock.

____ I get irritated when I am interrupted.

____ I stay busy and keep many irons in the fire.

____ I find myself doing two or three things at one time, such as eating lunch and writing a memo while talking on the telephone.

____ I over-commit by biting off more than I can chew.

____ I feel guilty when I am not working on something.

____ It is important that I see the concrete results of what I do.

____ I am more interested in the final results of my work than in the process.

____ Things just never seem to move fast enough or get done fast enough for me.

____ I lose my temper when things don't go my way.

____ I ask the same question, without realizing it, after I've already been given the answer.

Alleviating stress in the office

A growing body of research suggests that millions of Americans manage their stress in precisely the wrong way. They compartmentalize, stressing out all day and then pushing relaxation into isolated blocks of time like evening yoga classes and weekend getaways.

Ultimately, it's how you spend your days—not your downtime—that matters. People who handle stress well recover quickly when confronted by it. The goal is to train people to deal with stress as it happens, by changing how they react, rather than trying to eliminate stress or treat its symptoms. Some suggestions:

Breathe easy
When anxiety starts mounting, adjust the way you breathe (the more deeply the better), sit (drop your shoulders) or think (imagine yourself on the beach). Bringing the body back to a state of calm is what stress-resistant people do naturally.

The computer really is out to get you
Don't trust that ergonomic chair. Even if every piece of equipment is at the perfect height and angle, merely sitting at your desk produces physical reactions that can increase stress. About 95% of people raise their shoulders the moment they sit down at a computer, and 30% begin breathing more shallowly.

Enlighten up
A slew of studies suggest nearly every spiritual practice, including yoga and saying rosaries, induces relaxation simply by slowing your heart rate through breathing. And of course the old standbys— getting enough exercise and sleep— are still crucial.

Avoid emotional overeating
Stress sometimes makes people reach for high-calorie comfort food. When the urge hits, ask yourself if you're really hungry. If the need is to fill an emotional void rather than your stomach, try a healthy snack like raw carrots or a non-food activity like walking.

Keep your perspective
When stress hits, rate the situation on a scale of one to 10, with 10 being a catastrophic event, like death. It can help put inconveniences in perspective.

Keep expectations realistic
Shedding stress also involves cultivating a certain amount of pessimism to avoid constant disappointments. Don't expect to find a parking place immediately. Acknowledge in advance that computers crash.

If all else fails, try laughing. It opens up the blood flow.

Source: The Wall Street Journal.

It can make you sick or even kill you.

Prolonged, unmanaged stress can attack both body and mind. Perpetually stressed people are at increased risk of cardiovascular disease 75, musculo-skeletal and psychological disorders 61, injury at the workplace, suicide, cancer 87, ulcers and impaired immune systems.

Source: Encyclopaedia of Occupational Safety and Health.

In Japan, **10,000** workers a year drop dead at their desks as a result of 60- to 70-hour work weeks, a phenomenon known as *karoshi*.

Source: Encyclopaedia of Occupational Safety and Health.

TIP
Balance work and personal life. Maintain a support network of friends and co-workers. Keep a relaxed and positive outlook.

---

statement.

1 = Never   3 = Often true

2 = Sometimes true   4 = Always true

____ I prefer to do most things myself rather than ask for help.

____ I get impatient when I have to wait for someone or when something takes too much time.

____ I seem to be in a hurry and racing against the clock.

____ I get irritated when I am interrupted.

____ I stay busy and keep many irons in the fire.

____ I find myself doing two or three things at one time, such as eating lunch and writing a memo while talking on the telephone.

____ I over-commit by biting off more than I can chew.

____ I feel guilty when I am not working on something.

____ It is important that I see the concrete results of what I do.

____ I am more interested in the final results of my work than in the process.

____ Things just never seem to move fast enough or get done fast enough for me.

____ I lose my temper when things don't go my way.

____ I ask the same question, without realizing it, after I've already been given the answer.

____ I spend a lot of time planning and thinking about future events, while tuning out the here and now.

____ I find myself continuing to work after my co-workers have called it quits.

____ I get angry when people don't meet my standards of perfection.

Prescription (Rx) drugs

These common mistakes in using Rx drugs can have serious, even lethal, consequences.

Not anticipating drug-drug interactions

Drugs are chemicals—and when combined, undesirable reactions can occur. Any type of drug-drug combination—Rx-Rx, Rx-OTC, Rx-herbal—may carry these risks. That's why it's critical to tell your doctor and pharmacist every medicine and supplement you use.

Not following directions

"Take with food." "Avoid alcohol while using this medicine." "Take 3 times daily." Commonplace though they may be, instructions like these can be crucial to how well—and how safely—a medicine works.

Stopping the drug

Some people, not liking a drug's side effects, stop taking it altogether without informing their doctor. This can make the condition return or even worsen. Always make sure you check with your doctor or pharmacist before you stop taking the drug or decrease your dosage.

Poor monitoring

Some medicines require lab tests in the weeks or months after a person starts using them. If a doctor forgets to order these tests—or a patient fails to show up—serious problems could go undetected.

Improper storage

Your drug could increase in toxicity or cause unexpected side effects if stored improperly or kept past the expiration date.

> **CONSUMER ALERT:**
> Child-proof your medicine bottles—even if you don't have kids at home. 23% of oral Rx drugs ingested by children under 5 belonged to someone who didn't live with them. Common scenarios: Kids find medicines in guests' purses or, when visiting others, grab containers on bathroom sinks. Place your medicines out of children's reach and choose child-resistant bottles.

Non-prescription drugs

Over-the-counter (OTC) painkillers, perhaps the most popular OTC drugs, are used safely by millions of people. But they're also widely taken for granted, with many users either failing to read—or disregarding—the dosing instructions.

Aspirin and its cousins

The drugs **aspirin**, **ibuprofen** (Advil®, Motrin®, Midol IB®, Nuprin®) and **naproxen** (Aleve®, Naprosyn®, Anaprox®) belong to the category of drugs known as **NSAIDs** (pronounced EN-seds; **n**on-**s**teroidal **a**nti-**i**nflammatory **d**rugs)

- **The problem:** Exceeding recommended dose in amount or duration
- **The risks:** Stomach ulcers and bleeding that can lead to hospitalization, even death
- **Be aware:** Although aspirin's gotten the rap as a stomach irritant, the other NSAIDs carry the same risks.

Acetaminophen (Tylenol®, Panadol®)

- **The problem:** Exceeding the maximum daily dose; combining excessive dosing with alcohol use
- **The risks:** Liver damage
- **Be aware:** Some Rx and OTC pain relievers contain acetaminophen. Taking these drugs in addition to acetaminophen tablets could lead to overdose. Read ingredients labels.

OTC drugs and driving

Read the warning labels on all your OTC drugs.

- **The problem:** Sleepiness and slowed reactions
- **The risks:** Impaired ability to operate a car or other machinery
- **Be aware:** Having even a small amount of alcohol can increase the drowsiness caused by some OTCs.

ACTION ITEMS How to prevent mistakes

Ask questions

- What is this medicine supposed to do for me?
- What are the possible side effects?
- Are there any special instructions?
- Could this drug interact with any others I take?
- Should I avoid certain foods? any activities?

Keep track of your drugs

"Brown bag it" when you go to a new doctor or pharmacy: Dump all of your medicine vials—including herbal and vitamin supplements—into a bag (unless refrigeration is required). This way, your doctor and pharmacist can see exactly what you use and help you avoid possible drug interactions.

Help your loved ones

- Don't share your medications, even if a family member has a similar condition. Each person's body chemistry is different.
- See if older relatives need help using medicines properly. Hearing problems can prevent a person from comprehending a pharmacist's instructions; poor eyesight can result in misreading labels. Limited mobility or transportation problems can mean going without a prescription refill.
- Make sure your pre-teens and teens remember to take their medications. As kids become increasingly independent, they're out of your sight more often.

Drugs and other substances

Drugs can interact with some of the common things we eat and drink every day. Heed the warnings and instructions on your medicine bottles.

Drugs and alcohol

Drinking alcohol when you're taking drugs can make them more toxic or ineffective or cause an alcohol-drug interaction. And the consequences can be serious: breathing difficulties, heart problems, bleeding, fainting, even death. It's not just prescription drugs that carry these risks; mixing alcohol and OTC drugs can also be dangerous. And don't assume you can stagger your drinks and your medicines. Alcohol and drugs can interact harmfully even if you don't take them at the same time.

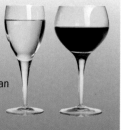

Drugs and food

Many prescription vials have stickers like **"take with food"** or **"take 3 hours after eating."** Some drugs, designed to act quickly, must be taken on an empty stomach so they can be absorbed into the body quickly. Others must be taken with food so that drug absorption is slowed, thereby reducing side effects. ■ Food-drug interactions can also be an issue. For example, if taken with certain blood pressure drugs, grapefruit juice can dangerously increase the drugs' levels in the blood. And calcium-rich dairy foods can make some antibiotics less effective.

Drugs and herbs

Just like "real drugs," herbal remedies have side effects and drug interaction risks. Patients should tell their doctors which herbal products and vitamin supplements they're taking. ■ **Particularly dangerous:** Taking herbals for a condition that's already being treated with a prescription drug (unless specified by one's doctor). People who take the widely used blood-thinning drug warfarin (**Coumadin®** and other brands) should not take **garlic pills** or **gingko biloba**, both of which thin the blood. Individuals taking antidepressants should not take **St. John's wort**, which can decrease the effectiveness of some drugs and cause negative side effffects with others.

What are the safety risks in using medicines?

Be careful.
About 100,000 Americans die each year because of adverse reactions to **prescription (Rx)** or **over-the-counter (OTC)** drugs. Another 2 million are hospitalized due to drug allergies or the unintentional combination of medicines.

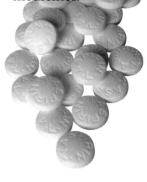

TIP

Ask your doctor to write the reason for the medication right on your prescription.

How to store your medicines

Don't use the medicine cabinet

● Bathrooms may be the worst possible place to store medicines. Heat, humidity and light can cause drugs to decompose. Instead, keep your medicines in a dark, dry place, such as a closet or dresser drawer.

● Don't refrigerate medicines unless directed.

● Don't leave medicines in your car. Interiors get too hot in the summer and too cold in the winter for most drugs.

Flush a medicine if:

● It smells foul, has changed color or become cloudy (liquids)

● It has cracked coatings (pills) or powdered rings (liquids)

● The expiration date has passed

Resources

● Drug interactions
The Center for Drug Evaluation and Research
www.fda.gov/cder/consumerinfo/druginteractions.htm

● List of prescription medicine sites
California Health Decisions
www.cahd.org

● National Poison Control Hotline
800.222.1222

Kathy never gave heart disease much attention. Afterall, women don't usually have heart attacks, or so she believed. At 45, she considered herself too young to have a "man's disease."

She'd recently quit smoking and joined a gym to lose a few pounds. It was while exercising that she first noticed a burning sensation in her lower chest. Kathy also felt short of breath, but chalked it up to being out of shape and overweight.

At work, she laughed about it with Kim, a co-worker. Kim, however, didn't laugh. "My mother died of a heart attack when she was 48," she confided. "It's far more common than you think and the symptoms aren't the same as a man's. You really should see a doctor."

Kathy agreed and made an appointment. After the visit she returned to work. "She told me to take a vacation," she told Kim. "She thinks it's stress."

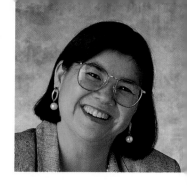

A stress test is the most common test for coronary artery disease. The patient walks on a treadmill while heartbeat and blood pressure is monitored. The speed and incline are gradually increased to a safe maximum for the patient's age and sex. Some doctors prefer a stress echocardiogram as a better test for heart disease in women.
Source: Women Are Not Small Men: Life-Saving Strategies for Preventing and Healing Heart Disease in Women.

Kathy got help after a friend pushed her to take her symptoms seriously.

"Did he do a stress test or any other cardiac tests?" Kim asked. The answer was no.

"You deserve better than that," she told her friend. "Get a second opinion and make sure you get those tests. If you're fine, great! But you need to know for sure."

Kathy called her doctor and requested a referral to a cardiologist. The doctor said it wasn't necessary, but Kathy wouldn't give up and she got her referral.

Kathy's new doctor asked lots of questions about her symptoms and her family's medical history. While on the treadmill during her stress test, Kathy felt the burning in her chest again and numbness in her arm.

The tests showed that Kathy had a major blockage in her coronary arteries and a heart attack was in her future if she didn't get care now. While absorbing this news, Kathy gave silent thanks to Kim.

A cardiologist is a medical doctor trained in internal medicine and specialty training in diseases of the heart and blood vessels.
Source: Online Medical Dictionary.

Coronary artery disease (CAD) causes the arteries that feed the heart to narrow, giving less blood to the heart. When the blood supply is cut off completely, the result is a heart attack. Risk factors for CAD include high blood pressure, high blood cholesterol, smoking, obesity and lack of exercise.

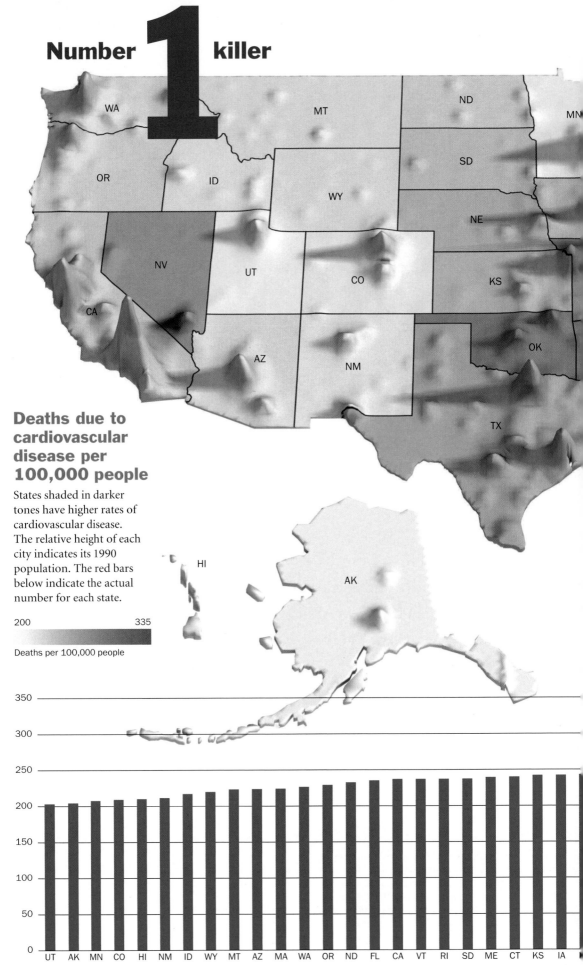

Number 1 killer

Deaths due to cardiovascular disease per 100,000 people

States shaded in darker tones have higher rates of cardiovascular disease. The relative height of each city indicates its 1990 population. The red bars below indicate the actual number for each state.

200   335

Deaths per 100,000 people

Cardiovascular disease accounted for
1 of every 2.5 deaths
in the US in 2000.

Across the nation, more than 260 per 100,000 people die from cardiovascular disease each year.

Utah, with its relatively young population, has a low cardiovascular disease death rate— only about 204 deaths per 100,000 compared with 334 for Mississippi.

Source: americanheart.org.

Although the death rate from cardiovascular disease declined by **17%** between 1990 and 2000, due to the rising population the actual number of deaths dropped only **2.5%**.

According to year 2000 estimates, almost

62,000,000

Americans have some form of cardiovascular disease (high blood pressure, coronary heart disease or stroke).

Risk factors

Your chance of dying from cardiovascular disease increases if your health and lifestyle includes any of these factors:

- Diabetes 121
- High cholesterol
- High blood pressure 111
- Obesity 127
- Physical inactivity 47
- Smoking 51

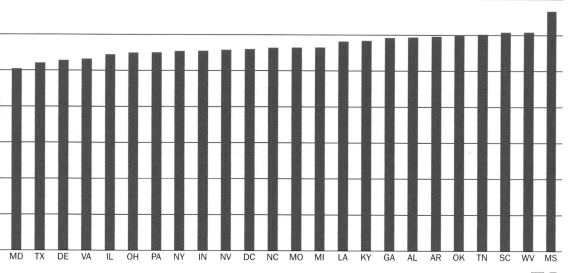

| MD | TX | DE | VA | IL | OH | PA | NY | IN | NV | DC | NC | MO | MI | LA | KY | GA | AL | AR | OK | TN | SC | WV | MS |

According to a report by the **World Health Organization,** cardiovascular diseases cause 12 million deaths in the world each year.

High blood pressure alone causes about 50% of the heart disease and stroke deaths worldwide. **High cholesterol** causes about 1/3 of the deaths.

Death rates attributable to CVD have risen by 60% in **Poland** and by 40% in **Hungary.**

CVD is emerging as a major health problem in the eastern **Mediterranean.**

In **China and India** alone, 5 million people die from CVD each year.

CVD is the leading cause of death in **Indonesia.**

Within South America, mortality rates from CVD are highest in **Argentina, Chile and Uruguay.**

The highest rate of heart disease in the Americas is in **Argentina, Canada, the United States and Uruguay.**

Sources: Merck Health Library, mercksource.com; Centers for Disease Control; American Heart Association; *USA Today.*

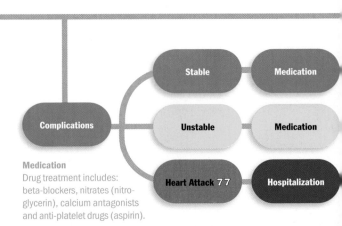

What treatments are commonly used for coronary artery disease?

Lifestyle Modifications Exercise & Dietary Changes

Treatment depends upon the severity and stability of the symptoms. When symptoms are stable and mild to moderate, reducing risk factors and using drugs may be most effective. If the symptoms don't improve with drug treatment and lifestyle changes, surgery may be necessary.

Complications

Stable — **Medication**

Unstable — **Medication**

Heart Attack 77 — **Hospitalization**

Medication Drug treatment includes: beta-blockers, nitrates (nitroglycerin), calcium antagonists and anti-platelet drugs (aspirin).

Congestive heart failure is the single most frequent cause of hospitalization for people aged 65 years and older.

More than 2,600 Americans die each day of CVD. That is an average of 1 death every 33 seconds.

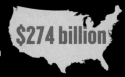

$274 billion

CVD costs the US $274 billion annually, including health expenditures and lost productivity.

ACTION ITEMS Stop these risky behaviors

Three health-related behaviors contribute markedly to heart disease. Modifying these behaviors is critical both for preventing and for controlling cardiovascular disease. Other steps that adults with cardiovascular disease should take to reduce their risk of death and disability include adhering to treatment for high blood pressure and cholesterol, using aspirin as appropriate and learning the symptoms of a heart attack.

1 Smoking 51
Smokers have twice the risk for heart attack as non-smokers. Nearly one-fifth of all deaths from cardiovascular disease, or about 190,000 deaths a year, are smoking-related. Every day, more than 3,000 young people become smokers.

2 Lack of physical activity 47
People who are not physically active have twice the risk for heart disease of those who are active. More than half of American adults do not achieve recommended levels of physical activity.

What are the risk factors for coronary artery disease?

- High cholesterol levels
- Poor physical fitness 47
- Tobacco use 51
- High-fat diet
- Low-fiber diet 43
- Poor stress management 67
- High blood pressure 111
- Obesity 127

How am I likely to be diagnosed with coronary artery disease?

Certain tests will help determine the presence and extent of the disease: Exercise tolerance (treadmill) test, radionuclide imaging, exercise echocardiography, coronary arteriography and electrocardiogram monitoring.

Normal Life

Normal Life

Additional Treatment
Bypass Surgery or Angioplasty

Normal Life

What can I expect as an outcome?

Age, the extent of coronary artery disease, the severity of symptoms and the degree of normal heart muscle function are key factors in determining outcome. The prognosis is good for a person with stable angina and normal pumping ability; reduced pumping ability and multiple blocked arteries worsen the outlook.

Cardiovascular disease (CVD) is a condition in which fatty deposits (atheromas or plaques) accumulate in the cells lining the wall of a coronary artery and obstruct the blood flow.

This gradual process is known as atherosclerosis. Plaques bulge into the arteries, narrowing them. As they grow, portions may rupture and enter the bloodstream, or small blood clots may form on their surfaces. The major complications of CVD are angina and heart attack.

 Two daily glasses of cranberry juice will help raise your level of HDL (good cholesterol) and lower your level of LDL (bad cholesterol).

More than 960,000 Americans die of CVD each year, accounting for over 40% of all deaths.

Among patients suffering acute myocardial infarction (heart attack) more than 70% are smokers.

3 Poor nutrition 43

People who are overweight have a higher risk for cardiovascular disease. Almost 60% of adults in the US are overweight or obese. Only 18% of women and 20% of men report eating the recommended five servings of fruits and vegetables each day.

 UNDERSTANDING ANGINA

Angina is a temporary chest pain or pressure that occurs when the heart muscle isn't receiving enough oxygen. Angina is typically triggered by physical activity and subsides with rest. Emotional stress may also cause angina. The pattern of symptoms is generally predictable.

Unstable angina refers to angina in which the pattern of symptoms suddenly changes, due to increased obstruction of a coronary artery caused by a ruptured atheroma, or blood clot.

It is estimated that approximately **1 million patients** visit the hospital each year with some type of heart attack as their principal diagnosis.

Angina (chest pain due to coronary heart disease) is almost always an indication that you are at risk for a heart attack sometime in the future.

Cholesterol comes from two sources. Your own liver produces cholesterol and it is found in foods, especially animal products such as meat, poultry, dairy products and eggs.

Inflammation of fatty buildups in the blood vessels is a central factor in CVD. Studies show that inflammation in the bloodstream is twice as likely as high cholesterol to trigger a heart atttack. Inflammation can be measured with a test that checks for C-reactive protein, a chemical necessary for fighting injury and infection.

Sources: Merck Health Library, mercksource.com.

What are the risk factors of a heart attack?

- Smoking 51
- Hypertension (high blood pressure) 111
- High-fat diet 43
- High blood cholesterol (LDL) levels
- Diabetes 121
- Male gender 31
- Age 133
- Family history 29
- Stress 67

What symptoms might suggest a heart attack?

- Chest pain below breastbone
- Back pain
- Sudden shortness of breath
- Fainting
- Sweating
- Nausea or vomiting
- Abdominal pain, sometimes experienced as bad indigestion
- Prolonged pain that lasts over 20 minutes
- Light-headedness/dizziness
- Dry mouth
- Feeling of "impending doom"
- Anxiety

According to *The Journal of the American Medical Association*, 650,000 new heart attacks each year could be prevented or delayed for decades by quitting smoking, reducing cholesterol and controlling hypertension and diabetes.

What treatments are commonly used after a heart attack?

Hospitalization
Emergency Treatment

Medication

Additional Treatment
Angioplasty or Bypass Surgery

Initial treatment includes aspirin to reduce the clot, beta-blockers to slow the heart rate and reduce the heart's workload, oxygen to minimize tissue damage, nitroglycerin to relieve pain and thrombolitic drugs to dissolve the clot.

Warning: Don't try to diagnose yourself. Because the most damage occurs during the first two hours of a heart attack, it is important to call for emergency medical service, or 911, if you are experiencing chest pain or other symptoms of a heart attack. Sit down and wait for the paramedics to arrive. Do not try to drive yourself to the hospital.

Being married reduces your risk of dying from a heart attack. An unmarried person is 3 times more likely to have a fatal outcome.

A high blood level of homocysteine, a naturally occurring amino acid, is thought to be a risk factor because it can irritate your arteries and lead to plaque buildup. Many doctors believe that taking folic acid and vitamins B6 and B12 may lower homocysteine levels.

ACTION ITEMS

Assessing your risk for a heart attack

You can reduce your risk of heart attack by becoming aware of your risk factors. Although some risk factors can't be changed, moderate daily changes can reduce or eliminate others. Use this quiz to learn where to focus your efforts.

Check all boxes in the quiz that apply to you. These factors may increase your risk of a heart attack. As always, see your healthcare provider for a complete assessment of your risks.

Your age may increase your risk if
- ☐ You are a man over 45 years old.
- ☐ You are a woman over 55 years old OR you have passed menopause OR had your ovaries removed and are not taking estrogen.

Your family history may increase your risk if
- ☐ Your father or brother had a heart attack before age 55 OR your mother or sister had one before age 65.
- ☐ You have a close blood relative who had a stroke.

Cigarette and tobacco smoke increases your risk if
- ☐ You smoke. 51
- ☐ You live or work with people who smoke.

When am I likely to show symptoms of a heart attack?

80% of people who die from the disease are 65 years or older. Men are at greater risk of heart attack than women. A man's risk typically begins between the ages of 35 to 40. Once a woman is postmenopausal, her risk is equal to that of a man.

Sources: A.D.A.M. Health Illustrated Encyclopedia, Best Practice of Medicine, Merck Health Library, mercksource.com; AOL Health News; Esquire; USA Today.

How am I likely to be diagnosed with a heart attack?

Only 10 to 20% of chest-pain patients admitted to emergency rooms are actually having a heart attack, so an evaluation and testing are conducted as soon as possible after you arrive. Your doctor will perform an electrocardiogram. 165

Heart Attack Timeline

00:00 - blood pressure, pulse, temperature taken

00:01 - heart rhythm and rate monitored

00:05 - electrocardiogram machine connected (if normal, doctor will look for other causes of the symptoms)

00:15 - oxygen, heparin, aspirin or beta-blockers may be administered

00:30 - transfer to cath lab for diagnostics

What can I expect if I have a heart attack?

A heart attack (myocardial infarction) occurs when an artery supplying the heart with blood carrying oxygen and nutrients suddenly becomes blocked, causing part of the heart muscle to die.

Such clots usually form in arteries that have been narrowed by a build-up of fats and plaques over time. This narrowing can exist and grow without symptoms. When the artery becomes blocked, your heart can not receive the blood and oxygen it needs to survive.

Lifestyle Modifications — **Normal Life**

How likely am I to die of a heart attack?

Complications Arrhythmia/Congestive Heart Failure — **Death**

The expected outcome varies with the amount and location of damaged tissue. Approximately one-third of cases are fatal. If the person is alive 2 hours after an attack, the probable outcome for survival is good, but may include complications. Patients with uncomplicated cases may recover fully and gradually resume normal activity.

Healthy heart habits include avoiding red meat, fried foods, high-fat dairy products and high-fat processed foods.

If you smoke cigarettes, cigars or pipe tobacco, your risk of heart attack is doubled.

TIP

Chew aspirin while waiting for the paramedics, unless you have serious trouble with stomach bleeding. It can decrease additional clot formation.

Your cholesterol levels may increase your risk if

☐ Your total cholesterol level is 240 mg/dL or higher.

☐ Your HDL cholesterol level is less than 35 mg/dL.

☐ You don't know your total cholesterol or HDL levels.

Your blood pressure may increase your risk if

☐ Your blood pressure is 120/80 or higher. 111

☐ You don't know what your blood pressure is.

Physical inactivity may increase your risk if

☐ You get less than a total of 30 minutes of physical activity most days. 47

Excess body weight may increase your risk if

☐ You are 20 pounds or more overweight. 127

Diabetes may increase your risk if

☐ You have diabetes. 21

☐ You have a fasting blood sugar of 126 mg/dL or higher.

☐ You need medicine to control your blood sugar.

Your medical history may increase your risk if

☐ You have cardiovascular disease. 75

☐ You've had a heart attack.

☐ You've had a stroke. 115

☐ You have a disease of the leg arteries.

77

*H*e'd planned on retiring from teaching soon, spending more time with his wife and grandchildren. Cancer wasn't part of the plan, but when Thomas, 55, found out he had prostate cancer, he used his skills as an educator to help him cope with this life-threatening challenge.

"I've had annual screening tests for the past 10 years." It was this test for prostate specific antigen (PSA) that revealed a problem. A biopsy confirmed that Thomas had cancer.

His first doctor recommended surgery. "It shook me," Thomas said. "I know I came across as angry, but I was really more scared than anything else."

Thomas decided to get opinions from other doctors.

"I felt like I was back in grad school again," Thomas said adjusting a pair of wire-rim glasses. "It was an exercise in research and discovery."

Prostate specific antigen (PSA) screening is a blood test that can detect prostate cancer in its early stages.

When you're considering treatment options, the American Cancer Society suggests taking into account:

  your age and expected life span

  your feelings about treatment side effects

  other serious health conditions you may have

  the stage and grade of your cancer

  the likelihood that treatment will be curative

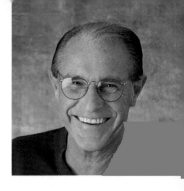

Watchful waiting is a treatment option for prostate cancer and simply means that the patient receives no treatment but is monitored by his doctor for problems.
Source: More Options, and Decisions, for Men with Prostate Cancer, New York Times, October 3, 2000.

Thomas met with a range of doctors from oncologists to urologists. He learned about alternatives to surgery, which included watchful waiting and radioactive seeds. Thomas preferred these options to surgery. He noticed that most specialists recommended their own treatment over others.

"It was so confusing," Thomas said. "How could I make a decision when the doctors couldn't agree?"

He turned to an online support group of cancer survivors. "It was a relief to get opinions from people who've been in my situation."

He learned how others weighed their options. On the minus side for surgery was the possibility of impotence. Radiation could bring impotence, fatigue and diarrhea.

Prostate cancer is often slow moving, but Thomas' cancer was aggressive and he decided his best option for recovery was surgery.

Thomas sought additional information and advice while deciding on a treatment plan for his prostate cancer.

A recent study shows that physicians' opinions about treatments tend to favor their own specialty. About 93 percent of urologists leaned toward radical prostatectomy (surgery) as the recommended treatment and 72 percent of radiation therapists felt radiation treatments were as effective as surgery in treating the disease.
Source: The Dartmouth Atlas of Health Care.

Radioactive seeds are one treatment for prostate cancer. The tiny seeds are injected into the prostate to kill cancer cells. There is a 10 to 20 percent chance of men developing impotence with this treatment, according to the American Cancer Association.
Source: More Options, and Decisions, for Men with Prostate Cancer, New York Times, October 3, 2000.

Source: American Cancer Society.

One in two men will get cancer.

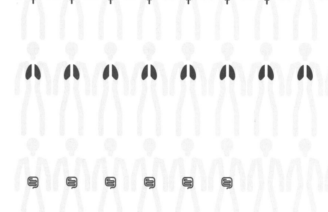

prostate
16.67% or 1 in 6

lung & bronchus
7.69 % or 1 in 13

colon & rectum
5.88% or 1 in 17

bladder
3.45% or 1 in 29

non-Hodgkin's lymphoma
2.08% or 1 in 48

melanoma of the skin
1.72% or 1 in 58

leukemia
1.43% or 1 in 70

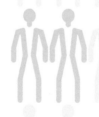

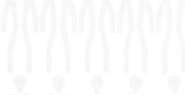

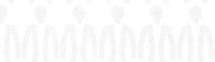

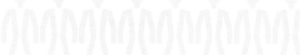

Figures above show approximate occurance of specified cancers in 100 men from birth to death.

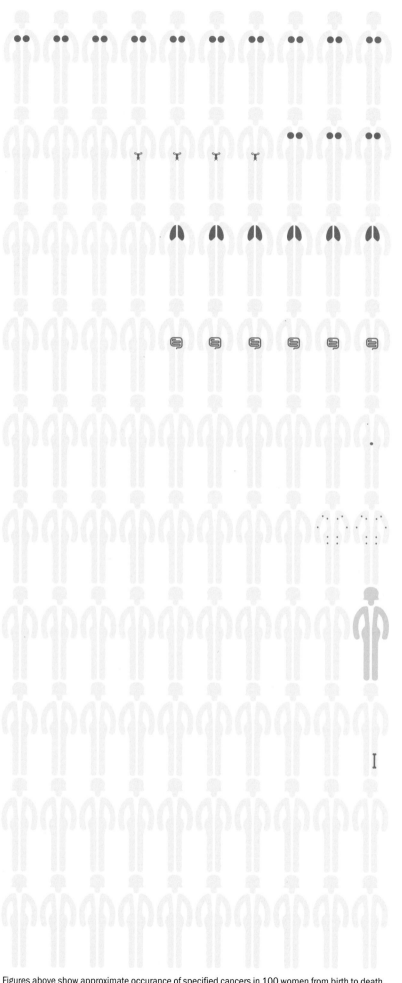

One in three women will get cancer.

●● *breast*
  12.5% or 1 in 8

Ⴢ *uterine, corpus and cervix*
  3.55% or 1 in 37 and 1 in 117

◖◗ *lung & bronchus*
  5.88% or 1 in 17

⊜ *colon & rectum*
  5.55% or 1 in 18

• *bladder*
  1.12% or 1 in 89

⠂⠂ *non-Hodgkin's lymphoma*
  1.75% or 1 in 57

☗ *melanoma of the skin*
  1.22% or 1 in 82

I *leukemia*
  1.04% or 1 in 96

Figures above show approximate occurance of specified cancers in 100 women from birth to death.

81

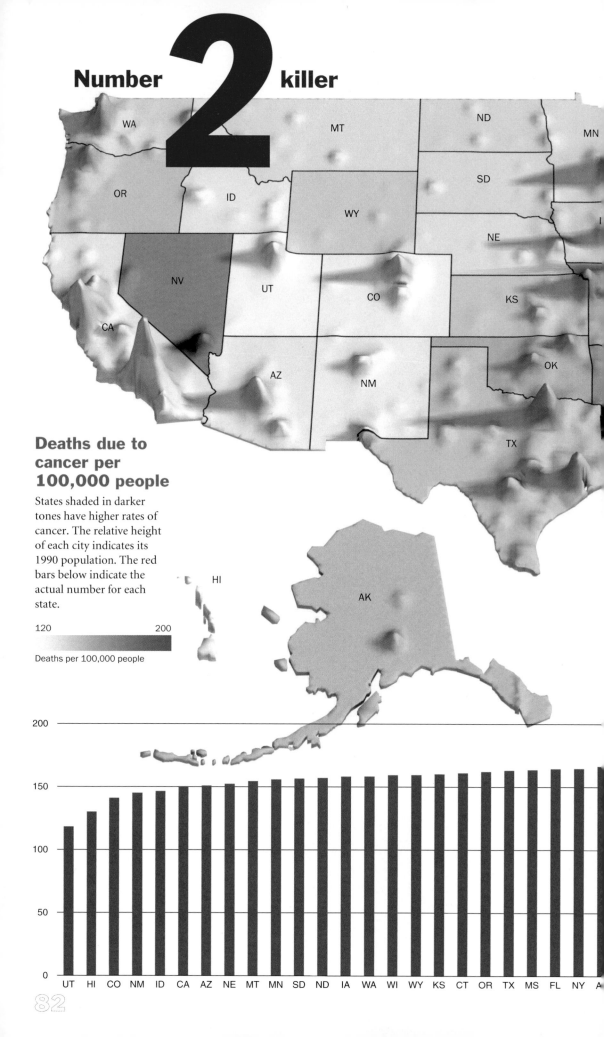

Number **2** killer

Deaths due to cancer per 100,000 people

States shaded in darker tones have higher rates of cancer. The relative height of each city indicates its 1990 population. The red bars below indicate the actual number for each state.

120 ———— 200

Deaths per 100,000 people

One of every four deaths
in the US is from cancer.

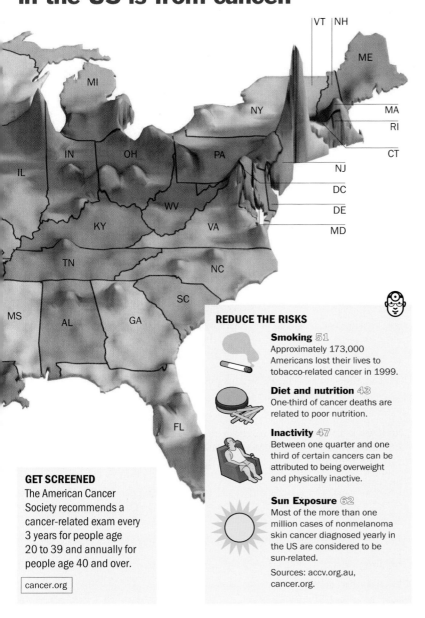

More than 550,000 Americans died of cancer in 2002.

Not surprising, considering the fact that cancer is the 2nd most common cause of death in the US. The National Cancer Institute estimates that approximately 8.2 million Americans alive today have a history of cancer.

Sources: ncbi.nlm.nih.gov, cdc.gov.

REDUCE THE RISKS

Smoking 51
Approximately 173,000 Americans lost their lives to tobacco-related cancer in 1999.

Diet and nutrition 43
One-third of cancer deaths are related to poor nutrition.

Inactivity 47
Between one quarter and one third of certain cancers can be attributed to being overweight and physically inactive.

Sun Exposure 62
Most of the more than one million cases of nonmelanoma skin cancer diagnosed yearly in the US are considered to be sun-related.

Sources: accv.org.au, cancer.org.

GET SCREENED
The American Cancer Society recommends a cancer-related exam every 3 years for people age 20 to 39 and annually for people age 40 and over.

cancer.org

The National Cancer Institute estimates that the overall annual cost of cancer in the United States is

$107 billion;
this estimate includes healthcare costs, costs of lost productivity and mortality costs.

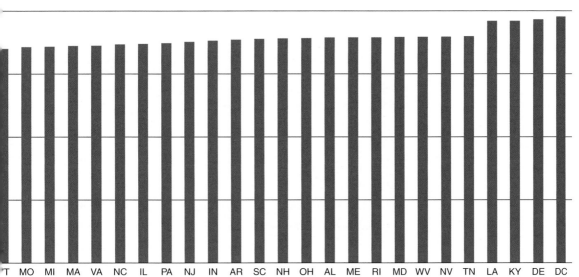

T | MO | MI | MA | VA | NC | IL | PA | NJ | IN | AR | SC | NH | OH | AL | ME | RI | MD | WV | NV | TN | LA | KY | DE | DC

Source: Mayo Clinic Family Health Book.

If you've been recently diagnosed with cancer, you're on a steep and fast learning curve. Take some of the mystery out of cancer by learning as much as you can about your type of cancer and treatment options.

Discovery 7

You find a suspicious lump or wonder why your voice is constantly hoarse. Your doctor notices something during an exam. Your spouse sees changes in a mole on your back. Here are some typical ways people discover they have a problem that needs to be checked for cancer:

- During a self-exam
- During a routine medical exam
- During a screening test

Diagnosis 153

Diagnosis means your doctor is figuring out what type of cancer you have and if it has spread. Ask your doctor how long diagnosis will take. It could take days or even weeks to get laboratory results. Generally, these results come from one of these two means:

- Studying tissue samples (biopsy)
- Studying x-rays, CTs, PET scans or other images

Type of Cancer

Once you know the type of cancer, you and your doctor can move forward on treatment decisions. There are over 100 types of cancer. Some of the more common types are:

- Breast cancer 93
- Cervical cancer
- Colorectal cancer 89
- Endometrial cancer
- Lung cancer
- Oral cancer
- Prostate cancer 95
- Skin cancer

Treatment Options

Your treatment options vary. Your doctor will most likely follow the treatment guidelines for your type of cancer. These guidelines take years to develop and are based on best practices for treatment of specific diseases and illnesses. Your treatment could include:

- Surgery 205
- Radiation Therapy
- Immunotherapy
- Chemotherapy
- Medication (oral or injection) to help tolerate chemotherapy
- Experimental: Gene therapy, lasers 267

You can check for the most current guidelines at the National Guideline Clearinghouse.

www.guideline.gov

Are all cancers the same?

No.

All cancers are not the same.

WHERE IS IT?

That's one reason cancer is such a difficult topic.

HOW WAS IT FOUND?

Each has it's own set of symptoms and treatment options.

WHAT TYPE IS IT?

Some cancers stay contained, while some spread.

HAS IT SPREAD?

Some cancers grow slowly.

Others grow rapidly.

Cancer is the **second leading cause of death** in the US, exceeded only by heart disease.

The **National Institutes of Health** estimates overall annual costs for cancer at $171.6 billion.

In 2000, about 552,000 Americans died from cancer, more than **1,500 per day.**

Treatment for **breast, lung and prostate cancers** costs around $18.5 billion a year.

Since 1990, nearly **17 million new cancer cases** have been diagnosed.

The **incidence of breast cancer** is highest among white women (113.2 per 100,000) and lowest among American Indian women (33.9 per 100,000).

Source: Cancer Facts and Figures 2001, American Cancer Society, cancer.org; cnn.com.

What are the most common forms of cancer?

The three most common cancers in men are prostate cancer, colon cancer and lung cancer. In women, the most frequently occurring cancers are breast cancer, colon cancer and lung cancer.

Certain cancers are more common in particular geographic areas. For instance, gastric (stomach) cancer is prevalent in Japan, while relatively rare in the US. Liver cancer occurs more often in countries with high rates of viral infections from Hepatitis B or C.

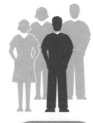

In the US, 1 in every 4 deaths is from cancer. 13

What are the treatment options for cancer?

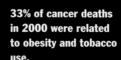

Surgery

Surgery is the oldest form of treatment and offers the greatest chance for cure in many types of cancer. About 60% of people with cancer will have some type of surgery or operation.

Radiation

Radiation therapy uses high-energy particles, such as x-rays or gamma rays, to destroy or damage cancer cells. It is the primary treatment for many kinds of cancer, and is used in almost any part of the body.

Chemotherapy

Chemotherapy is the use of drugs to treat cancer. Anticancer drugs destroy cancer cells by stopping them from multiplying or growing.

All cancers caused by cigarette smoking and heavy use of alcohol can be prevented completely.

33% of cancer deaths in 2000 were related to obesity and tobacco use.

Blacks are 33% more likely to die of cancer than whites, and 2 times more likely to die of cancer than Asians, American Indians and Hispanics.

ACTION ITEMS Coping with chemotherapy

Chemotherapy can bring major changes to a person's life. It can affect overall health, threaten a sense of well-being, disrupt day-to-day schedules and put a strain on personal relationships. Here are some tips to help yourself while you are getting chemotherapy.

① Stay focused.
Try to keep your treatment goals in mind. This will help you keep a positive attitude on days when the going gets rough.

② Eat well. 43
Remember that eating well is very important. Your body needs food to rebuild tissues and regain strength.

③ Stay informed. 323
Learn as much as you want to know about your disease and its treatment. This can lessen your fear of the unknown and increase your feeling of control.

④ Record your thoughts.
Keep a journal or diary while you're in treatment. A record of your activities and thoughts can help you understand the feelings you have as you go through treatment, and highlight

What is the chance I'll get cancer?

In the US, men have about a 1 in 2 lifetime risk of developing cancer, and women have about a 1 in 3 risk. 81

About 5% to 10% of cancers are hereditary, which means that a person may inherit a faulty gene that predisposes that person to a particular cancer. But most cancers result from damage to genes (mutations) that occurs as people age. Damaging agents can include sunlight, chemicals, radiation or hormones.

How is cancer staged?

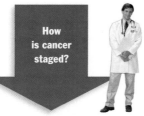

A cancer's stage is based on the extent of the primary tumor, the absence or presence of regional lymph node involvement and the absence or presence of any metastases, which is the spreading of the disease. This information then determines the stage of the cancer.

What can I expect if I have cancer?

What is cancer?

Cancer is a group of diseases that are characterized by an uncontrolled growth of abnormal cells that have mutated from normal tissues. All cancers involve the malfunction of genes that control cell growth and division.

Sources: Cancer Facts and Figures 2001 and Cancer Resource Center, American Cancer Society, cancer.org; cnn.com; National Cancer Institute, cancer.gov; A.D.A.M. Illustrated Health Encyclopedia, Merck Health Library, mercksource.com.

Hormone Therapy

Hormone therapy uses hormones, or drugs that interfere with hormone production or action. It can also include the surgical removal of hormone-producing glands. This can help kill cancer cells or slow their growth.

Immunotherapy

Immunotherapy is the use of treatments that promote or support the body's immune system response to a disease such as cancer.

What is the chance of surviving cancer?

Surviving cancer and its prognosis (prospect of recovery) varies widely depending on the type of cancer and the stage at which treatment begins. However, the 5-year relative survival rate for all cancers combined is about 62%. This represents people living five years after diagnosis who are disease-free, in remission or under treatment with evidence of cancer.

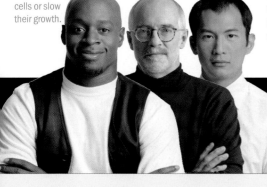

The number of Americans with cancer is expected to double from 1.3 million in 2000 to 2.6 million in 2050.

 2000   2050

TIP

Regular screening examinations for cancer can result in early detection and treatment that is more likely to be successful.

questions you need to ask your doctor or nurse. You also can use your journal to record the steps you take to cope with side effects and how well those steps work. That way, you'll know which methods worked best for you in case you have the same side effects again.

5 Don't try to overdo it.

Set realistic goals and don't be too hard on yourself. You may not have as much energy as usual, so try to get as much rest as you can, let the "small stuff" slide, and only do the things that are most important to you.

6 Try to stay active. 47

Try new hobbies and learn new skills. Exercise if you can. Using your body can make you feel better about yourself, help you get rid of tension or anger, and build your appetite. Ask your doctor or nurse about a safe and practical exercise program.

Source: National Institutes of Health.

According to the **American Cancer Society**, in 2003, some 147,500 new cases of colon cancer were diagnosed in the US, with 56,300 resulting deaths.

Medical studies have found that a daily multivitamin with **folic acid** and increased **calcium** intake can lower your risk.

Aspirin and ibuprofen may cut the risk of colon cancer.

Having colorectal polyps, ulcerative colitis, Crohn's disease or a family history of colorectal cancer puts you at **increased risk.**

A **low-fat, high-fiber diet** may reduce your risk for colon cancer. Try to eat 5 to 6 servings of fruits, vegetables and high-fiber grains every day.

Source: National Center for Biotechnology Information, National Library of Medicine, National Institutes of Health, ncbi.nlm.nih.gov; A.D.A.M. Illustrated Health Encyclopedia, Best Practice of Medicine, Merck Health Library, mercksource.com.

What symptoms might suggest colon cancer?

In its earliest stages, colorectal cancer has few or no symptoms, so it is extremely important to undergo routine screening tests beginning at age 50. More advanced colorectal cancer can produce changes in bowel habits and bloody stools. If you experience constipation, diarrhea or pencil-thin stools for more than 10 days, you should see your doctor.

Stage 1, 2 and 3 cancers are considered curable, based on the chance of living at least 5 years after diagnosis. In most cases, stage 4 cancer is incurable.

Stage 1 has a 90% 5-year survival. Stage 2 has a 75-85% 5-year survival, and Stage 3 a 40%-60% 5-year survival.

What treatments are commonly used for colon cancer?

The main treatment for colorectal cancer is surgical removal of a large segment of the affected intestine and the associated lymph nodes.

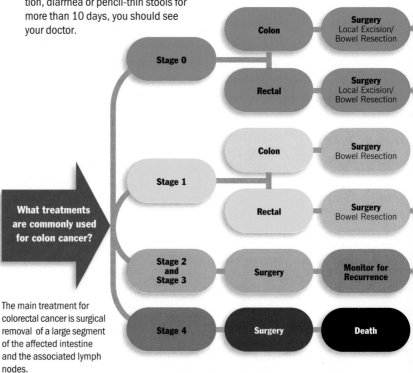

Stage 0 → Colon → **Surgery** Local Excision/ Bowel Resection

Stage 0 → Rectal → **Surgery** Local Excision/ Bowel Resection

Stage 1 → Colon → **Surgery** Bowel Resection

Stage 1 → Rectal → **Surgery** Bowel Resection

Stage 2 and Stage 3 → **Surgery** → **Monitor for Recurrence**

Stage 4 → **Surgery** → **Death**

 Throughout the world, people at highest risk for colon cancer tend to live in cities. 63

Colon cancer occurs most often in older adults. Incidences of cancer begin to rise around age 40 and peak at age 70.

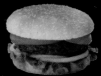 A diet high in calories and fat (animal fat, in particular) may increase colorectal cancer risk. 43

ACTION ITEMS
Questions to ask before surgery

Never hesitate to ask your doctor any question. Keep a written list of issues as they come up so you won't forget to bring something up at an office visit.

1 **Should I have a CEA test?**
A CEA blood test can detect chemicals produced by some colon cancers and can help in early diagnosis. Almost all physicians urge patients to get a CEA test before surgery as well as afterwards, and you should ask about that.

2 **What is the stage of my cancer, and what does that mean in my case?**

3 **Where is the cancer located? Has it spread beyond the place where it began?**

4 **What tests will you perform before and after the surgery to determine how far advanced my cancer is?**

5 **What should I do to be ready for treatment?**

6 **Will I need a colostomy?**

7 **When should I see an oncologist?** 15

How am I likely to be diagnosed with colon cancer?

Physical examination rarely shows abnormalities, though an abdominal mass may be present. To check signs of colon cancer, the doctor typically conducts certain tests 180:

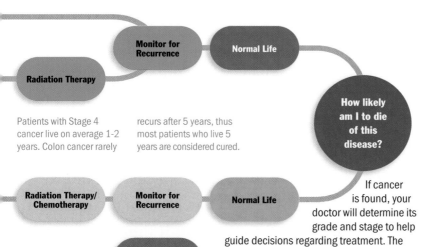

- Colonoscopy, which provides a look at the entire colon.
- Fecal occult blood test (FOBT), which may detect small amounts of blood in the stool, a possible indicator of colon cancer.
- Blood test, which may reveal evidence of anemia with low iron levels.
- CT scan, which may show an abdominal mass.

Colorectal cancer is unchecked cell growth in the large intestine (colon) or rectum that results in tumors that can spread to other parts of the body.

The majority of cases occur in the lower part of the colon or rectum. A quarter of cancers show up in the rectum. Colorectal cancer tends to develop slowly over many years, and starts out as precancerous lesions or polyps. When detected and treated early enough, it is usually curable.

Radiation Therapy → **Monitor for Recurrence** → **Normal Life**

Patients with Stage 4 cancer live on average 1-2 years. Colon cancer rarely recurs after 5 years, thus most patients who live 5 years are considered cured.

How likely am I to die of this disease?

Radiation Therapy/ Chemotherapy → **Monitor for Recurrence** → **Normal Life**

Normal Life

If cancer is found, your doctor will determine its grade and stage to help guide decisions regarding treatment. The stage will fall between 0 and 4, depending on the extent of cancer spread within the intestinal wall, whether cancer has invaded neighboring tissue and whether it has spread to lymph nodes, liver, lungs or elsewhere in the body.

Family tree

Aunt
Sister
Uncle
Father
At Risk
Grandfather

Colon cancer is one of the most common inherited cancer syndromes known. 29

Colorectal cancer is the 3rd leading cause of cancer-related death in the US, accounting for about 11% of cancer deaths.

Colon cancer is more common in women. Rectal cancer is more common in men. 31

TIP

Regular screening can detect colorectal polyps and cancer very early on before symptoms are apparent, and when cancer can be prevented or cured.

8. **What if I don't have surgery?**

9. **Will I need any treatment before surgery?**

10. **Will treatment be needed after surgery?**

11. **How long will I be in the hospital?** 239

12. **If I'm in pain, what will you give me to make me feel better?** 221

13. **What are the chances my cancer will come back with this treatment plan?**

The American Cancer Society recommends that all Americans undergo yearly colon cancer screenings beginning at age 50. 7

Source: ccalliance.org.

A was incredibly shocked when my doctor told me I had breast cancer," said Diane, a 33-year-old mother of three from Texas. "None of the women in my family have had it. I just couldn't believe it."

Diane's gynecologist found a lump during a regular visit. "I could tell by her face that she'd found something," Diane said. "Her face just kind of fell."

The next surprise was how quickly the biopsy was scheduled. "The next day I was in an operating room." But then events slowed. "I thought I'd know the results right away, but the doctor said it would take two to three days. Waiting was so hard."

She was sure the biopsy would come back negative. But it didn't. "I spent a day in bed crying."

The surgeon suggested a modified radical mastectomy, removing most of the breast. "I was stunned—too stunned to ask about alternatives."

A day at the library gave Diane a wealth of infor-

There are several methods of breast biopsy including:

Fine-needle aspiration biopsy: A thin needle is inserted into the lump to remove cells.

Core needle biopsy: A large needle with a special tip collects a section of tissue.

Sterotactic biopsy: An x-ray tool locates the lump and an incision is made in the breast, then the tool guides a needle to the right spot, often used when a lump is seen on a mammogram but can't be felt by hand.

Open biopsy: An incision is made in the breast and a sample or the entire lump is removed. The sample is rushed to the lab and if it is cancerous, the surgeon may proceed to remove the entire lump.

Source: Laurus Health.

For many years radical mastectomy (removal of the breast, chest muscles and under arm lymph nodes) was the standard treatment for breast cancer.

A medical oncologist specializes in diagnosing and treating cancer using chemotherapy, hormonal therapy and biological therapy. Studies show that women referred to a medical oncologist prior to surgery to discuss treatment options are more satisfied with their treatment selection.
Sources: National Cancer Institute; Discussion of Treatment Options for Early-Stage Breast Cancer, Medical Care, July 2001.

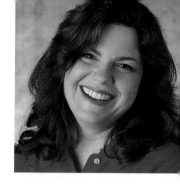

mation, but she was still confused. "Talk to an oncologist," said a friend. "I'll go with you."

At the appointment Diane's friend Jill took notes as they discussed treatment options including surgery that would remove less tissue (lumpectomy), chemotherapy, and radiation therapy. "I learned there were a lot of options and combinations of treatments. We also talked about complementary therapy, which was great because I like knowing that there are some things that I can do to help myself."

She took a few days to think over her options, possible side-effects and after care. "Ultimately, because my cancer was caught early and studies show positive results from breast-conserving surgery, I chose to have a lumpectomy," Diane said. "I know I still have a lot to go through, but I'm confident that I'll be a cancer survivor."

Diane made a decision on treatment for her breast cancer after a second opinion and some help from a friend.

Complementary therapies help boost your immune system, reduce stress and help you relax. They don't take the place of traditional treatment but are used to enhance your wellbeing. Yoga, massage and meditation are examples.
Source: Abramson Cancer Center of the University of Pennsylvania.

A surgeon removes the cancer and some tissue during a lumpectomy and preserves as much of the breast as possible. In 1998, doctors performed 340,000 lumpectomies on an out-patient basis in the US.
Source: Ambulatory Surgery in the United States, National Center for Health Statistics.

TESTING FOR CHEMOTHERAPY RESISTANCE

Resistance to chemotherapy is a major cause of failure in treating breast cancer patients. Italian researchers have developed a test that can predict the effectiveness of this treatment. Knowing that a tumor is likely to be resistant allows doctors to prescribe drugs that can boost the body's responsiveness.

Who is most at risk?

All women are at risk for breast cancer. However, certain factors appear to result in a higher incidence of the disease.

- Genetic factors (in 5% to 10% of breast cancer cases) 29
- Early menarche or late menopause
- First full-pregnancy after age 30
- Long-term estrogen therapy, high-fat diet and alcohol use

What symptoms might suggest breast cancer?

Regular self-examination often detects early symptoms when the chance for cure is highest. Report any of the following symptoms immediately to your physician:

- A breast or axillary (armpit) lump or thickening
- Breast pain

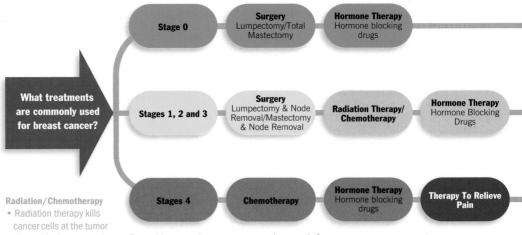

What treatments are commonly used for breast cancer?

| Stage 0 | Surgery Lumpectomy/Total Mastectomy | Hormone Therapy Hormone blocking drugs |

| Stages 1, 2 and 3 | Surgery Lumpectomy & Node Removal/Mastectomy & Node Removal | Radiation Therapy/ Chemotherapy | Hormone Therapy Hormone Blocking Drugs |

| Stages 4 | Chemotherapy | Hormone Therapy Hormone blocking drugs | Therapy To Relieve Pain |

Radiation/Chemotherapy
- Radiation therapy kills cancer cells at the tumor site and in the surrounding lymph nodes.
- Chemotherapy and hormone-blocking drugs suppress cancer growth throughout the body.

Even with appropriate treatment, breast cancer often spreads to other parts of the body. The recurrence rate is 5% after total mastectomy and removal of non-cancerous armpit lymph nodes. The recurrence rate is 25% when the lymph nodes are cancerous.

In more than 80% of breast cancer cases, the woman detects the lump herself.

Asian/Pacific Islander and Hispanic women have 2/3rds the risk of white women.

1 woman out of 8 develops breast cancer in her lifetime.

ACTION ITEMS
Performing a breast self-exam

Women should perform this procedure once a month, 2 or 3 days after the end of each menstrual cycle.

1 In the shower, raise your left arm. With the fingers of the right hand, carefully examine the left breast. In a circular pattern, starting from the outer top, press firmly enough to feel the tissue inside the breast. Complete 1 full circle, then move toward the center and circle again. Continue until you reach the nipple. Then check the area above the breast and the armpit. Repeat the examination on your right breast.

2 In front of a mirror, place your hands at your sides and check your breasts for any changes in color, shape or size. Also look for any dimpling or scaling of the skin.

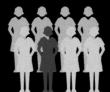

Sources: A.D.A.M. Illustrated Health Encyclopedia, Merck Health Library, mercksource.com; National Cancer Institute, cancer.gov; Centers for Disease Control, cdc.gov; HealthScout, healthscout.com; Mayo Clinic, mayoclinic.com; University of Pennsylvania, oncolink.upenn.edu.

How and when am I likely to be diagnosed with breast cancer?

Doctors rely on mammography 169 (breast x-ray) to detect abnormalities or lumps and recommend getting a mammogram every 1-2 years for women between ages 40-49 and annually thereafter or if there is a family history of breast cancer. Although not foolproof, mammograms usually detect breast cancer before it can be felt. A breast lump usually warrants a needle aspiration or surgical biopsy to study the suspicious tissue more closely.

- Nipple scaling, retraction, thickening or discharge
- Skin dimpling or erythema (reddening)
- Edema (swelling)
- Ulceration
- Distended veins in an irregular pattern

Monitor for Recurrence

Normal Life

Breast Reconstruction

Monitor for Recurrence

Normal Life

How likely is my condition to improve? How likely am I to die of this disease?

Normal Life

Death

Five-year survival rates for women with breast cancer are:
95% for Stage 0
88% for Stage 1
66% for Stage 2
36% for Stage 3
7% for Stage 4

What can I expect if I have breast cancer?

Breast cancer is a malignant growth that begins in the tissues of the breast.

It is the 2nd leading cause of cancer death for women in the US, with an estimated 203,500 new cases and 39,600 deaths occurring in 2002. From 1973 to 1998, female breast cancer incidence rates increased by more than 40%. On the other hand, mortality rates showed a significant drop, probably due to earlier detection and improved treatment.

White and black women have the highest levels of breast cancer.

Less than 1% of all breast cancer cases occur in men.

In the US, breast cancer accounts for 29% of all cancers in women.

3 Still in front of the mirror, place your hands on your hips. Press your shoulders and elbows forward to flex the chest muscles. Then raise your hands and clasp them behind your head. Check again for any changes in color, shape, size or texture.

4 Lie down and place a pillow under your left shoulder. Raise your left arm above your head. Using the circular method described in step 1, examine your left breast. Repeat the process for your right breast.

5 Gently squeeze each nipple to check for discharge.

6 Report any changes to your doctor.

The following organization can provide more information about early detection.

- The National Breast and Cervical Cancer Early Detection Program (NBCCEDP), Centers for Disease Control
  www.cdc.gov/cancer/nbccedp/

What symptoms might suggest prostate cancer?

- Difficulty starting urination or holding back urine
- Weak or interrupted flow of urine
- Painful or burning urination
- Difficulty in having an erection
- Painful ejaculation
- Blood in urine or semen
- Frequent pain or stiffness in the lower back, hips or upper thighs

Early prostate cancer often does not exhibit any symptoms, but it can cause any of these problems:

- A need to urinate frequently, especially at night

What is BPH?

Benign Prostatic Hyperplasic is the abnormal but benign growth of prostate cells. In BPH the prostate grows larger and presses against the urethra and bladder, interfering with the normal flow of urine. More than half of the men in the US show symptoms of BPH by ages 60 to 70, and about 90% show signs of BPH between ages 70 to 90.

What treatments are commonly used for prostate cancer?

Treatment for prostate cancer depends on the stage of the disease and the grade of the tumor (which indicates how abnormal the cells look, and how likely they are to grow or spread). Other factors are the man's age and general health and his feelings about the treatments and possible side effects.

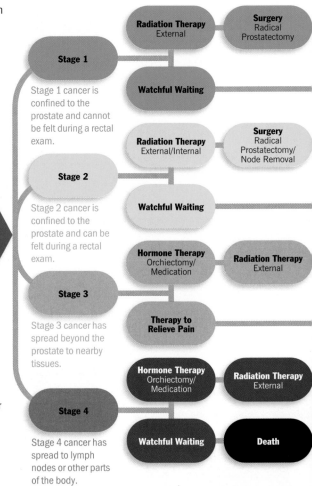

Stage 1

Stage 1 cancer is confined to the prostate and cannot be felt during a rectal exam.

- Radiation Therapy — External → Surgery — Radical Prostatectomy
- Watchful Waiting

Stage 2

Stage 2 cancer is confined to the prostate and can be felt during a rectal exam.

- Radiation Therapy — External/Internal → Surgery — Radical Prostatectomy/ Node Removal
- Watchful Waiting

Stage 3

Stage 3 cancer has spread beyond the prostate to nearby tissues.

- Hormone Therapy — Orchiectomy/ Medication → Radiation Therapy — External
- Therapy to Relieve Pain

Stage 4

Stage 4 cancer has spread to lymph nodes or other parts of the body.

- Hormone Therapy — Orchiectomy/ Medication → Radiation Therapy — External
- Watchful Waiting → Death

 83% of all prostate cancers are discovered in the local and regional stages.

 The average age of death from prostate cancer is 71.

 In 2002, 1 new case of prostate cancer was diagnosed every 3 minutes.

 Prostate cancer is the 2nd leading cause of cancer death in men.

ACTION ITEMS

Performing a testicular self-exam

Because testicular cancer often produces no symptoms, many doctors recommend monthly self-exams. Although most are not cancer, any lumps or other symptoms should be checked by a physician immediately.

1 The best time to examine your testicles is during or right after a warm bath or shower. The heat causes the skin of the scrotum to soften and relax. And, soapy skin may make it even easier to feel any lumps underneath.

2 Examine each testicle separately with both hands by rolling the testicle between the thumbs and fingers. You'll feel a cord-like structure (the epididymis which stores and transports sperm) on the top and back of the testicle. Gently separate this tube from the testicle with your fingers to examine the testicle itself.

3 Feel for any swelling, lumps or any change in the size, shape or consistency of the testes.

Sources: National Cancer Institute, cancer.gov.; Best Practice of Medicine, Merck Health Library, mercksource.com.

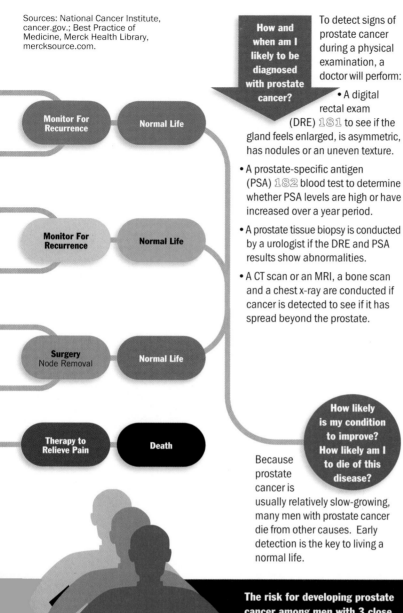

How and when am I likely to be diagnosed with prostate cancer?

To detect signs of prostate cancer during a physical examination, a doctor will perform:

- A digital rectal exam (DRE) 181 to see if the gland feels enlarged, is asymmetric, has nodules or an uneven texture.

- A prostate-specific antigen (PSA) 182 blood test to determine whether PSA levels are high or have increased over a year period.

- A prostate tissue biopsy is conducted by a urologist if the DRE and PSA results show abnormalities.

- A CT scan or an MRI, a bone scan and a chest x-ray are conducted if cancer is detected to see if it has spread beyond the prostate.

Monitor For Recurrence → Normal Life

Monitor For Recurrence → Normal Life

Surgery Node Removal → Normal Life

Therapy to Relieve Pain → Death

How likely is my condition to improve? How likely am I to die of this disease?

Because prostate cancer is usually relatively slow-growing, many men with prostate cancer die from other causes. Early detection is the key to living a normal life.

What is a prostate?

The prostate is a walnut-sized gland that produces a thick fluid that forms the major part of semen. It is located below the bladder, in front of the rectum, and surrounds the upper part of the urethra, the tube that empties urine from the bladder. If the prostate grows too large, the flow of urine can be slowed or stopped. To work properly, the prostate needs male hormones—primarily, testosterone—which is made mainly by the testicles. Some male hormones are produced in small amounts by the adrenal glands.

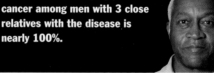

The risk for developing prostate cancer among men with 3 close relatives with the disease is nearly 100%.

Black men have the highest prostate cancer incidence rate worldwide.

Here are some questions a patient may want to ask his doctor before prostate cancer treatment begins:

- What is the stage of the disease?
- What is the grade of the disease?
- What are my treatment choices? Is watchful waiting a good choice for me?
- Are new treatments under study? Would a clinical trial be appropriate for me?
- What are the expected benefits of each kind of treatment?

- What are the risks and possible side effects of each treatment? How can the side effects be managed?
- Is treatment likely to affect my sex life?
- Am I likely to have urinary problems?
- Am I likely to have bowel problems, such as diarrhea or rectal bleeding?
- Will I need to change my normal activities? If so, for how long?

What are the most common respiratory problems?

Respiratory disorders are primarily due to acute or chronic airflow obstruction. Asthma, chronic bronchitis, emphysema, bronchiolitis and cystic fibrosis are some common diseases. The term chronic obstructive pulmonary disease (COPD) describes chronic bronchitis and emphysema, in which the airway obstruction is irreversible.

Asthma is found in 5% of adults and 10% of children. Half of the people with asthma develop it before age 10 and most develop it before age 30. Asthma symptoms can decrease over time, especially in children.

What are the risk factors for asthma?

- Family tendency 29
- Viral respiratory infections
- Allergens 125, tobacco 51, certain foods or drugs
- Intense exercise, especially when performed in cold air
- Environmental hazards 63, occupational exposure to certain workplace materials.
- Medical conditions, such as GERD 123, sleep apnea, thyroid problems, sinusitis

What symptoms might suggest asthma?

Asthma attacks vary in frequency and severity. They may last minutes or days. Symptoms often occur at night or early in the morning.

- Coughing
- Chest tightness
- Wheezing
- Shortness of breath

What treatments are commonly used for asthma?

Lifestyle Modifications
Reduce expose to allergens

Medication

Short-Term: Widen airways

Long-Term: Reduce inflammation

Severe Attack
Oxygen/Intravenous Fluid/Anti-biotics

Lifestyle Modifications
- Avoid exposure to allergens (see Action Items).
- Attacks triggered by exercise can be avoided by taking medication beforehand.

Medication
- Drug treatments allow most people with asthma to lead relatively normal

lives. There are two main kinds of medicines: those used to prevent attacks and those used to provide immediate relief. Bronchodilators such as adrenaline, albuterol and theophylline relieve sudden attacks. Corticosteroids, cromolyn and nedocromil provide long-term control.

In severe cases, asthma attacks can be life-threatening. Your skin will turn a bluish color. Emergency treatment is required.

More than 95% of all deaths from COPD occur in people over age 55.

15% of long-term smokers will develop COPD.

The asthma death and hospitalization rate for blacks is 3 times the rate of whites.

30% of people with severe COPD die in 1 year; 95% die in 10 years.

ACTION ITEMS
Avoiding asthma triggers

You can help prevent asthma attacks by staying away from things that make your asthma worse.

1 Tobacco Smoke
If you smoke, ask your doctor for ways to help you quit. Ask family members to quit, too. Do not allow smoking in your home or around you.

2 Dust Mites
Many people with asthma are allergic to dust mites. To reduce the dust mites in your bedroom, encase your mattress and pillows in a special dust-proof cover, wash bedding weekly in hot water, reduce indoor humidity to less

than 50% and try not to sleep or lie on cloth-covered cushions or furniture.

3 Animal Dander
Some people are allergic to the flakes of skin or dried saliva from animals with fur or feathers. Keep furred or feathered pets out of your home or, at least, keep the pet out of your bedroom and keep your bedroom door closed.

4 Vacuum Cleaning
Try to get someone else to vacuum for you once or twice a week, if you can. Stay out of rooms while they are being vacuumed and for a short while afterward while the dust settles. If you must vacuum yourself, use a dust mask.

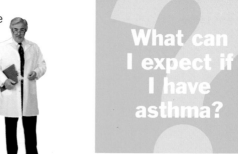

How am I likely to be diagnosed with asthma?

Your doctor will make a diagnosis based upon symptoms and a physical examination. These tests may also be performed:

- Lung function tests

- Spirometry to assess the severity of the airway obstruction
- Peak expiratory flow to measure the rate at which air can be exhaled
- Allergy and blood tests, chest x-ray

Asthma is a chronic respiratory disease that causes difficulty breathing.

It is caused by inflamed and constricted airways brought on by an allergic reaction or an environmental trigger and is characterized by periodic attacks of wheezing, coughing, shortness of breath and excessive mucous.

Sources: A.D.A.M. Health Illustrated Encyclopedia, Best Practice of Medicine, Merck Health Library, mercksource.com; Geriatric Services of America, geriatric services.com; US Department of Health and Human Services, National Heart, Lung and Blood Institute.

How likely is my condition to improve?

There is no cure for asthma, though symptoms sometimes decrease over time. With proper self management and medical treatment, most people can lead normal lives.

Normal Life

Lung Failure

How likely am I to die of this disease?

Although rare, uncontrolled asthma can lead to lung failure. Make an action plan with your doctor so that you know when to take your medicine and what to do if symptoms get worse.

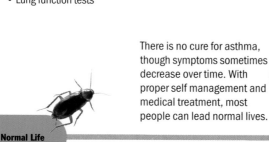

The number of Americans with asthma increased 42% since 1982.

1982   1992

---

5 Indoor Mold
Fix leaky faucets, pipes or other water sources. Clean moldy surfaces with a bleach cleanser.

6 Pollen and Outdoor Mold
During allergy season (when pollen or mold spore counts are high), try to keep your windows closed. If you can, stay indoors with windows closed during the midday and after-noon when pollen and some mold spore counts are highest.

7 Smoke, Strong Odors and Sprays
If possible, do not use a wood-burning stove, kerosene heater or fireplace. Try to stay away from strong odors and sprays, such as perfume, talcum powder, hair spray and paints.

8 Exercise, Sports, Work or Play
See your doctor if you have asthma symptoms when you are active—like when you exercise, do sports, play, or work hard. Try not to work or play hard outside when air pollution or pollen levels are high.

9 Sulfites
Do not drink beer or wine or eat shrimp, dried fruit or processed potatoes if they cause asthma symptoms.

10 Cold air
Cover your nose and mouth with a scarf on cold or windy days.

Source: National Institutes of Health, National Heart Lung and Blood Institute.

How Viruses Reproduce

To survive, viruses must reproduce inside living cells. The genetic material from the virus uses the host cell to make new virus particles. The new viruses leave the host by bursting out of the cell or by budding out from the cell surface.

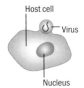
Host cell
Virus
Nucleus

1. The virus attaches to the host cell.

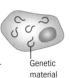
Genetic material

2. Once inside the cell, the genetic material of the virus reproduces, using substances from inside the cell.

New virus

3. The genetic material each form a new virus cell.

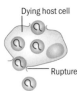
Dying host cell
Rupture

4. The viruses leave the cell, either by rupturing the cell membrane, or by budding out from the surface.

Source: *Your Body and Disease, Infections and Infestations.*

❓ How often do most people get a common cold?

About half of the population of the United States and Europe develops at least one cold a year. Children are more susceptible to colds than adults because they have not yet developed immunity to the most common viruses and also because viruses spread very quickly in communities such as child care centers and schools.

What treatments are helpful for a cold?

Only symptomatic treatment is available for uncomplicated cases of the common cold:

Symptomatic Treatment
- Bed rest
- Plenty of fluids
- Gargling with warm salt water
- Petroleum jelly for a raw nose
- Aspirin or acetaminophen to relieve headache or fever

Over-the-Counter Medication
- Nonprescription cold remedies, including decongestants and cough suppressants, may relieve some symptoms, but will not prevent, cure or even shorten the duration of the illness.

What symptoms might suggest a cold virus?

Symptoms of the common cold usually begin 2 to 3 days after infection and often include nasal discharge, obstruction of nasal breathing, swelling of the sinus membranes, sneezing, sore throat, cough and headache. Fever is usually slight but can climb to 102° F in infants and young children. 143

Sources: National Institute of Allergy and Infectious Disease, niaid.nih.gov; Merck Health Library, mercksource.com.

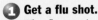

Rhinoviruses cause an estimated 30% to 35% of all adult colds.

To prevent the spread of germs, wash hands often with soapy water for at least 15 seconds.

Colds occur year-round, but are most prevalent in the spring and fall.

ACTION ITEMS
Lower your chance of viral infection

1 Get a flu shot.

The flu vaccine remains the best way to prevent and control the flu.

Flu season in the US runs from November to April. October to November is the usual vaccination time. You need a new flu shot every year because the predominant flu viruses change.

The flu vaccine is made of killed virus and can't cause the flu. Although some people get a low-grade fever and muscle aches for a day or two, the most common side effect is soreness at the injection site. The flu shot is not recommended for certain people, including those allergic to eggs since the viruses for flu vaccines are grown in eggs.

2 Wash your hands.

Both colds and flu can be passed through coughing, sneezing and touching surfaces such as doorknobs and telephones. So it's wise to make a habit of washing your hands and teach children to do the same. This helps you prevent spreading respiratory infections and picking them up from someone else.

The CDC recommends regular scrubbing of your hands with warm, soapy water for about 15 seconds. Touching your nose, mouth, and eyes with contaminated hands makes it easy for cold and flu viruses to enter the body. Others can become ill by just coming in contact with

When should you suspect that the cause is allergy 125, not a cold?

DOES COLD WEATHER CAUSE A COLD?

Although many people are convinced that a cold results from exposure to cold weather, or from getting chilled or overheated, research has shown these conditions have little or no effect on the development or severity of a cold. Nor is susceptibility apparently related to factors such as exercise, diet or enlarged tonsils or adenoids. Research, however, does suggest that psychological stress, allergic disorders affecting the nasal passages or throat and menstrual cycles may have an impact on a person's susceptibility to colds.

An allergy is actually an immune response to a substance in the environment that is normally harmless, while a cold is caused by a virus. However, they share many of the same symptoms—watery eyes, runny nose, congestion, sneezing. If symptoms occur often or last longer than two weeks, they may be the result of an allergy rather than a cold.

A virus is a small infectious organism—much smaller than a fungus or bacterium—that needs a living cell in order to reproduce.

There are at least 200 highly contagious viruses that can cause the common cold. Rhinoviruses (from the Greek rhin, meaning "nose")—a viral infection of the lining of the nose, sinuses, throat, and large airways—account for the largest percentage of all adult colds.

How quickly can I expect to get better?

Cold symptoms can last from 2 to 14 days, but two-thirds of people recover in a week.

- Nonprescription antihistamines may have some effect in relieving inflammatory responses such as runny nose and watery eyes.
- It is important to remember that antibiotics do not kill viruses, and will not prevent secondary bacterial infections.

Achoo!
Sniffle

Sniffle

Achoo!
Achoo!
Achoo!

On average, children have 6-8 colds per year; adults have 2-4; and the elderly have 1.

someone who has become infected with a cold or flu virus or who has come in contact with a contaminated area.

3 Limit exposure to infected people.

Sometimes people infected with a virus don't know it because they haven't experienced symptoms yet. If possible, avoid people who you know have colds and flu. Keep infants away from crowds for the first few months of life.

If keeping your distance is too difficult—say in the case of parents who can't help but hold and kiss their sick kids—then, in addition to washing your hands frequently, you can keep surfaces clean with a virus-killing solution of 1 part bleach mixed with 10 parts water.

4 Practice healthy habits.

Eating a balanced diet, getting enough sleep and exercising can help the immune system better fight off the germs that cause illness.

Because smoking interferes with the mechanisms that keep bacteria and debris out of the lungs, those who use tobacco or who are exposed to secondhand smoke are more prone to respiratory illnesses and more severe complications than nonsmokers.

If you've been feeling run down, try to get some extra rest. If you are feeling particularly stressed, some stress management might help keep you healthy.

Source: US Food and Drug Administration.

In 2000, 8,800 cases of severe **Group A streptococcal disease** were reported in the US.

Bacteremia (blood stream infections), toxic shock syndrome and necrotizing fasciitis (flesh-eating disease) are considered three of the **most severe types of streptococcal infection.**

Bacteria from raw meats, poultry and fish can contaminate other foods. **Wash cutting boards, utensils and counter tops** in hot, soapy water between the different steps in meal preparation to avoid cross-contamination.

Half of the 100 million **antibiotic prescriptions** written each year are unnecessary.

More than **120 different strains** of Group A streptococci exist, each producing its own unique proteins.

Sources: CDC; National Institute of Allergy and Infectious Diseases, National Institutes of Health, niaid.nih.gov; College of American Pathologists, cap.org.

? Why can antibacterial products be a problem?

Antibacterial products may cause long-term problems because they kill weaker strains of bacteria, leaving stronger, more resistant germs to flourish. Drug-resistant germs are on the rise in the US and experts predict a sharp jump in the strains of a dangerous form of strep that can overcome two common antibiotics.

Researchers warn that by the summer of 2004, as many as 40% of the strains of streptococcus pneumoniae could be resistant to both penicillin and erthromycin. That form of strep causes thousands of cases of meningitis, sinusitis, ear infections and pneumonia every year.

To prevent the spread of germs, experts recommend following common-sense cleaning practices: washing hands thoroughly, washing cutting boards, knives and other utensils after working with raw meats and cleaning and changing dishtowels and sponges often.

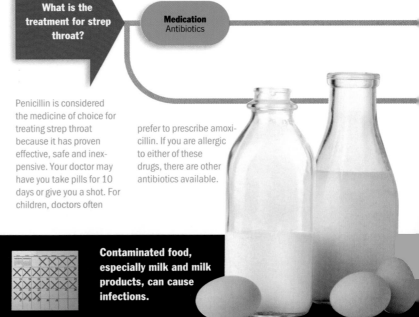

What is the treatment for strep throat?

Medication Antibiotics

Penicillin is considered the medicine of choice for treating strep throat because it has proven effective, safe and inexpensive. Your doctor may have you take pills for 10 days or give you a shot. For children, doctors often prefer to prescribe amoxicillin. If you are allergic to either of these drugs, there are other antibiotics available.

Infected people can pass the germ to others for up to two to three weeks even if they don't have symptoms.

Contaminated food, especially milk and milk products, can cause infections.

ACTION ITEMS — Preventing the spread of infection

Some diseases have become immune to the antibiotics we use. As a result, controlling diseases and preventing infections from spreading are more crucial than ever, and doing so begins with measures every individual can take. Here are 10 tips to remember.

1. Wash your hands frequently, especially before preparing food, before eating and after using the restroom. Insist that your health care providers wash their hands and use gloves, especially before any invasive treatment or procedure.

2. Don't insist that your physician give you antibiotics if you don't need them. Antibiotics have no effect on illnesses caused by viruses.

3. Take prescribed antibiotics exactly as instructed. Do not stop taking them without checking with your physician, even if the medicine makes you feel better, or worse.

4. Keep your immunizations and those of your children up to date. 149

5. Don't send your child to a child care center or to school with symptoms of an infection such as vomiting, diarrhea or fever.

What symptoms might suggest a strep throat?

People with strep throat infections have a red and painful sore throat with white patches on their tonsils. The person may also have swollen lymph nodes in the neck, run a fever and have a headache. Nausea, vomiting and abdominal pain can occur but are more common in children than in adults.

How do I know it's not just a cold?

The surest way to tell is by having a doctor take a throat culture and run it through a rapid strep test, which takes from 10-20 minutes. Most sore throats are caused by viral infections, which don't respond to antibiotics.

What can I expect if I get a strep throat?

Strep throat is caused by a bacteria called streptococcus.

Group A streptococci are the most virulent species for humans, who are their natural hosts, and can cause strep throat, tonsillitis, wound and skin infections, blood infections, scarlet fever, pneumonia, rheumatic fever, Sydenham's chorea (St. Vitus Dance) and kidney inflammation.

Sources: Merck Health Library, mercksource.com; National Institute of Allergy and Infectious Diseases, National Institute of Health, niaid.nih.gov.

Normal Life

Complications
Rheumatic Fever/ PSGN

Untreated Group A strep infection can result in rheumatic fever and post-streptococcal glomerulonephritis (PSGN). Rheumatic fever develops about 18 days after a bout of strep throat and causes joint pain and heart disease. Less common is PSGN, which leads to an inflammation of the kidneys.

With treatment, how quickly can I expect to get better?

An antibiotic treatment may help you feel better within 4 days, but be sure to finish all the medicine to prevent complications.

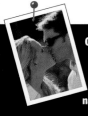

Group A strep infections can spread from person to person by direct contact with saliva or nasal discharge.

Hand washing with soap gets rid of germs by cleansing the skin of potentially transmittable microorganisms, dissolving the membranes on the surface of some viruses and rubbing away skin cells that may contain organisms.

6. **Follow safe sex practices.** 55

7. **Do not use I.V. drugs** 53**. If you do, never share needles.**

8. **Don't share personal items such as razor blades, tooth brushes, combs and hairbrushes, and don't eat or drink from others' utensils, plates or glasses.**

9. **Keep kitchen surfaces clean and disinfected, especially when preparing meat, chicken and fish.**

10. **Keep hot foods hot and cold foods cold, especially when they will be left out for a long time.**

Germs can thrive in sponges and towels. Soak sponges in a bleach and water solution or run them through the dishwasher. Change hand and dishtowels daily and launder them in hot water.

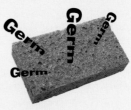

Source: Association for Professionals in Infection Control and Epidemiology, apic.org.

According to the **United Nations 14th International AIDS Conference,** roughly 3 million people died of AIDS in 2001.

Acute respiratory failure accounts for 50-75% of HIV intensive care admissions.

The number of **infants born in the US with HIV** has declined by 80% during the last decade.

$7 to $10 billion are needed each year to fight HIV/AIDS in low- and middle-income countries.

About half of the 5 million new HIV infections world-wide in 2001 appeared in **females under 25.**

The **annual cost** of treating HIV-positive patients in the US ranges from $14,000–$34,000 depending on the stage of the illness.

68 million will die of AIDS worldwide between 2000 and 2020—5 times the number of deaths from 1980 to 2000.

What symptoms might suggest HIV/AIDS?

Typically, HIV progresses through four stages: primary infection, asymptomatic disease, symptomatic disease and AIDS.

During the primary HIV infection stage, a person may have no symptoms, or experience a brief flu-like illness within 2 to 6 weeks of exposure. There may be no additional symptoms for 8-10 years.

Eventually, there may be additional symptoms such as:

- Mild infections
- Diarrhea
- Weight loss
- Fever
- Shortness of breath
- Cough

AIDS is diagnosed when the patient has developed at least one of the following:

- Serious infection such as pneumonia
- CD4 cell count of 200 or less

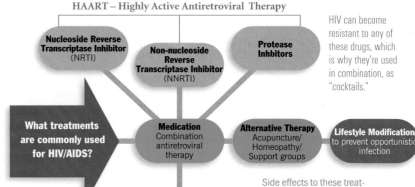

HAART – Highly Active Antiretroviral Therapy

Nucleoside Reverse Transcriptase Inhibitor (NRTI)

Non-nucleoside Reverse Transcriptase Inhibitor (NNRTI)

Protease Inhbitors

HIV can become resistant to any of these drugs, which is why they're used in combination, as "cocktails."

What treatments are commonly used for HIV/AIDS?

Medication Combination antiretroviral therapy

Alternative Therapy Acupuncture/ Homeopathy/ Support groups

Lifestyle Modification to prevent opportunistic infection

Other Drug Therapy to treat/prevent infection

NRTI inhibitors interrupt early stages of viral duplication and delay the start of opportunistic infections.

NNRTIs also interfere with viral replication, but at a different cellular site.

Protease inhibitors interrupt virus replication at a later stage of the HIV cycle, and are used in combination with RT inhibitors for a more effective treatment.

Side effects to these treatments include:

- Nausea
- Diarrhea
- Gastrointestinal symptoms
- Decreased red or white blood cells
- Nerve and bone marrow damage
- Inflammation of the pancreas

 Intravenous drug use accounts for 30% of HIV infections in the US.

 1/3 of new cases of HIV in the US appear in women, and the majority are Black and Latina.

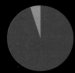 An estimated 95-100% of people infected with HIV will go on to develop AIDS.

ACTION ITEMS
Nutrition tips for people with HIV

Although the food pyramid 43 **works well for a basic approach to eating, modifications may be needed for HIV-positive people. Talk to your doctor about what is right for you. For additional assistance, ask for a referral to a registered dietitian who knows HIV and AIDS.**

1 Eat more.
Your total nutritional needs are increased by a chronic viral infection like HIV since your revved up immune system is constantly burning up calories. Any opportunistic infections

that you develop will only increase these needs. Weigh yourself regularly and keep a food diary to try to keep your weight at a healthy level.

2 Limit or eliminate milk products.
HIV-positive people, especially those with more advanced disease, often develop lactose intolerance. If this occurs, reduction or elimination of milk and milk products (cheese, ice cream, yogurt, etc.) may be necessary.

3 Limit fat.
Poor fat absorption, another cause of diarrhea and gas common in HIV-positive people, may necessitate keeping the fat content of your diet moderately low.

At this point the immune system is seriously damaged causing additional symptoms such as:

- Fatigue
- High fever
- Drenching night sweats
- Lesions on the tongue or in the mouth
- Headaches
- Blurred vision

Some people also develop AIDS Dementia Complex (ADC). Early symptoms include:

- Confusion
- Depression
- Forgetfulness
- Difficulty learning new things

Later symptoms can include:

- Problems with speech and balance
- Incontinence
- Difficulty walking
- Mania
- Psychosis

How and when am I likely to be diagnosed with HIV/AIDS?

Once exposed to the HIV virus, the body makes antibodies but they do not reach detectable levels in the blood for about 1 to 3 months and it may take as long as 6 months for antibodies to be measured in standard blood tests—ELISA and Western Blot. Both tests deliver the findings in 1 to 2 weeks.

Once diagnosed with HIV, a doctor will determine the health of the immune system by measuring CD4 cells in the blood and testing for HIV viral load. Both tests help physicians choose the appropriate therapy regime.

Human immuno-deficiency virus (HIV) gradually destroys the body's immune system. AIDS, or acquired immunode-ficiency syndrome, is the final and most serious stage of HIV disease.

The virus targets white blood cells known as helper T-cells or CD4 cells and begins to destroy them and impair the immune system's ability to fight infection.

Sources: Best Practice of Medicine, A.D.A.M. Illustrated Health Encyclopedia, Merck Health Library, mercksource.com; National Institutes of Health, niaid.nih.gov.

Complications (from opportunistic infection)

Death

What can I expect as an outcome?

Opportunistic infections include pneumonia, toxoplasmosis, tuberculosis, gastrointestinal infections and cytomegalovirus of the retina (resulting in blindness). In severe cases late in the course of the disease, some people need urgent care for respiratory failure or neurological complications.

Only a few people with AIDS die from the direct effects of HIV infection. Usually death is caused by the cumulative effects of many opportunistic infections.

Exposure to HIV does not always lead to infection and many people with the virus remain well for years. However, HIV is a chronic medical condition that can be treated, but not yet cured. While effective drug therapies help prevent complications, most HIV infections advance to AIDS.

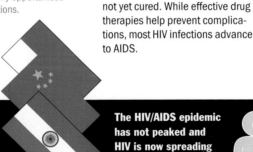

More than 10% of new AIDS cases in the US occur in people over the age of 50.

The HIV/AIDS epidemic has not peaked and HIV is now spreading to China, India and Indonesia.

Women can transmit HIV to their babies during pregnancy or birth. HIV can also be spread to babies through breast milk.

4 Reduce protein intake if needed.
If you have advanced liver disease due to coinfection with hepatitis, you may need to reduce your protein intake. Although protein consumption is important, too-high levels will produce an overabundance of ammonia in your system which is difficult for a damaged liver to process.

5 Follow nutritional drug requirements.
Some HAART regimens require certain dietary adjustments. Ask your physician if you need to follow any dietary restrictions.

6 Drink lots of water.
Your body needs lots of water to stay properly hydrated, especially when you are suffering from diarrhea, nausea, vomiting, fever or night sweats.

7 Try warm liquids.
Warm liquids like soup and herbal teas can be nutritious and less demanding on your body than icy cold fluids because our body doesn't have to expend energy to warm them up.

According to the **National Institute of Allergy and Infectious Diseases,** there are 15.3 million new cases of STD in the US each year.

The **annual cost of STD** in the United States exceeds $10 billion.

650,000 cases of **gonorrhea** occur annually in the US.

Cervical cancer is linked to genital warts. It is the second most common cancer among women.

Three million cases of **chlamydia** occur annually in the US.

One in five Americans has **genital herpes.**

Less than half of adults have ever been tested for an STD other than **HIV/AIDS.**
103

Source: National Institute of Health, niaid.nih.gov; National Woman's Health Information Center, US Department of Health and Human Services, 4woman.gov; coolnurse.com.

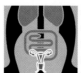

What is an STD?

Sexually-transmitted diseases (STDs) are infections that are often, if not always, passed from person to person through sexual contact. 55

Once called venereal diseases, STDs are among the most common infectious diseases in the United States. They are most prevalent among teenagers and adults under the age of 25.

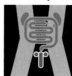

What symptoms might suggest a sexually transmitted disease?

Most of the time, STDs cause no symptoms, particularly in women.

Symptoms vary with the particular disease.

- Gonorrhea: Abnormal genital discharge or difficulty urinating for both men and women.
- Syphilis: The initial symptom is a chancre, a painless open sore in the genital area. More advanced stages include a rash, and heart and nervous system damage.

What treatments are commonly used for chlamydia?

Medication
Antibiotics

Abstain/ Notify & Test Partner(s)

No Medical Treatment

Pelvic Inflammatory Disease
In women

Lifestyle Modifications
- Antibiotics. Azithromycin or doxycylicine are the most commonly used treatments.
- Finish all of your medicine.

Abstain/Test Partners
- Make sure your partner(s) are tested.
- Avoid sexual activity while being treated.

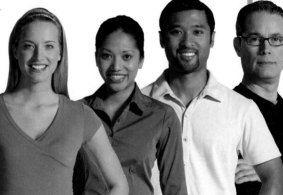

By age 30, 50% of sexually active women have had chlamydia.

3 of every 4 cases of chlamydia occur in people under age 25.

ACTION ITEMS
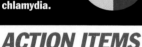

Preventing chlamydia

1 Abstain.
The best way to prevent chlamydia or any sexually-transmitted disease (STD) is to practice abstinence (don't have sex). Delaying having sex for the first time is another way to reduce your chances of getting an STD. Studies show that the younger people are when having sex for the first time, the more likely it is that they will get an STD. The risk of getting an STD also becomes greater as the number of sex partners increases, and the more a person has unprotected sex.

2 Be faithful.
Your next best bet: Have a sexual relationship with one partner who doesn't have any STDs (Get tested to be sure.). Have sex with each other and no one else.

3 Be selective.
If you do have sex with more than one partner, at least be selective. Your risk of getting chlamydia increases with the number of partners you have.

4 Use condoms.
Practice "safer sex." This means protecting yourself with a condom EVERY time you have vaginal, anal or oral sex. Be aware that condoms don't provide complete protection. They only

- **Genital Herpes:** Painful blisters in the genital area; tingling in the legs or genital region.
- **Genital Warts:** Small, painless bumps in the genital area. If untreated, they may develop a fleshy appearance.

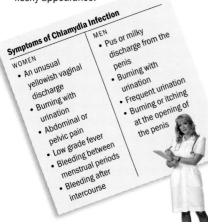

Symptoms of Chlamydia Infection

WOMEN	MEN
• An unusual yellowish vaginal discharge	• Pus or milky discharge from the penis
• Burning with urination	• Burning with urination
• Abdominal or pelvic pain	• Frequent urination
• Low grade fever	• Burning or itching at the opening of the penis
• Bleeding between menstrual periods	
• Bleeding after intercourse	

How and when am I likely to be diagnosed with chlamydia?

The infection is often not diagnosed until there are complications.

Your doctor will ask for a thorough sexual history and conduct a physical examination to look for sores or discharge in your genital and rectal areas. He will check your groin for swelling, and obtain samples of genital secretions for laboratory tests. A urine test may be performed, and, if you are a woman, a pelvic exam.

Lab tests will confirm the diagnosis.

Regular STD Examinations

Lifestyle Modifications
Prevent reinfection

What can I expect as an outcome?

Chlamydia is usually completely curable, especially when treated in the early stages. If untreated, it can lead to serious complications, such as infertility in both men and women. In infected mothers, it can lead to premature delivery and infections in newborns.

Chlamydia can increase the risk of acquiring HIV or developing Reiter's syndrome, a form of arthritis.

Infertility
In both sexes

Ectopic Pregnancy
In pregnant women

Death
If untreated

Common sexually transmitted diseases are chlamydia, gonorrhea, HIV and AIDS, syphillis, hepatitis B, genital herpes and genital warts.

Chlamydia is the most common sexually transmitted disease in the United States. Untreated, it can lead to pelvic inflammatory disease (PID), infertility, and ectopic pregnancy.

Sources: National Institute of Health, niaid.nih.gov; National Woman's Health Information Center, US Department of Health and Human Services, 4woman.gov; coolnurse.com.; Best Practice of Medicine, Merck Health Library, mercksource.com.

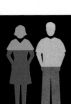

Chlamydia is called the silent disease. 75% of infected women and 50% of infected men have no symptoms.

40% of all PID cases are the result of a chlamydia infection.

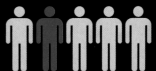

1 in 5 people in the US has an STD.

decrease your chances of getting an STD. Know also that other methods of birth control, like birth control pills, shots, implants or diaphragms don't protect you from STDs. If you use one of these methods, be sure to also use a condom every time you have sex.

5 Don't douche.
Douching removes some of the normal bacteria in the vagina that protects you from infection. This can increase your risk for getting chlamydia.

6 Talk about it.
Learn how to talk with your partner about STDs and using condoms. It's up to you to make sure you are protected.

7 Get routine medical exams.
When you are sexually active, especially if you have more than one partner, get regular exams for STDs from a health care provider. Tests for STDs can be done during an exam. And, the earlier an STD is found, the easier it is to treat.

8 Be informed.
Learn the common symptoms of chlamydia and other STDs, but remember that chlamydia often has no symptoms. Seek medical help right away if you think you may have chlamydia or another STD.

Source: The National Women's Health Information Center.

How does osteoarthritis differ from rheumatoid arthritis?

Rheumatoid arthritis is an autoimmune disorder in which the body's defense system attacks the joints. The thin layer of cells called the synovium that line and lubricate the joints becomes inflamed. Rheumatoid arthritis usually hits people between ages 30 and 50, but can strike at any age, including childhood.

What are the risk factors for osteoarthritis?

The precise causes of osteoarthritis are not known, but certain factors increase your risk of developing the disease:

- Age 133. After age 40 in women and after age 50 in men, the incidence of osteoarthritis increases dramatically.

- Gender 31. More women than men develop osteoarthritis, particularly in the hand and knee. Men are more prone to affliction in the hip.

- Obesity 127. Excess weight contributes to osteoarthritis of the knee and to some extent the hip.

- Heredity 29. Some forms of this disease, especially in the fingers, appear to run in families.

- Repetitive use 117. Jobs or recreational activities that require repetitive bending or continuous "wear and tear" of a joint adds to the risk.

- Severe trauma. A fracture or ligament tear can accelerate osteoarthritis.

What treatments are commonly used for osteoarthritis?

Lifestyle Modifications
Weight Management
Regular Exercise

Nutritional Supplements
Glucosamine/Chondroitin

Painkillers

Alternative Therapy
Physical Therapy/Acupuncture

Surgery
Arthroscopy/Joint Replacement

Lifestyle Modifications
- Exercise therapies include: water workouts, recumbent bicycle, walking and low-impact aerobics.

Medication
- For mild pain, try over-the counter medications such as acetaminophen, aspirin or ibuprofen.
- Steroid shots can provide short-term relief from more severe joint pain.

Arthroscopy works best when a joint is still mechanically sound. If it is damaged beyond repair, then joint replacement may be the only option. The hip is the most commonly replaced joint.

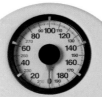

Losing as little as 10 lbs. can improve osteoarthritis symptoms.

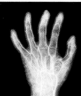

X-rays are considered the best, most accurate tests for diagnosing osteoarthritis. 187

1/3 of all Americans suffer from some type of joint disease.

ACTION ITEMS
Coping with osteoarthritis

Osteoarthritis can damage your joints. There are things you can do to keep the damage from getting worse and help make yourself feel better.

1 Maintain a healthy weight.
Try to keep your weight down. Too much weight can make your knees and hips hurt.

2 Exercise.
Moving all of your joints may help you reduce the stiffness in your joints. The doctor or nurse can show you how to move more easily. Going for a walk every day will help, too.

3 Take your medicine.
Take your medicines when and how you are supposed to. They can help reduce pain and stiffness.

4 Warm up with a soothing shower.
Try taking a warm shower in the morning to loosen up your joints.

What symptoms might suggest osteoarthritis?

Osteoarthritis manifests itself through many symptoms, and you cannot diagnose it on your own. Some warning signs include stiffness when you awake; one or more joints that don't move normally and may be swollen; and joint pain. Early in the disease, the pain may last only a couple of hours and come on after physical exercise. As the disease progresses, the pain may persist for longer periods.

How and when am I likely to be diagnosed with osteoarthritis?

Osteoarthritis may first appear without symptoms between 30 and 40 years of age and is present in almost everyone by the age of 70. Before the age of 55, symptoms occur equally in both sexes. After 55, the incidence is higher in women. A physical exam can show limited range of motion, grating of a joint with motion, joint swelling and tenderness, but an x-ray of affected joints is needed to determine loss of the joint space, and, in advanced cases, wearing down of the ends of the bone and bone spurs.

What can I expect if I have osteoarthritis?

Osteoarthritis is a chronic joint disorder that occurs when cartilage, the tissue that cushions the ends of the bones in a joint, degenerates.

This causes the smooth, slippery surface of the cartilage to become rough and pitted, so that the joint can no longer move smoothly. The result is often disabling pain and stiffness, particularly in the joints of the fingers, spine, hips, knees and feet.

Normal Life

What preventative measures can I take?

Maintaining a healthy weight and exercising regularly are the best ways to keep your cartilage healthy.

Only exercise a joint that is tender after talking to your doctor.

Common Pain Sites

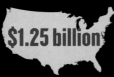

- Neck
- Spine
- Fingers
- Knees
- Feet

Sources: Merck Health Library, Best Practice of Medicine, A.D.A.M. Health Illustrated Encyclopedia, mercksource.com; *Time*, 2002; *Arthritis*, Johns Hopkins Health, TimeLife Books.

Musculoskeletal conditions such as osteoarthritis cost the US economy nearly $125 billion per year in direct expenses and lost wages and production.

$1.25 billion

In 2002, an estimated 20 million Americans were afflicted with osteoarthritis; by 2020, that number is expected to reach 40 million.

 2002
 2020

5 See your doctor.
It is important to make and keep regular check ups so you and your doctor can keep your osteoarthritis under control.

6 Seek information that can help you.
For more information on arthritis and musculoskeletal and skin diseases, contact any of the following organizations:

- National Institute of Arthritis and Musculoskeletal and Skin Diseases (NIAMS)
  877.22.NIAMS
  TTY 301.565.2966
  www.niams.nih.gov/hi
  www.niams.nih.gov/hi

- Arthritis Foundation
  800.283.7800
  www.arthritis.org

- American Academy of Orthopaedic Surgeons
  800.824.BONE (2663)
  www.aaos.org

- American College of Rheumatology
  404.633.3777
  www.rheumatology.org

Sources: National Institute of Arthritis and Musculoskeletal and Skin Diseases, National Institutes of Health.

How Alzheimer's Damages the Brain

AMYLOID PLAQUES

APP is a protein that aids in the growth and maintenance of neurons. Enzymes called secretases clip it into shorter pieces that can build up to form sticky deposits called plaques. A protein called A-beta is formed during the process.

Most A-beta dissolves quickly in the fluid surrounding the neuron, but some of it survives and forms clusters.

The clusters of A-beta expand to create large plaques, which displace brain cells and kill them.

NEUROFIBRILLARY TANGLES

The branches that sprout from the neurons house structures called microtubules. Each microtubule is held together by tau proteins.

In a healthy brain, tau are tightly fastened to the microtubule. During Alzheimer's disease, tau break loose to form tangles.

Lacking tau proteins to hold them together, the microtubules start to disintegrate. The neurons shrink and die.

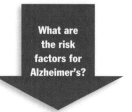

What are the risk factors for Alzheimer's?

Although Alzheimer's usually begins after age 60 and the risk goes up as people grow older, it is not a normal part of aging. A rare form of AD has a genetic link and runs in families. It tends to affect people between 30 and 60 years of age. Other risk factors have been suggested but not clinically proven, including head trauma, low educational level and environmental factors such as mercury, viruses and infectious proteins.

Sources: Alzheimer's Association, alzheimers.org; Reuters Limited; Best Practice of Medicine, Merck Health Library, mercksource.com; *Technology Review.*

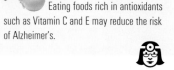

REDUCING YOUR RISK
Eating foods rich in antioxidants such as Vitamin C and E may reduce the risk of Alzheimer's.

What treatments are commonly used for Alzheimer's?

Therapies for Alzheimer's are advancing rapidly, but no cure is yet available. Researchers believe that the onset of AD is a decades-long process involving numerous steps. Treatments now target slowing the disease and reducing behavioral symptoms.

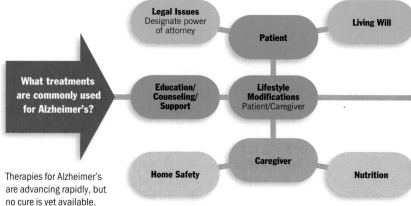

Legal Issues
Designate power of attorney

Living Will

Patient

Education/ Counseling/ Support

Lifestyle Modifications
Patient/Caregiver

Home Safety

Caregiver

Nutrition

Lifestyle Modifications
• Establish daily routines to provide a consistent environment for a person with Alzheimer's.

• Monitor and test the ability of a person with AD to drive safely.
• Encourage exercise and social interaction to improve mental and physical functioning, and morale.

70% of people with Alzheimer's live at home. 3 out of 4 caregivers 237 are women.

A 21-year study in Finland found that high cholesterol and high blood pressure 111 seem to increase Alzheimer's risk.

People with 1 afflicted parent are 3 times more likely to develop Alzheimer's than those with no family history.

ACTION ITEMS

Warning signs of Alzheimer's disease

To help family members and health care professionals recognize warning signs of Alzheimer's disease, the Alzheimer's Association has developed a checklist of common symptoms.

1 Memory loss
One of the most common early signs of dementia is forgetting recently learned information. While it's normal to forget appointments or names, sometimes those with dementia will forget such things more often and not remember them later.

2 Difficulty performing familiar tasks
People with dementia often find it hard to complete everyday tasks, like preparing a meal or using a household appliance, that are so familiar we usually do not think about how to do them.

3 Problems with language
Everyone has trouble finding the right word sometimes, but a person with Alzheimer's disease often forgets simple words or substitutes unusual words, making his or her speech or writing hard to understand.

What other forms of dementia have similar symptoms?

Alzheimer's-like symptoms sometimes result from clogged arteries in the brain, a buildup of fluid within the brain, normal-pressure hydrocephalus, vitamin deficiencies, certain hormonal disorders, drug toxicity and dementia associated with Huntington's disease, HIV infection, Parkinson's disease and syphilis. Many are treatable.

How is Alzheimer's disease diagnosed?

At specialized centers, physicians can diagnose AD accurately about 90% of the time. Diagnostic tools include:

- A focused evaluation of cognitive problems
- A complete medical history to rule out other treatable forms of dementia
- A physical and neurological exam
- Medical tests of blood, urine and spinal fluid
- Neuropsychiatric tests to measure memory, problem solving, attention, counting and language
- Brain imaging 159

Supplements
Vitamin E

Medication

Nursing Home

What can I expect as an outcome?

Medication
- Several drugs are available for people in the early and middle stages of the disease, and scientists are testing new anti-inflammatory drugs aimed at slowing AD progression. Additionally, vitamin E has been shown to impede AD progression by about 7 months. Other antioxidant vitamins also show promise.

Moving patients to an assisted living facility early, when they are still able to form new memories, may help reduce confusion and maximize self-care.

Although the disease progresses differently in different individuals, a person with Alzheimer's can expect progressive deterioration of memory and mental functioning.

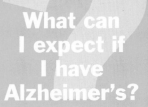

What can I expect if I have Alzheimer's?

Alzheimer's disease (AD) is a progressive brain disease that causes loss of memory and other cognitive functions, such as judgement, problem solving, orientation and attention. It is the most common form of dementia among older people.

Scientists believe Alzheimer's is most likely due to the destructive accumulation of a protein called beta amyloid around nerve cells in the brain.

People taking cholesterol drugs called statins reduced their risk of developing Alzheimer's by 79%, according to a Boston University School of Medicine study.

Alzheimer's strikes at least 35% of those over age 85. 133

People with AD live an average of 8-10 years after diagnosis; some may live for 20 years or more.

4 Disorientation to time and place
People with Alzheimer's can become lost on their own street and not know how to get back home.

5 Poor or decreased judgment
Those with Alzheimer's may dress without regard to the weather or show poor judgment about money, giving away large amounts to telemarketers or paying for home repairs they don't need.

6 Problems with abstract thinking
Balancing a checkbook may be hard when the task is more complicated than usual. Someone with Alzheimer's disease could forget completely what the numbers are and what needs to be done with them.

7 Misplacing things
Anyone can temporarily misplace a wallet or key. A person with Alzheimer's disease may put things in unusual places: an iron in the freezer or a wristwatch in the sugar bowl.

8 Changes in mood or behavior
Everyone can become sad or moody from time to time. Someone with Alzheimer's disease can show rapid mood swings—from calm to tears to anger—for no apparent reason.

Reprinted with permission from the Alzheimer's Association.

What are the risk factors for high blood pressure?

- Age and gender. Hypertension usually develops between the ages of 35-55 in men, and increases with age for both sexes.

- Ethnicity 35. Blacks are at highest risk.
- Obesity 127. 33%-50% of all people with hypertension are overweight.
- Diabetes 121.
- Heredity 29. 30%-60% of all cases are inherited.
- Sedentary lifestyle 47.
- Excessive alcohol consumption 49.
- High-salt diet .
- Smoking 51.

What symptoms might suggest hypertension?

Hypertension is called the "silent killer" because it rarely causes symptoms until your condition becomes severe, which typically takes years.

DASH (Dietary Approaches to Stop Hypertension) Diet Guidelines

7-8 servings of grains and grain products per day

4-5 servings of vegetables per day

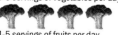

4-5 servings of fruits per day

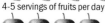

2-3 servings of low-fat or nonfat dairy foods per day

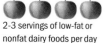

2 or fewer servings of meats, poultry and fish per day

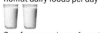

4-5 servings of nuts, seeds and legumes per week

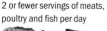

Limited intake of fats and sweets

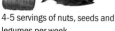
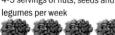

What treatments are commonly used for hypertension?

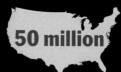
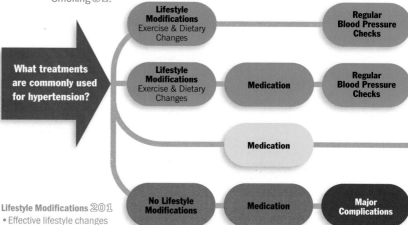

Lifestyle Modifications 201
- Effective lifestyle changes (see Action Items) can help you maintain your blood pressure at a normal level, and may help you avoid a lifelong commitment to medication .

Medication
- Drug treatment should be tailored to the individual. Different types of drugs reduce blood pressure by different mechanisms. Diuretics help the kidneys eliminate salt and water, thus decreasing blood volume and lowering pressure. Beta blockers block the part of the nervous system that raises pressure in response to stress. ACE inhibitors, calcium blockers and ACE II blockers lower pressure by dilating the arteries. People who currently have hypertension may need more than one type of medication to control the disease.

Only 2 out of 3 Americans with high blood pressure have been diagnosed with the disease.

There is a 90% risk of developing hypertension between the ages of 55-65.

50 million

More than 50 million Americans have high blood pressure.

ACTION ITEMS   Preventing high blood pressure

You can take steps to prevent high blood pressure by adopting these heart-healthy behaviors.

1 Eat Healthy.
A healthy eating plan can reduce the risk of developing high blood pressure and lower an already elevated blood pressure. Try an eating plan that emphasizes fruits, vegetables and low-fat dairy foods and is low in saturated fat, total fat and cholesterol.

2 Reduce Salt and Sodium in Your Diet.
Most Americans consume more salt than they need. The current recommendation is to consume less than 2.4 grams (2,400 milligrams[mg]) of sodium a day. That equals 6 grams (about 1 teaspoon) of table salt a day. The 6 grams include ALL salt and sodium consumed, including that used in cooking and at the table.

3 Maintain a Healthy Weight.
Blood pressure rises as body weight increases. Losing even 10 pounds can lower blood pressure—and it has the greatest effect for those who are overweight and already have hypertension.

Being overweight also increases your chance for developing high blood cholesterol and diabetes—two more major risk factors for heart disease.

How and when am I likely to be diagnosed with hypertension?

If your blood pressure 190 reads 140/90 or higher on repeated visits to your doctor, you may have hypertension. Multiple readings are needed to confirm diagnosis because blood pressure can be influenced by factors such as stress, medication, diet or exercise.

Your doctor will take your medical history and conduct a physical examination.

He will check your eyes to see if you have any hypertension-related damage in your retina. He will listen to your heart for abnormal rhythms and may check for an enlarged thyroid gland or any signs of kidney disorder.

Lab tests will confirm the diagnosis and reveal any damage to the heart or other organs. Tests include: CBC 190, urinalysis, potassium/glucose/cholesterol levels and electrocardiogram 164.

High blood pressure is controllable with treatment. It requires lifelong monitoring and may require periodic adjustment of treatment.

What can I expect as an outcome?

Normal Life

Normal Life

Minor Complications

Normal Life

Death

Untreated high blood pressure increases your risk of developing heart disease, kidney failure and stroke.

High blood pressure (hypertension) is a mostly symptomless condition of elevated blood pressure.

It is characterized by a systolic pressure (generated when the heart beats) of 140 or more, or a diastolic pressure (generated when the heart is at rest) of 90 or more. High blood pressure can increase your risk of stroke, aneurysm, heart failure, heart attack and kidney damage.

Sources: Best Practice of Medicine, Merck Health Library, mercksource.com; American Heart Association.

Optimal blood pressure is 115/75.

		SYSTOLIC	DIASTOLIC
☐	Normal		
☑	Pre-hypertensive	Below 120	Below 80
	HYPERTENSION	120-139	80-89
☐	Stage 1 (mild)	140-159	90-99
☐	Stage 2 (moderate)	160-179	100-109
☐	Stage 3 (severe)	180-209	110-119
☐	Stage 4 (very severe)	210+	120+

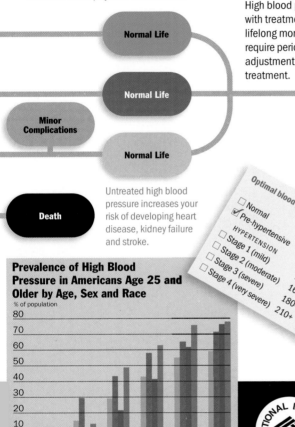

Prevalence of High Blood Pressure in Americans Age 25 and Older by Age, Sex and Race

% of population

Ages	25-34	35-44	45-54	55-64	65-74	75+

White Men ■ Black Men ■ White Women ■ Black Women
Source: Third National Health and Nutrition Examination Survey

In 2003, NIH reclassified normal blood pressure as below 120 over 80—and readings from 120 over 80 to 140 over 90 as prehypertensive. Based upon these new levels, 45 million Americans are prehypertensive.

NATIONAL INSTITUTE OF HEALTH

TIP

Studies show the DASH diet can lower high blood pressure by the same extent as hypertensive medication.

4 Be active.
Physical activity helps to prevent or control high blood pressure, and reduce your risk of heart disease. Even a moderate walking routine can have a positive effect.

5 Limit Alcohol.
Drinking too much alcohol can raise blood pressure and harm the liver, brain and heart. Alcoholic drinks also contain empty calories, which can add up if you are trying to lose weight. If you do drink alcoholic beverages, have only a moderate amount—one drink a day for women; two drinks a day for men.

6 Quit Smoking.
Smoking injures blood vessel walls and speeds up the process of hardening of the arteries. This applies even to filtered cigarettes. So even though it does not cause high blood pressure, smoking is bad for anyone, especially those with high blood pressure. If you smoke, quit. If you don't smoke, don't start. Once you quit, your risk of having a heart attack is reduced after the first year. You have a lot to gain by quitting.

What counts as a drink?
12 ounces of beer
5 ounces of wine
1.5 ounces of 80-proof liquor

Source: National Institutes of Health.

Number 3 killer

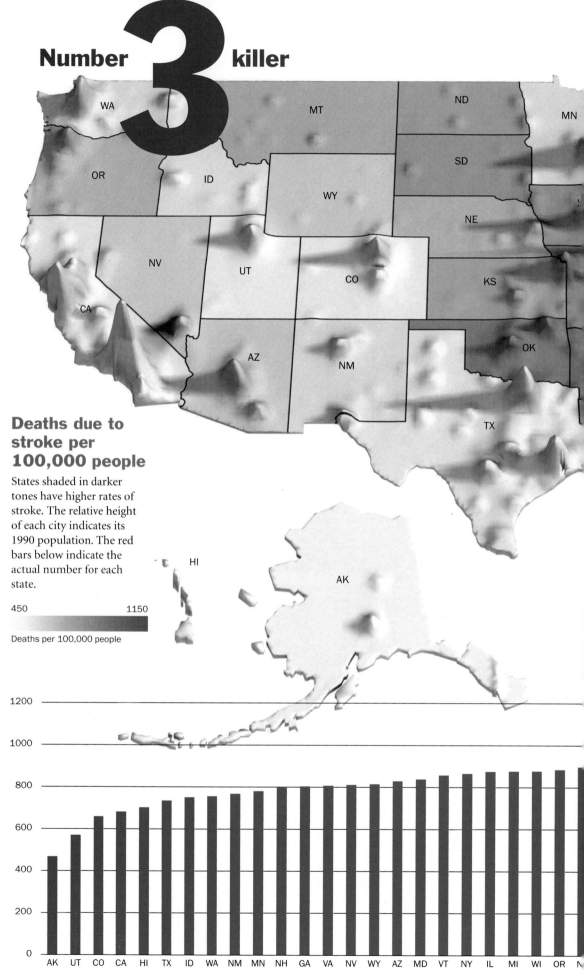

Deaths due to stroke per 100,000 people

States shaded in darker tones have higher rates of stroke. The relative height of each city indicates its 1990 population. The red bars below indicate the actual number for each state.

450   1150

Deaths per 100,000 people

May is National Stroke Awareness Month.

Visit www.strokeassociation.org for more information about stroke-related issues.

How many people die from strokes?

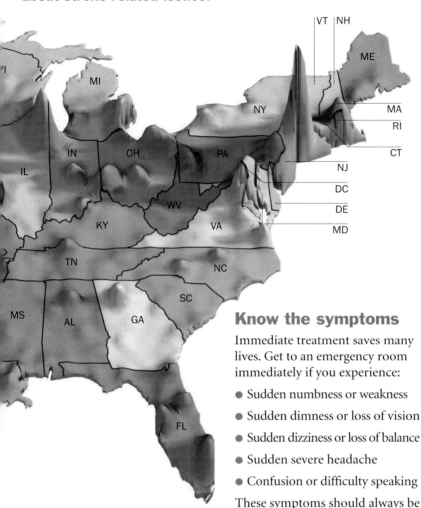

More than 167,000 people suffer stroke-related deaths each year.

About 500,000 US residents suffer their first stroke annually. While stroke has many causes, you can reduce your risk by controlling these factors: high blood pressure, diabetes, high cholesterol and smoking.

Source: cdc.gov.

Know the symptoms

Immediate treatment saves many lives. Get to an emergency room immediately if you experience:

● Sudden numbness or weakness

● Sudden dimness or loss of vision

● Sudden dizziness or loss of balance

● Sudden severe headache

● Confusion or difficulty speaking

These symptoms should always be taken seriously. Even if they are short lived, they could indicate a *transient ischemic attack*, or a "mini stroke." TIAs don't damage the brain, but they increase your risk of having a full-blown stroke.

Who is affected?

Blacks are much more likely to suffer strokes than whites; men are at a slightly higher risk than women.

Children can have strokes, too. Intrauterine stroke affects fetuses; childhood, or pediatric, stroke affects infants and children.

MT MA CT KS IN NC ND LA SC SD OH IA ME KY MO TN RI AL MS OK FL PA AR DC WV

Source: National Vital Statistics Report, Vol 50, NO 15, September 16, 2002.

❓ What are common types of stroke?

A stroke can occur in two ways. In an ischemic stroke, a blood clot blocks a blood vessel or artery in the brain. A clot that forms in the brain is a thrombus; one that travels to the brain from another location is an embolism. About 80% of all strokes are ischemic. Thrombotic stroke is more common in the elderly and may occur at any time.

Embolisms are most commonly caused by heart disorders and can cause severe damage to the brain.

In a hemorrhagic stroke, a blood vessel in the brain breaks and bleeds into the brain. It is often associated with hypertension, but can be caused by an aneurysm (weak spot in the artery wall). About 20% of strokes are hemorrhagic.

What are the risk factors for a stroke?

- Family history 29.
- Race 35.
- Age 133.
- Smoking 51.
- Hypertension 111 (increases risk of stroke 4 to 6 times).
- Gender 31. Women are particularly at risk during pregnancy, childbirth and menopause.
- Certain medical conditions such as artherosclerosis, heart disease or diabetes 121.
- Alcohol 49 or substance abuse 53.

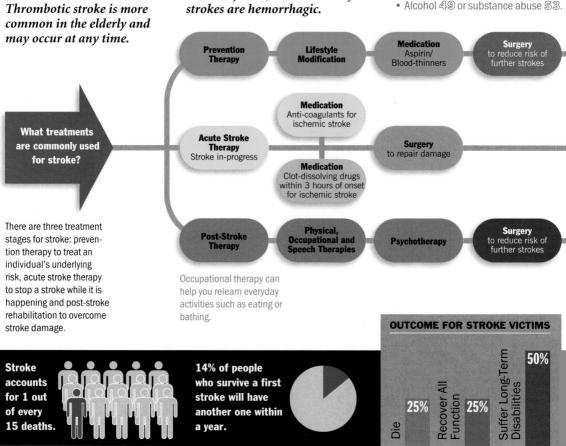

What treatments are commonly used for stroke?

Prevention Therapy → Lifestyle Modification → Medication Aspirin/Blood-thinners → Surgery to reduce risk of further strokes

Acute Stroke Therapy Stroke in-progress → Medication Anti-coagulants for ischemic stroke → Medication Clot-dissolving drugs within 3 hours of onset for ischemic stroke → Surgery to repair damage

Post-Stroke Therapy → Physical, Occupational and Speech Therapies → Psychotherapy → Surgery to reduce risk of further strokes

There are three treatment stages for stroke: prevention therapy to treat an individual's underlying risk, acute stroke therapy to stop a stroke while it is happening and post-stroke rehabilitation to overcome stroke damage.

Occupational therapy can help you relearn everyday activities such as eating or bathing.

Stroke accounts for 1 out of every 15 deaths.

14% of people who survive a first stroke will have another one within a year.

OUTCOME FOR STROKE VICTIMS

Die 25%
Recover All Function 25%
Suffer Long-Term Disabilities 50%

ACTION ITEMS

Recognizing a stroke

Only a fraction of stroke patients get to the hospital in time to receive a treatment that makes the difference between disability and full recovery. Thousands more could benefit from drug treatment called tissue plasminogen activator (t-PA)—but do not, because they often do not know the symptoms of stroke or do not get to the hospital within the drug's 3-hour window of effectiveness. The National Institute of Neurological Disorders and Stroke (NINDS) is launching a national public education campaign, "Know Stroke: Know the Signs. Act in Time," to help people overcome these barriers and to get medical help in time.

A key component of the campaign is educating bystanders—family members, co-workers, friends—who may be the first to recognize a stroke in progress.

"Stroke is an unmistakable event," said John R. Marler, MD, associate director for clinical trials at NINDS. "Few other medical conditions come on so suddenly or are so noticeable to a bystander. The sooner the stroke is recognized and the patient begins receiving treatment, the better are the chances for a complete recovery."

Because stroke injures the brain, the person having the stroke may not be able to recognize the symptoms and take action. An alert bystander can help a stroke patient get to the hospital quickly enough

What symptoms might suggest a stroke?

Symptoms vary depending upon the location of the bleeding, the amount of brain tissue affected and the cause of the stroke. See Action Items (below) for common symptoms.

Normal Life

Steps you can take to reduce risk of stroke:
- Monitor your blood pressure.
- Track your cholesterol level.
- Stop smoking.
- Exercise regularly.
- Find out if you should be taking a drug to reduce blood clotting.

How and when am I likely to be diagnosed with a stroke?

Diagnosis is based upon the history of events and a physical examination. Your doctor will look for specific neurologic, motor, sensory and vision deficits, because these often correspond to the location of the injury. He will try to determine the cause of the stroke. If it is caused by an embolism, another stroke is likely to follow unless corrective measures are taken.

CT or MRI scans will confirm the diagnosis and define the extent of the stroke.

Other possible tests include: electrocardiogram, echocardiogram, blood tests, angiography, ultrasound and cerebral arteriography.

What can I expect as an outcome?

Disabilities include pain, paralysis, cognitive and speech deficits, emotional difficulties and daily living problems. Neurologic losses that remain after 6 months are likely to be permanent.

Many people who suffer a stroke recover all or most function and enjoy years of normal life. Others are physically and mentally devastated and unable to move, speak or eat normally.

Lifestyle Modifications for physical disabilities

Normal Life

Death

20% of stroke victims die in the hospital.

Sources: National Institute of Neurological Disorders and Stroke, ninds.nih.gov; American Heart Association Heart and Stroke 2000

What can I expect if I have a stroke?

A stroke is the death of brain tissue resulting from lack of blood flow and insufficient oxygen to the brain.

A stroke occurs when the blood supply to part of the brain is suddenly interrupted (ischemic) or when a blood vessel in the brain bursts, spilling blood into the spaces surrounding the brain cells (hemorrhagic). Most strokes begin suddenly, develop rapidly, and cause brain damage within minutes.

Statistical Update, American Heart Association, americanheart.org; A.D.A.M. Illustrated Encyclopedia, Merck Health Library, mercksource.com.

 Someone has a stroke every 45 seconds.

 72% of stroke victims are 65 years or older.

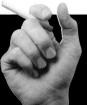 Risk of stroke in heavy smokers is twice that of light smokers.

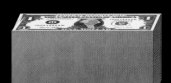

---

to receive treatments that can drastically reduce disability caused by stroke. A breakthrough study by NINDS found that stroke patients who received t-PA within 3 hours of their initial symptoms were at least 30% more likely to recover with little or no disability. t-PA dissolves the clots that cause most strokes.

"It is really worth the effort it takes to call 911," says Dr. Marler. "Treating stroke as an emergency pays back in terms of going home and living your life."

Stroke symptoms appear suddenly:

1. **Sudden numbness or weakness of the face, arm, or leg (especially on one side of the body).**

2. **Sudden confusion or trouble speaking or understanding speech.**

3. **Sudden trouble seeing in one or both eyes.**

4. **Sudden trouble walking, dizziness or loss of balance or coordination.**

5. **Sudden severe headache with no known cause.**

Source: National Institutes of Health.

❓ What are the most common injuries?

The leading causes of work-related injury are overexertion, equipment-related injury and falls. Food, medical and manufacturing industries experience the largest number of injuries. The US Department of Labor, Occupational Safety and Health Administration states that repetitive strain injuries are the nation's most common and costly occupational health problem, costing more than $20 billion a year in workers compensation.

What are the risk factors for carpal tunnel syndrome?

- Overuse of the wrists due to repetitive tasks. High-risk repetitive tasks include typing, sewing, playing a musical instrument, using scissors, driving, assembly-line work, painting, writing, overuse of small-hand tools or tools that vibrate and sports activities such as racquetball or handball.
- Age. The condition occurs most often in people 30 to 60 years old.
- Wrist area fractures or sprains.
- Hormonal changes. Pregnancy and menopause can put women at risk.
- Certain medical conditions, such as arthritis, thyroid imbalance, diabetes or acromegaly (excessive production of growth hormones).

What treatments are commonly used for carpal tunnel syndrome?

Wrist Brace → **Lifestyle and Workplace Modifications** → **Medication**
Anti-inflammatory Drugs/ Steroid Injections → **Alternative Medication**
Dietary Changes/ Herbal Medication

Dietary Changes
Include whole grains, liver, salmon and other vitamin B6-rich foods in your diet. Limit protein intake and avoid sugar, caffeine and processed grains.

Herbal Medication
Herbs known for their anti-inflammatory properties, such as meadowsweet and willow bark, may be recommended.

Lifestyle Modifications
- Take frequent short rests from your repetitive tasks.
- Avoid or reduce the number of repetitive wrist movements.
- Use tools and equipment designed to reduce the risk of injury.

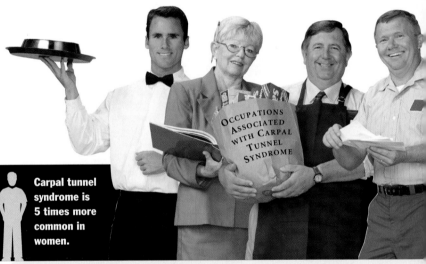

OCCUPATIONS ASSOCIATED WITH CARPAL TUNNEL SYNDROME

Carpal tunnel syndrome is 5 times more common in women.

ACTION ITEMS — Preventing carpal tunnel syndrome

Because carpal tunnel syndrome is so frequently job-related, both employees and employers should be concerned about prevention.

1 Use proper equipment.

People at risk for carpal tunnel syndrome should ask their employers for equipment that is designed to reduce stress on their arms and wrists. Tools and their handles can be designed or modified so that the wrist is not required to bend or twist into awkward positions, and computer keyboards should be lowered so that they are positioned just slightly above your legs.

2 Practice good posture.

Make sure you are working in a comfortable position. Your wrists should not be bent any more than they would be to hold a pencil for writing, and your elbows should be bent to a 90° angle.

3 Warm up.

Do a 5-minute warm-up before you start a repetitive task. The American Academy of Orthopaedic Surgeons recommends the following:

- Hold your arms straight out in front of you. Extend your hands, fingers pointing up, in the stop position. Hold for a count of 5.

What are the symptoms of carpal tunnel syndrome?

- Tingling in the hands is an early sign. It involves the thumb, index, and middle fingers.
- Weakness or numbness in the hands and intense shooting pain that travels up the arm.
- Night pain.
- Decreased hand strength and dexterity. Inability to firmly grip an object or make a fist.
- Trouble using touch to distinguish between hot and cold.

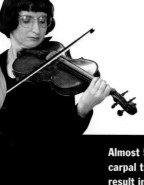

Median nerve is compressed at the wrist, resulting in numbness or pain.

How am I likely to be diagnosed with carpal tunnel syndrome?

Your doctor will conduct tests that include these simple tests:

- Tinel's sign. Tapping over the affected wrist nerve will cause pain to shoot from the wrist to the hand.
- Phalen's sign. Flexing your wrists, palms down, for a minute will cause pain or tingling.
- Electromyography, nerve conduction velocity tests, wrist x-rays or an MRI may be recommended.

Carpal tunnel syndrome, which refers to a passage formed by the wrist bones and the carpal ligament, is a painful condition caused by pressure on the nerve that supplies sensation to the fingers and palm.

Tendons which flex the fingers and the median nerve pass through the carpal tunnel. Swelling and inflammation in this area can cause compression of the median nerve, which leads to pain and weakness in the hand.

Surgery
Carpal Tunnel Release

50% of cases eventually require surgery. It is often successful but full healing can take months.

What can I expect as an outcome?

Most patients respond well to treatment. Patients can prevent recurrence by changing or avoiding the action(s) that has led to the original condition. If untreated, permanent weakness and numbness may result.

Sources: Best Practice of Medicine, A.D.A.M. Health Illustrated Encyclopedia, Merck Health Library, mercksource.com; US Department of Labor; NIOSH.

Almost 50% of all carpal tunnel cases result in 31 days or more of work loss.

50% of all computer operators may have carpal tunnel syndrome.

- Straighten your wrists and relax your fingers.
- Make a tight fist with both hands.
- Bend both wrists down while keeping the fists and hold for a count of 5.
- Straighten wrists and relax fingers for a count of 5.
- Repeat this exercise 10 times, then let your arms hang loosely at your sides and shake them for a few minutes.

4 Take breaks.

Rest frequently and stretch to ease strain on your arms and wrists, and try to avoid long periods of uninterrupted repetitive movement.

Rotate jobs with another employee so that you can take a longer break from a repetitive task. If you work on an assembly line, ask your employer to vary your tasks over the course of the workday.

5 See your doctor.

See your doctor for a professional diagnosis if pain is severe and numbness persists even after rest, or if your grip becomes weak. It is important to diagnose and treat carpal tunnel syndrome. The symptoms of the disorder may lead to permanent loss of hand function if prolonged.

*J*ose loved to eat. His favorites, ice cream and cookies, were part of his daily diet. When he was younger the physical demands of his construction job burned off extra calories. Later, managing crews from an office, the pounds piled on.

When Jose turned 50, the father of four teens suspected something was wrong with his health. He was constantly thirsty, and felt tired and weak. Since his mother had type 2 diabetes, Jose knew he was at risk for the condition and that his extra weight didn't help. As he feared, the results of a diabetes-screening test came back positive.

Jose resisted the idea of making lifestyle changes. 201 "Give up ice cream? Live on vegetables? No way," he complained to his doctor, who gently, but firmly, explained that he needed to make changes, and in fact, might like the way he felt and looked after he started taking better care of his health.

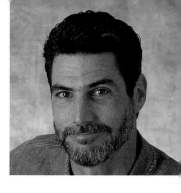

Jose and his wife, Theresa, attended a diabetes management education class where they learned how to prepare delicious meals with less fat and sugar. They left the class with a cooking video and an exercise plan designed to fit their family's lifestyle. Later, Jose received additional information from his health plan. He also looked up diabetes on the Internet 325 and found more helpful resources.

At first, Jose controlled his diabetes with insulin, diet 43 and exercise. 47 Jose, now 30 pounds lighter, is managing his condition without insulin.

Jose credits his wife and doctor, along with all the information he gathered, with giving him the support he needs. "Everybody is different, so just learn what works for you," he suggests. "It's like learning to play baseball; people can teach you the fundamentals, but you have to learn the rest yourself."

Jose got serious and made the lifestyle changes needed to control his diabetes.

The main purpose of insulin is to keep blood sugar levels within their normal range. Although some people can maintain healthy blood sugar levels through diet and exercise, others need insulin to avoid extreme blood sugar levels.

If you take insulin to manage your diabetes you should see a doctor at least four times a year. Otherwise, see your doctor two to four times a year.
Source: American Diabetes Association.

119

A 2002 **National Center for Chronic Disease Prevention and Health Promotion** report states that diabetes is the 6th leading cause of death in the US. It accounts for nearly $132 billion in direct and indirect medical costs and lost productivity each year .

17 million Americans have diabetes; about 1/3 of the cases are **undiagnosed.**

About **2,200 new cases** are diagnosed every day in the United States.

More than 200,000 people die of related **complications** each year.

Diabetes is the leading cause of end-stage **kidney disease, lower extremity amputations** and new cases of **blindness** among adults aged 20-74 years.

Diabetes increases the risk of **heart attack and stroke** two to four times.

Source: United States Department of Health and Human Services Centers for Disease Control and Prevention.

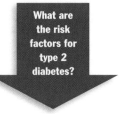

? What are the main types of diabetes?

Type 1 diabetes most often appears during childhood or adolescence.

Type 2 diabetes is more commonly associated with adults. It tends to develop gradually after age 40, but it is now being diagnosed in many overweight children and young adults.

What are the risk factors for type 2 diabetes?

- Heredity 29
- Ethnicity 35
- Age 133
- Being overweight or obese 127
- Hypertension 111

Type 1
Type 2

90% of all diabetes cases are type 2.

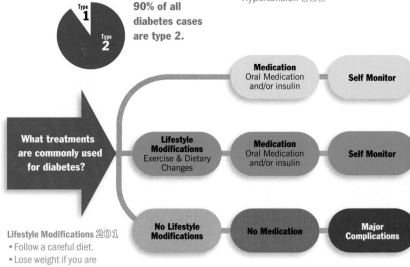

What treatments are commonly used for diabetes?

Medication
Oral Medication and/or insulin → **Self Monitor**

Lifestyle Modifications
Exercise & Dietary Changes → **Medication**
Oral Medication and/or insulin → **Self Monitor**

No Lifestyle Modifications → **No Medication** → **Major Complications**

Lifestyle Modifications 201
- Follow a careful diet.
- Lose weight if you are overweight.
- Maintain a regular exercise regimen.
- If you smoke, quit. Cigarette smoking is a major risk factor for cardiovascular diseases related to diabetes.

Self Monitor 265
- Check your feet for sores and avoid infections.
- Get your eyes checked yearly.
- Get an annual flu vaccine and the pneumonia vaccine.

- Monitor your blood sugar at least daily.
- Contact your doctor if you experience symptoms of low blood sugar.

 People with diabetes who walk at least 2 hours per week had a 39% lower death rate from all causes.

 The majority of people with type 2 diabetes are obese.

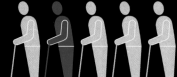 **1 in 5 adults over age 65 has diabetes.**

ACTION ITEMS
Resources for more information

The following organizations may help in your search for more information on diabetes

Federal Government Organizations

- Department of Veterans Affairs
  www.va.gov/diabetes

- National Diabetes Education Program
  800.438.5383
  www.cdc.gov/diabetes/projects/ndeps.htm

- National Institute of Diabetes and Digestive and Kidney Diseases
  800.438.5383
  www.niddk.nih.gov

- Educating People with Diabetes Kit
  (Sponsored by the National Eye Institute)
  www.nei.nih.gov/nehep/diabkit.htm

Non-Federal Government Organizations

- American Diabetes Association
  800.342.2383 or 800.DIABETES
  www.diabetes.org

- American Dietetic Association Consumer Nutrition Hotline
  800.366.1655 (Spanish speaker available)
  www.eatright.org/

What symptoms might suggest type 2 diabetes?

You can have diabetes without showing any symptoms. However, common symptoms include:

- Frequent urination
- Increased thirst
- Weight loss
- Fatigue
- Numbness or tingling in the hands or feet
- Blurred vision

How am I likely to be diagnosed with diabetes?

Doctors will take a medical history, conduct a physical exam, and do an eye exam 161 to look for damage to the blood vessels supplying the retina.

Your doctor will run blood tests 177 to confirm a diagnosis of diabetes.

What can I expect if I have type 2 diabetes?

Diabetes is a chronic disease 219 in which the body makes little or no insulin, or is unable to use insulin.

Insulin is a hormone produced by the pancreas that helps your body use the energy from sugar and other foods. When insulin is missing or ineffective, sugar (glucose) levels build up in your blood. Over time, high blood sugar levels can damage blood vessels and nerves, leading to serious health problems such as blindness, kidney failure, lower extremity amputation, heart disease and stroke.

Normal Life

Minor Complications

Normal Life

Death

Sources: United States Department of Health and Human Services Centers for Disease Control and Prevention, cdc.gov; Merck Health Library, mercksource.com; National Diabetes Information Clearinghouse, niddk.nih.gov.

What can I expect as an outcome?

Type 2 diabetes is a serious condition that can have long-term complications. Better nutrition, physical activity and control of blood glucose can reduce or delay progression of the disease.

THE DIABETES DIET DO'S AND DON'TS

~~Alcohol~~, Fish, Lean Meat, ~~Fruit Juice~~, ~~Pasta~~, Vegetables, Peanut Butter, Non-fat Milk, ~~White Rice~~, ~~Cake~~, Whole Wheat Bread

The number of Americans with diabetes has increased 49% since 1990.

1990

2000

TIP

Moderate, consistent physical activity and a healthy diet can reduce a person's risk for developing type 2 diabetes by nearly 60%.

- American Heart Association National Center
  214.373.6300
  www.americanheart.org

- American Optometric Association
  800.262.3947
  www.aoanet.org

- International Diabetic Athletes Association
  800.898.IDAA
  www.diabetesnet.com/diabetes_resources/idaa.html

- Juvenile Diabetes Foundation International
  800.JDF.CURE or 800.223.1138
  www.jdf.org

- National Diabetes Information Clearinghouse
  301.654.3327
  www.niddk.nih.gov/health/diabetes/ndic.htm

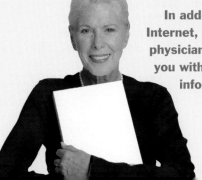

In addition to the Internet, your personal physician can connect you with customized information.

Most Common Digestive Disorders

Number of people affected by a disease in a year (in millions).

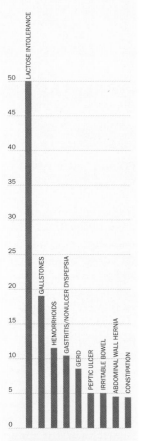

- LACTOSE INTOLERANCE
- GALLSTONES
- HEMORRHOIDS
- GASTRITIS/NONULCER DYSPEPSIA
- GERD
- PEPTIC ULCER
- IRRITABLE BOWEL
- ABDOMINAL WALL HERNIA
- CONSTIPTION

Source: National Institute of Diabetes and Digestive and Kidney Diseases.

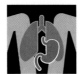

The digestive system includes the stomach, intestines and liver. Digestive diseases affect 60 to 70 million people a year, and account for 13% of all hospitalizations. According to the US Department of Health and Human Services, costs related to this disease exceeded $100 billion in 1992.

What are the risk factors for GERD?

- Diet 43 and lifestyle.
- Illness. Asthma 97, Crohn's disease, diabetes 121 or trauma to the chest.
- Medication. Asthma and hypertension drugs, pain killers, antibiotics and the hormone progesterone.
- Family history 29. Pre-existing medical conditions, such as a faulty esophageal sphincter or hiatal hernia.

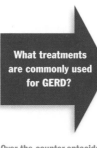

What treatments are commonly used for GERD?

Lifestyle Modifications
Exercise & Dietary Changes

Over-the Counter Antacids
Neutralize Stomach Acids

Medication
Oral medication and/or insulin

Histamine blockers decrease the amount of stomach acid

Foaming agents cover your stomach to prevent reflux

Proton pump inhibitors can relieve symptoms in most GERD sufferers

Prokinetic drugs strengthen the sphincter

Antibiotics make your stomach empty faster

Over-the-counter antacids
- Taking an antacid 1 to 3 hours after meals can reduce symptoms.
- Common antacids: Alka-Seltzer, Maalox, Mylanta, Pepto-Bismol, Rolaids.
- Calcium carbonate antacids, such as Tums, can also be a supplemental source of calcium.

Foaming agents
- Gaviscon is a common foaming agent.

Histamine blockers
- Common histamine blockers: Tagamet HB, Pepcid AC, Zantac 75.

Proton pump inhibitors
- Proton inhibitors include: Prilosec, Prevacid, Nexium.

10% of patients with GERD will eventually develop Barrett's esophagus.

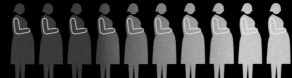

Between 30% and 80% of pregnant women experience symptoms of GERD.

ACTION ITEMS

Take heartburn seriously

1 Heartburn, also called acid indigestion, is the most common symptom of GERD. Anyone experiencing heartburn twice a week or more may have GERD.

2 You can have GERD without having heartburn. Your symptoms could be excessive clearing of the throat, problems swallowing, the feeling that food is stuck in your throat, burning in the mouth or pain in the chest.

3 In infants and children, GERD may cause repeated vomiting, coughing and other respiratory problems. Most babies grow out of GERD by their first birthday.

4 If you have been using antacids for more than two weeks, it is time to see a doctor. Most doctors can treat GERD. Or you may want to visit an internist, a doctor who specializes in internal medicine, or a gastroenterologist, a doctor who treats diseases of the stomach and intestines.

What symptoms might suggest GERD?

The most common symptoms are heartburn and regurgitation. Other symptoms include:

- Chest pain or tightness
- Asthma
- Chronic nausea and vomiting
- Blood in the stool or vomit
- Hoarseness (laryngitis)
- Trouble swallowing
- Chronic cough

How and when am I likely to be diagnosed with GERD?

If heartburn and acid regurgitation are present and antacids seem to help, GERD is diagnosed based on symptoms alone.

If you have chest pain or other symptoms and antacids do not help, your doctor may order the following tests: barium swallow radiograph, endoscopy, pH monitoring or manometry.

Surgery is an option for patients with severe GERD. It can stop regurgitation and improve asthma symptoms.

Surgery Fundoplication

Barrett's Esophagus

Surgery Esophagectomy

A serious complication of GERD, Barrett's esophagus, can increase the risk of cancer.

What can I expect as an outcome if I have GERD?

Most patients with GERD respond well to lifestyle changes and drug therapy. Symptoms can return quickly, however, if treatment is stopped. It is important to continue to take your medication and change your habits for good.

Gastroesophageal reflux disease (GERD) causes food or liquid in the stomach to back up into the esophagus (food pipe).

This partially digested material is acidic and can irritate the esophagus, causing heartburn and acid indigestion. It occurs when the lower esophageal sphincter (LES) valve does not close properly, allowing stomach contents to splash back (reflux) into the esophagus.

Sources: Merck Health Library, mercksource.com; National Digestive Diseases Information Clearinghouse, niddk.nih.gov.

Foods to avoid: caffeinated drinks, chocolate, spicy foods, garlic, onions, peppermint, tomato-based foods, fatty foods, citrus.

24% of adults have had persistent heartburn symptoms for over 20 years. **24%**

50% of patients with asthma also have GERD.

5 **Doctors usually recommend the following lifestyle and dietary changes to relieve heartburn. Many people with GERD also need medication or surgery.**

- If you smoke, stop. 51
- Do not drink alcohol. 49
- Lose weight if needed. 127
- Eat small meals.
- Wear loose-fitting clothes.
- Avoid lying down for 3 hours after a meal.
- Raise the head of your bed 6 to 8 inches by putting blocks of wood under the bedposts – just using extra pillows will not help.

 Barrett's esophagus is caused by chronic, severe exposure to acid and bile reflux. Cellular changes in the inner lining of the esophagus occur that can increase the risk of cancer. This type of cancer is one of the most rapidly increasing cancers in North America. Patients who develop GERD at an early age and whose symptoms last longer than average are at a higher risk for developing Barrett's esophagus. Patients with this condition must be monitored periodically with endoscopy and biopsy in order to detect cancer early.

A report by the **American Academy of Allergy, Asthma and Immunology** states that allergies are the 6th leading cause of chronic disease in the United States, costing the health care system $18 billion annually.

Allergies tend to run in families. More than half of hay fever sufferers have a close relative with a history of allergies.

Each year more than **50 million Americans** suffer from allergic diseases.

Nine million office visits to physicians each year are attributed to hay fever.

Chronic sinusitis is the most commonly reported chronic disease, affecting 12.6% of people (approximately 38 million) in the US.

Source: Best Practice of Medicine, Merck Health Library; The Allergy Report: Science Based Findings on the Diagnosis & Treatment of Allergic Disorders, American Academy of Allergy, Asthma and Immunology; US Department of Health and Human Services, Centers for Disease Control and Prevention.

What are the risk factors for allergies?

- Family tendency 29
- Environmental conditions 63
- Geographic location
- Exposures to allergen
- Illness
- Abnormal immune system

What symptoms might suggest allergic rhinitis?

- Coughing
- Headache
- Itching of the nose, mouth, eyes, throat, skin or any area
- Runny nose (rhinitis)
- Impaired smell
- Frequent sneezing
- Nasal congestion
- Tearing
- Sore throat

What treatments are commonly used for allergic rhinitis?

- Short-acting antihistamines (Benedryl)
- Decongestants
- Lifestyle Modifications
- Medication
- Long-acting antihistamines (Allegra/Claritin)
- Nasal corticosteroid spray (Flonase/Nasonex)
- Cromolyn sodium (Nasalcrom)

Lifestyle Modifications
- Avoid or reduce exposure to allergens (see Action Items).
- People with strong seasonal allergies may consider moving to a region where the allergen doesn't exist.

Medication
- Short-acting antihistamines relieve mild to moderate symptoms, but can cause drowsiness. They can also cause confusion, light-headedness, dry mouth, constipation, difficulty with urination and blurred vision in the elderly.

Allergies usually develop before age 20. The average age that allergies begin is 10 years.

Pollen count peaks between 5 am and 10 am each day. Try to stay indoors during those hours.

Peanut or nut allergies affect 3 million Americans and cause the most severe food-induced allergies.

ACTION ITEMS Make your home allergy friendly

Since avoidance is the best treatment for allergies, you may want to consider some of the following tips for allergy-proofing your home.

1 Concentrate on the bedroom.
Since the bedroom harbors the greatest number of dust mites and since most people spend about a third of their day there, it can be effective to concentrate your allergy-proofing efforts here. Start with a switch to synthetic bedding and cover your mattress and pillows with dust-proof covers. Washing your bedding with hot water (at least 130 degrees) will help kill the dust mites.

Replace soft surfaces with hard surfaces.
2 If possible, replace the flooring in carpeted rooms with wood, tile or linoleum which is much easier to keep clean. If carpet is your only choice, pick something with a low pile. Wood, leather and vinyl furniture make better choices than upholstered.

Vacuum properly.
3 If carpeting can't be removed, remember to vacuum it frequently. And, don't forget to vacuum the other fabric surfaces in your home—like upholstered furniture and draperies—that can't be washed. Try fitting your vacuum with

? What are common forms of allergies?

Common types of allergies include seasonal allergic rhinitis (hay fever), perennial allergic rhinitis, allergic conjunctivitis, food and drug allergies, insect allergies and physical allergies (cold, heat).

Immunotherapy may be recommended if the allergen cannot be avoided. It is most commonly used for allergies involving pollen, dust mites, insect venom and animal dander. Regular injections of the allergen in increasing doses may help desensitize the body. Too high a dose, however, can cause anaphalaxis. Treatment may take years, and can cause uncomfortable side effects. It is effective in about two-thirds of cases.

Immunotherapy
Allergy Shots

How am I likely to be diagnosed with allergic rhinitis?

Your doctor will take your medical history and conduct a physical examination. He may examine your nasal passages for evidence of obstruction.

Allergy skin tests can help determine which allergens are responsible for your symptoms. This may include interdermal, scratch, patch or other skin tests.

What can I expect as an outcome if I have allergic rhinitis?

Allergic rhinitis tends to improve with age, possibly because the immune system becomes less responsive with age.

Sources: A.D.A.M. Health Illustrated Encyclopedia, Merck Health Library, mercksource.com; Medline, US National Library of Medicine, National Institute of Health, nlm.nih.gov; National Institute of Allergy and Infectious Diseases, National Institute of Health, naid.nih.gov.

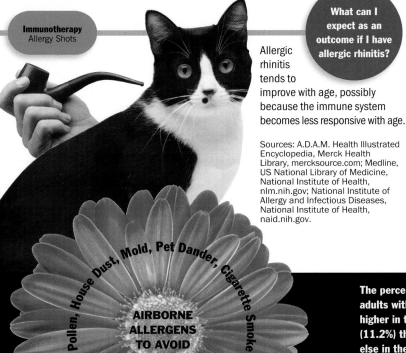

Pollen, House Dust, Mold, Pet Dander, Cigarette Smoke

AIRBORNE ALLERGENS TO AVOID

? What can I expect if I have allergies?

An allergy is an exaggerated immune response.

An allergy is an exaggerated immune response or reaction to substances (allergens) that are generally not harmful. The misdirected response triggers production of antibodies that bind to cells that contain histamine, which when released causes itching, swelling of affected tissues, mucous production, muscle spasms, hives, rash and other symptoms. Allergies can cause life-threatening reactions (anaphylaxis) or discomfort without being life-threatening.

The percentage of adults with hay fever is higher in the West (11.2%) than anywhere else in the US.

TIP
In many people, milk protein (casein) stimulates mucus production, irritating conditions such as asthma, bronchitis and sinusitis. Avoiding milk products may help.

a bag that is made to prevent allergens from escaping or buy a new vacuum equipped with a HEPA (High Efficiency Particulate Air) filter. Since vacuuming will temporarily stir up the allergens in your home, it is a good idea to keep allergic persons out of the area during vacuuming and for at least an hour after.

4 Minimize mold.
Keep mold to a minimum by using a dehumidifier (and cleaning it regularly) to lower the humidity level in your home. Use fans for ventilation and stay on top of any visible mold on walls and ceilings. Visible mold should be treated with fungicides (available from your local hardware store).

5 Filter your air.
Keep windows closed in warm weather while staying cool with central air or window air conditioning units. Invest in a HEPA filter and keep the filters clean. These can make a huge difference in removing pollen, mold and animal dander. Remember that they are not effective in keeping your home dust mite-free since dust mite allergens do not easily become airborne.

6 Don't smoke.
Don't allow anyone to smoke in your home—no excuses. Smoke will sabotage your anti-allergen efforts and it greatly increases the chance that children in the home will develop asthma.

Male/Female Weight Comparison

Percentage of men and women considered to be at a healthy weight, by age group.

■ Men
■ Women

[Bar chart with y-axis from 0 to 50 (increments of 5), x-axis labeled: 20-34, 35-44, 45-54, 55-64, 65-74, 75+]

Source: Centers for Disease Control and Prevention, USA Today.

What risk factors contribute to becoming obese?

- Family history 29
- High sugar/fat diets 43
- Stress and emotional disturbances
- Sedentary lifestyle 47
- Aging, which slows down metabolism 133
- Some medications
- Poverty 37

What kinds of symptoms result from obesity?

Excess fat below the diaphragm and in the chest wall may put pressure on the lungs, causing difficulty in breathing and shortness of breath, even with minimal exertion. Difficulty breathing may seriously interfere with sleep, causing momentary cessation of breath (sleep apnea), leading to daytime sleepiness and other complications.

Obesity may cause various orthopedic problems including low back pain and worsening of osteoarthritis, particularly

---

What can I do to get my weight under control?

To lose weight, obese people must consume fewer calories than they expend.

[Flow diagram:]
Lifestyle Modifications — Exercise & Dietary Changes → Surgery — Stomach Stapling & Gastric Bypass

No Lifestyle Modifications → Medical Complications — Diabetes, Gallbladder Disease, Arthritis → Cardiovascular Disease

Lifestyle Modifications 201
- A slow weight loss of 1 or 2 pounds a week, until the desired body weight is reached, is best. One pound of fat contains about 3,500 calories, so to lose
- 1 pound a week, a person should decrease calorie intake by 500 calories each and every day.
- Aerobic physical activity will assist in increasing muscle tissue and burning calories.

60% of Americans are overweight. 1 in 4 are obese.

People with an apple shape are at increased risk for diabetes and heart disease. Those with a pear shape (large hips and thighs) have a much lower risk.

30.3% of children (ages 6-11) are overweight and 15.3% are obese.

ACTION ITEMS

Are you at a healthy weight?

In the 1980's, our government, concerned about the impact of weight on health, created a formula, the BMI (body mass index), to define healthy weight, overweight and obesity, using a formula that combines both height and weight. It works for both men and women. To calculate your BMI use the following formula. Or, go online for a calculator.

www.nhlbisupport.com/bmi

Source: National Institutes of Health.

1. Weigh yourself.
   _____pounds

2. Have your height measured.
   _____ inches

3. Multiply your weight in pounds by .45.
   Step 1 x .45 = _____

4. Multiply your height in inches by .025.
   Step 2 x .025 = _____

5. Square the answer to Step 4 (multiply it by itself).
   Step 4 x Step 4 = _____

in the hips, knees and ankles. Skin disorders are particularly common because obese people have relatively little body surface for their weight and can't get rid of body heat efficiently. Swelling of the feet and ankles is also common.

What health problems am I likely to encounter if I am obese?

Obesity refers to having an excessive amount of body fat, regardless of what your actual body weight is.

People can be obese and still weigh an appropriate amount for their height because a large percentage of their weight is from fat. Obesity may be classified as mild (20% to 40% overweight), moderate (41% to 100% overweight) or severe (more than 100% overweight). Extremely muscular people may be described as "overweight" but are not fat.

What can I expect if I am obese?

Being obese shaves seven years off a person's life. Just being overweight shortens a person's life by three years.

Being overweight contributes to several serious, chronic conditions that can lead to death or disability. These include high blood pressure, blood cholesterol abnormalities, adult onset diabetes (type 2), heart disease, stroke, gallbladder disease, arthritis of the knees and hips, sleep apnea, respiratory problems and certain types of cancer.

Normal Life

Death

What can I expect as an outcome if I remain obese?

Being seriously overweight plays a role in nearly 70% of the diagnosed cases of cardiovascular disease and doubles the chance of developing high blood pressure.

Sources: Mayo Clinic Health Information, mayoclinic.com; A.D.A.M. Health Illustrated Encyclopedia, Merck Health Library, mercksource.com; Centers for Disease Control and Prevention; American Obesity Association, obesity.org.

Sweets: 75 calories

Fats: 3 to 5 servings

Protein/Dairy: 3 to 7 servings

Carbohydrates: 4 to 8 servings

Food Pyramid Recommended Daily Servings

Fruit: unlimited (at least 3 servings)

Vegetables: unlimited (at least 4 servings)

Overweight-related conditions result in some 300,000 deaths every year in the US, and are second only to smoking as a cause of preventable death.

300,000

6 **Divide the answer to Step 3 by the answer to Step 5.**
Step 3 / Step 5 = _____
This is your BMI.

BMI	
18.5 to 25	**Healthy**
25 to 30	**Overweight**
30+	**Obese**

Not all adults who have "healthy" BMI are at their most healthy weight. Some may have lots of fat and little muscle and, therefore,

be at risk. Others may be above the healthy range, but may be fine with lots of muscle and little fat.

Percentage of Obese Americans

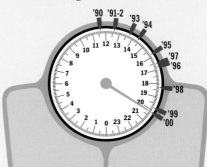

Source: Wired.

❓ What are common types of depression?

Major depression is characterized by a combination of symptoms that interfere with the ability to work, sleep and eat. Symptoms must be present for at least 2 weeks. If very severe, the depression may be accompanied by suicidal thoughts or behavior. Major depression may occur only once, but more commonly occurs several times over one's lifetime.

Low-grade depression, also known as dysthymia, is characterized by long-term, chronic symptoms that do not disable, but keep one from functioning well or from feeling good. People who suffer from dysthymia are at increased risk for episodes of major depression.

Bipolar disorder (manic-depressive illness) is characterized by cycling mood changes of severe highs (mania) and lows (depression). Sometimes the mood switches are dramatic and rapid, but most often they are gradual.

Source: *Plain Talk About Depression,* Margaret Strock; National Institute of Mental Health.

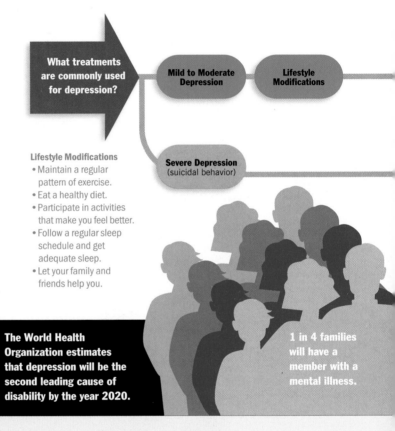

What are the risk factors for depression?

- Family tendency 29.
- Medical illness. Stroke 115, heart attack 77, cancer 87 or Alzheimer's disease 109.
- Hormones. Some women experience depression associated with menstrual cycles and childbirth 209.
- Medication. Side effects of certain drugs such as tranquilizers, blood pressure medication or steroids.
- Substance abuse 53.
- Low self-esteem.
- Stress 67. Emotionally upsetting events, particularly those involving loss of a spouse or family member. Change in life pattern, such as divorce, losing a job, moving from a home to a retirement facility.
- Age 133. Chronic pain 221, loss of mobility or memory loss can trigger depression in the elderly.

What treatments are commonly used for depression?

Mild to Moderate Depression → **Lifestyle Modifications**

Severe Depression (suicidal behavior)

Lifestyle Modifications
- Maintain a regular pattern of exercise.
- Eat a healthy diet.
- Participate in activities that make you feel better.
- Follow a regular sleep schedule and get adequate sleep.
- Let your family and friends help you.

The highest suicide rates in the US are found in white men over age 65.

#2 The World Health Organization estimates that depression will be the second leading cause of disability by the year 2020.

1 in 4 families will have a member with a mental illness.

ACTION ITEMS

Recognizing depression

A person with depression has several of the following symptoms. Keep in mind that some people experience only a few symptoms while others may experience many. The severity of symptoms varies with individuals and also varies over time. If someone you know seems to be depressed reassure them that depression is treatable and encourage them to seek professional help. Help them make arrangements and be sure they follow through. Take any references to suicide seriously.

1. Persistent sad, anxious or "empty" mood

2. Feelings of hopelessness or pessimism

3. Feelings of guilt, worthlessness or helplessness

4. Loss of interest or pleasure in hobbies and activities that were once enjoyed, including sex

5. Decreased energy

6. Difficulty concentrating, remembering or making decisions

What symptoms might suggest depression?

Symptoms typically develop gradually over days or weeks. Detecting depression in the elderly may be complicated by several factors. Symptoms such as fatigue or sleeping problems are often associated with the aging process rather than a depressive disorder. See Action Items for common symptoms.

How am I likely to be diagnosed with depression?

A complete medical history, psychiatric interview and physical examination will be performed to determine whether the cause is physical or psychological. Certain medications and conditions can cause the same symptoms as depression, and your doctor should rule out these possibilities.

Sleep studies and blood tests may be indicated.

What can I expect if I suffer from depression?

Depression is a psychiatric illness characterized by overwhelming feelings of sadness, discouragement and worthlessness.

These feelings may follow a recent loss or sad event but are out of proportion to that event and persist beyond an appropriate length of time. Severe depressions may affect health and interfere with work and relationships.

Sources: A.D.A.M. Health Illustrated Encyclopedia, Merck Health Library, mercksource.com; National Institute of Mental Health, nimh.nih.gov; National Mental Health Association, nmha.org.

Psychotherapy alone may be as effective as drug therapy for mild depression.

Counseling/Psychotherapy Interpersonal and cognitive therapy

Medication Anti-depressants

ECT can relieve depression quickly in individuals who are at risk for suicide.

Counseling/Psychotherapy

Electroconvulsive Shock Treatment (ECT)

Medication Anti-depressants

Depressed people have higher death rates.

Hospitalization May be Needed

What can I expect as an outcome if I have depression?

Treatment alleviates depression in 80% of cases. However, people who have had a major depression are at risk for future episodes. Major depression may last for years, if untreated.

 An episode of depression typically lasts for 6 to 9 months, but in 20% of the cases, it lasts for 2 years or more.

 9.5% of American adults suffer from a depressive disease in a given year.

 Women experience depression twice as often as men.

7 **Insomnia, early-morning awakening or over-sleeping**

8 **Decreased appetite leading to weight loss or overeating leading to weight gain**

9 **Restlessness or irritability**

10 **Persistent physical symptoms that do not respond to treatment such as headaches, digestive disorders and chronic pain**

11 **Thoughts of death or suicide or suicide attempts**

Some people become depressed each fall and winter when hours of sunlight are reduced. These people typically experience extreme fatigue, sleep excessively, have sugar cravings and gain weight. This type of depression is called seasonal affective disorder (SAD).

Menopause symptoms differ between cultures. 80% of American women experience hot flashes, vs. 9% in Japan and 16% in Thailand.

After menopause, **annual bone loss** occurs at a rate of 1 to 1.5% per year.

Women age 40 are 1/3 less likely to have a **heart attack** than men of the same age. But by age 75, both women and men are equally at risk.

Six million women in the US take **estrogen** and **progesterone** for relief from menopausal symptoms and prevention of heart disease and osteoporosis.

Thin Asian and Caucasion women are at highest risk for developing **osteoporosis.**

75% of women have **hot flashes** lasting anywhere from 30 seconds to 5 minutes.

Sources: *All About Menopause,* Frank Murray; *Natural Menopause,* Miriam Stoppard; Merck Health Library, mercksource.com; cnn.com.

When does menopause begin?

The average woman reaches menopause around age 51, although some may experience it earlier.

Approximately 4 to 6 years before menopause, you may begin to notice irregularity in your monthly periods due to decreasing estrogen levels. This stage is known as perimenopause. Symptoms are most bothersome during this time.

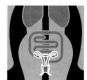

Do I need medical treatment while I'm going through menopause?

Lifestyle Modifications
Exercise & Dietary Changes

Lifestyle Modifications
Exercise & Dietary Changes

Alternative Therapies

Lifestyle Modifications
Exercise & Dietary Changes

Alternative Therapies

Alternative Therapies
- Alternative therapies include herbs, acupuncture and yoga.
- Dong quai, black cohash, and chasteberry are common herbal remedies for controling hot flashes.

Menopause itself requires no treatment. Lifestyle modifications, Hormone replacement (HRT) and other therapies can help minimize the symptoms that accompany menopause.

Lifestyle Modifications
- Eat a low-fat, high-fiber diet **43** that includes plenty of fruits and vegetables. Citrus fruits have natural estrogenic properties.
- Limit intake of caffeine, alcohol **49** and chocolate.

- Avoid tobacco **51**.
- Exercise regularly **47**. Include aerobic, weight-training and flexibility exercises.
- Learn ways to minimize or deal with stress **67**.

By the time a woman is 80, she will have lost 40% of her bone mass.

The best sources of calcium are milk and dairy products, canned salmon and sardines, broccoli and calcium-fortified juices.

Dress in layers to minimize the effects of hot flashes and night sweats.

ACTION ITEMS Using alternative therapies

Deciding whether to use hormone replacement therapy (HRT) after menopause is a difficult decision many women face as they age. Research has shown that HRT is very effective for relieving menopausal symptoms such as hot flashes and vaginal dryness. It can also reduce the risk of osteoporosis. However, there are also known health risks and uncertainties about long-term use. Recent research has demonstrated that long-term use of estrogen in combination with progestin results in more risks than benefits.

Many women may now be considering using alternatives to conventional HRT to relieve menopausal symptoms and to lower the risk of conditions such as osteoporosis and heart disease. At this time, there is not enough scientific evidence to determine whether alternate therapies like natural estrogen(s), acupuncture and herbal supplements are beneficial. In addition, we do not have sufficient information to show whether these therapies are as safe or safer than conventional drugs being used for menopausal symptoms, osteoporosis or heart disease.

What are the symptoms of menopause?

Symptoms can range from nonexistent to severe:

- Hot flashes or night sweats
- Mood swings
- Vaginal dryness
- Osteoporosis
- Increase in heart disease (elevated cholesterol and blood pressure)
- Insomnia
- Loss of bladder control
- Forgetfulnesss.

What causes the symptoms of menopause?

Estrogen affects many parts of the body. In addition to maintaining reproductive tissues, it stimulates the growth of bone cells, relaxes the arteries, aids the brain in regulating body temperature, reduces cholesterol, and helps the skin retain water. Fluctuating estrogen levels can have a wide range of effects. Hot flashes, the brain's response feeling overheated, are caused by decreased estrogen levels.

Water-soluble gels and greater attention to foreplay may relieve vaginal dryness.

Medication
Hormone Replacement Therapy

Medication
- Combination treatment of estrogen and progesterone is called hormone replacement therapy (HRT). It is effective in relieving hot flashes and may reduce the risk of osteoporosis.

Is hormone replacement treatment a safe way to treat menopause?

- Taking estrogen alone increases your risk of developing uterine cancer.
- HRT is available in a variety of forms: pills, patches, vaginal creams.
- Side effects include; headaches, breast tenderness, fluid retention, bleeding, weight gain.
- ACE inhibitors and biphosphates are effective drug treatments for heart disease and osteoporosis.

HRT is an effective short-term treatment for controlling acute symptoms of menopause. Once symptoms subside, you should ask your doctor whether you need to continue therapy. Risks associated with long-term use include increased incidence of blood clots, gall bladder disease, breast cancer and heart disease.

What can I expect as I go through menopause?

Menopause is the natural cessation of menstrual periods that marks the end of a woman's reproductive life.

The body decreases its production of the female hormones, estrogen and progesterone, the ovaries stop producing eggs and menstrual activity ceases. Menopause occurs at the end of a woman's last period and is defined by no menstruation for at least 12 months.

Sources: All About Menopause, Frank Murray; Natural Menopause, Miriam Stoppard; Perimenopause, Bernard Cortese; Woman's Health Source, Mayo Clinic.; Best Practice of Medicine, Merck Health Library, mercksource.com; TIME Magazine; cnn.com.

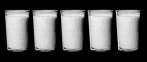

The recommended daily calcium intake for women over 50 is 1,500 mg. This is equivalent to 5 cups of milk.

Your adrenal glands release estrogen each time you exercise. Four 30-minute exercise sessions per week will keep you supplied with estrogen and lower your risk of osteoporosis.

TIP
Consumption of soy products may help reduce hot flashes, preserve bone mass and protect against breast cancer

1 Ask your doctor.
Postmenopausal women should consult their health care provider about their personal risks and benefits of using HRT, as well as the use of alternative therapies. Herbal therapies may have adverse side effects or exhibit harmful interactions with other medications. Consumers should always discuss their use of herbs and dietary supplements with their health care provider.

2 Try lifestyle changes first 201.
Certain lifestyle changes—including quitting smoking, eating well and exercising regularly—can also offer benefits and should be considered for promoting healthy aging and reducing the risk of heart disease.

3 Consider the risks.
Alternative therapies may or may not be helpful in relieving menopausal symptoms. More research is needed to define the benefits and risks.

4 Pay attention to the costs.
The cost of alternative therapies such as dietary supplements is usually not covered by insurance.

Laboratory studies show that cutting back on calories can increase your lifespan. **Caloric restriction** preserves bone mass, skin thickness and brain function, and provides resistance to heat, toxic chemicals and traumatic injury.

Studies show that people who **eat meals,** particularly breakfast, **at regular intervals** stay younger longer. Non-breakfast eaters have a mortality rate 1.5 times higher than those who eat breakfast regularly.

The **Framingham Heart Study** found that expending 2,000 calories a week in physical activity (the equivalent of walking one hour a day) increases life expectancy by two years.

If science cured every known disease of the elderly, it would add only 15 years to the current **life expectancy** ⑨ of 75.

Source: *Newsweek: Health for Life, Your Body,* 2001; *Time,* January 2002; *U.S. News and World Report,* March 2002; drkoop.com; realage.com.

What issues am I likely to face as a result of aging?

The study of aging (gerontology) shows that as people grow old, the body functions less efficiently, which includes a reduction in the ability to fight infection. Chronic illnesses like diabetes, kidney problems or heart disease tend to disable the elderly by impairing other body functions like blood pressure or circulation. And as the elderly tend to suffer from more than one disease, this can affect their response to multiple medications. Recuperation from acute illnesses or accidents such as heart attacks, pneumonia and hip fractures takes longer and can incapacitate the aged. This may result in a temporary or permanent loss of independence, which can trigger depression or dementia-like behavior. The elderly also experience more sleep disorders and sleep deprivation. These problems can be misdiagnosed as depression or dementia as well.

Economic factors and a loss of income also impact the way older people seek health care. The elderly may conceal or ignore problems because of budgetary constraints, but these health issues can become potentially fatal.

Body Composition
Percentage of total weight

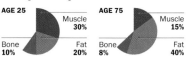

AGE 25		AGE 75	
	Muscle 30%		Muscle 15%
Bone 10%	Fat 20%	Bone 8%	Fat 40%

Source: *Newsweek: Health for Life, Your Body,* 2001.

What are our prospects for beating the aging process?

In the last century, the average life span for men and women has increased by 25 years. However, people still age. And while there is no known way to beat the aging process, people can maintain their health and quality of life.

The Aging Brain

Though the brain decreases in weight and loses the ability to process abstract problems quickly with age, it retains most of its cells (neurons). And engaging in mental as well as physical aerobic exercise helps maintain cognitive function.

The Aging Heart & Arteries

Cardiovascular disease ⑦⑤ is best prevented by regular exercise ④⑦ and eating fruits, vegetables and whole grains daily. People who work out regularly (20 minutes three times a week) can cut their age-related decline in half.

Arthritis affects 50% of all Americans over 64.

Oral problems are a leading cause of poor nutrition among the elderly.

The brain shrinks by 10% between the ages of 30 and 90.

Women will live an average of 6 years longer than men.

ACTION ITEMS
Ten tips for healthy aging

No known substance can extend life, but the chances of staying healthy and living a long time can be improved. Here are ten ways to help.

① Eat a balanced diet, including 5 helpings of fruits and vegetables a day ④③.

② Exercise regularly (check with a doctor before starting an exercise program) ④⑦.

③ Get regular health check-ups ⑤⑦.

④ Don't smoke ⑤① (it's never too late to quit).

⑤ Practice safety habits ⑥⑤ at home to prevent falls and fractures. Always wear your seatbelt in a car.

⑥ Stay in contact with family and friends. Stay active through work, play and community.

⑦ Avoid overexposure to the sun and the cold.

Eight Signs That You're Getting Old

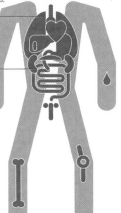

Brain. Loses cells, but adapts by increasing the number of connections between cells and by regrowing branch-like extensions that carry messages.

Hearing. Difficulty hearing higher frequencies.

Lungs. Maximum breathing capacity declines.

Kidneys. Become less efficient at extracting wastes from the blood. Bladder capacity declines and urinary incontinence increases.

Sight. Difficulty in focusing on close objects, and seeing in lowlight levels as well as detecting moving objects.

Heart. It grows larger and oxygen consumption during exercise declines.

Body Fat. Increases and redistributes to abdominal area and hips and thighs.

Muscles. Decline in size and weight.

The human body changes profoundly with age.

Muscle mass decreases as body fat increases, the skin wrinkles and becomes thin, bones lose density and people decrease in height. Internal organs (heart, lungs, brain) function less efficiently and the body's senses (sight, taste, smell, sensation and hearing) as well as its systems (circulation, respiration) begin to fail.

Sources: Merck Health Library, mercksource.com; *Newsweek: Health for Life, Your Body,* 2001; *Esquire,* May 2002.

Aging Bones & Cartilage

Retaining muscle mass, power and flexibility will keep aging bones strong and pain-free. Thus, doing weight-bearing exercise such as walking and lifting weights will help reduce bone loss and reverse the depletion of lean body mass.

Aging Skin

Anti-wrinkle creams, skin treatments and surgery 205 do not prevent skin from aging or repair damage from sunlight. The best prevention for aging skin and skin cancer is to use sunblock and cover-up.

Aging Sexual Function

Getting daily exercise 47, eating a balanced diet 43 and stopping smoking 51 contribute greatly to men and women's sexual energy, confidence and enjoyment.

 33% of seniors experience some urinary incontinence.

Every hour spent in vigorous exercise as an adult is repaid with 2 hours of additional life span.

 Nearly 1/3 of people over 65 have hearing problems. Hearing declines more quickly in men than in women.

TIP

Don't skip meals. If possible, eat dinner before 6 pm. Early meals keep your brain sharp and prevent food from being deposited as fat.

8 If you drink 49, moderation is the key. When you drink, let someone else drive.

9 Keep personal and financial records in order to simplify budgeting and investing. Plan long-term housing and money needs 305.

10 Keep a positive attitude toward life. Do things that make you happy 61.

Source: National Institute on Aging.

 DO WE NEED LESS SLEEP AS WE GET OLDER?
The elderly tend to sleep less as they get older. However, it is a myth that the need for sleep decreases with age. Many elderly have underlying sleep disorders that disrupt their sleep. Sleep disorders include sleep apnea and periodic limb movement disorder (kicking your feet while asleep). In addition, older people often take naps during the day, which makes it harder to sleep through the night.

? What is a herniated disk?

The vertebrae of the spinal column are separated by disks made of cartilage. Each disk has a strong outer layer and a soft inner layer that act as a shock absorber to cushion the vertebrae during movement. If the disk degenerates following injury or aging, the inner part of the disk can bulge or rupture through the outer layer (herniated disk). The ruptured inner part of the disk can compress or irritate a nerve root.

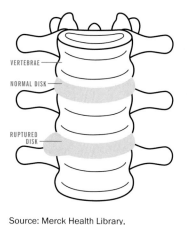

VERTEBRAE
NORMAL DISK
RUPTURED DISK

Source: Merck Health Library, mercksource.com

What symptoms can I expect if I am disabled due to back problems?

The location of the herniated disk determines where a person will feel pain. How badly the nerve root is damaged determines how severe the symptoms will be.

Most herniated disks occur in the lower back and affect only one leg.

The rupture can cause pain not only in the lower back but also down the sciatic nerve, which runs from the spinal column to the heel.

Symptoms include:
- Severe low back pain
- Pain radiating to the buttocks, legs and feet
- Pain made worse with movement, coughing, straining or laughing
- Tingling or numbness in legs or feet
- Muscle spasms and stiffness
- Muscle weakness or atrophy in later stages

Symptoms may appear suddenly, disappear and return at intervals or be constant and long-lasting

What can I do to improve my life if I am disabled by a back problem?

Rest

Lifestyle Modification

Rest
- Discomfort usually subsides in 6 to 8 weeks with proper rest and relaxation.

Lifestyle Modifications
- A firm, supportive mattress is helpful for sleeping. Pillows under the waist, shoulder or knees may help.
- Use safe work and play practices and proper lifting techniques.
- Weight control can help reduce the stress on your back.

Being overweight can put you at risk for back problems.

80% of all Americans will have at least one backache.

Disk herniation occurs more frequently in middle-aged men.

ACTION ITEMS Am I eligible for disability benefits?

Social Security pays disability benefits under two programs: the Social Security disability insurance program and the Supplemental Security Income (SSI) program.

1 After helping you complete an application, the Social Security office will review your case to see if you meet the basic requirements for disability benefits. They will look at your work history, your age and, if you are applying for benefits as a family member, your relationship to the worker. The office then will send your application to the Disability Determination Services (DDS) office in your state.

2 The DDS will consider medical evidence from your doctors and institutions where you have been treated and all the other information they have.

Your doctors or other sources are asked for a medical history of your condition:
- what is wrong with you
- when it began
- how it limits your activities
- what the medical tests have shown
- what treatment you have received

If the DDS needs more medical information they may ask you to go to a special examination called a "consultative examination."

What can I expect if a back problem disables me?

Your doctor will take your medical history and conduct a physical examination. He will check your spine for tenderness and test sensation, coordination, muscle strength and reflexes. He will perform a straight-leg test to reveal leg pain and may also assess muscle tone in the rectum.

Your doctor will order MRI or CT scans to help identify spinal compression. A myelogram may be performed to determine the size of the herniation.

Disability is any limitation in social or other activity caused by a chronic health disorder, injury, or impairment.

Approximately 38 million Americans suffer from disabilities. Heart disease and back problems are the two most common causes of disability, followed by arthritis, lower extremity orthopedic impairment and diabetes.

Sources: Disability Statistics Rehabilitation Research and Training Center, University of California; National Institute on Disability and Rehabilitation Research; A.D.A.M. Health Illustrated Encyclopedia, Merck Health Library, mercksource.com; *Your Body and Disease, Bones, Joints and Muscles.*

If there is severe pain, muscle weakness or impaired bladder or bowel function, surgery 205 may be necessary.

Exercise/ Physical Therapy

Medication Aspirin/Non-steroid anti-inflammatory drugs

Surgery Chemonucleosysis, Diskectomy or Open Surgery

What can I expect as an outcome if I am disabled?

Most people improve with treatment. It may take several months to a year or more to resume all activities without pain or strain to the back. Occupations that involve heavy lifting or back strain may need modification to avoid recurrent back injury.

- Better posture can promote beneficial changes in the back.

Exercise/Therapy
- Exercises are recommended to reduce muscle spasms and pain and to speed recovery.
- A physical therapist 213 can prescribe a specific program to meet your needs.

People who are injured on the job recover less well than those whose disability is non-injury related.

Injuries cause 13.4% of all disabling conditions.

Lifting heavy objects incorrectly increases your risk of injury.

TIP

Try this beneficial exercise: Lying down on the floor, pull each knee alternately up to the chest. Perform in sets of 10, 2 or 3 times a day.

How do they determine disability?

- Are you working? If you are and your earnings average more than $780 a month, you generally cannot be considered disabled.

- Is your condition "severe"? Your condition must interfere with basic work-related activities for your claim to be considered.

- Is your condition found in the list of disabling impairments? The DDS maintains a list of impairments for each of the major body systems that are so severe they automatically mean you are disabled.

- Can you do the work you did previously? If your condition is severe, but not at the same or equal severity as an impairment on the list, then the DDS must determine if it interferes with your ability to do the work you did previously.

- Can you do any other type of work? If you cannot do the work you did in the past, the DDS sees if you are able to adjust to other work.

For More Information

- Social Security Administration
  www.ssa.gov
  800.772.1213
  TTY 800.325.0778

What is an advance directive?

An advance directive consists of a living will and a medical power of attorney (durable power of attorney). It is a written legal document that ensures a patient's health care wishes will be followed in the event that the patient becomes unable to speak, communicate or make decisions. Talking with a doctor will assure that the advance directive reflects the patient's needs and medical circumstance.

A living will presents a patient's specific wishes including the type of care and end-of-life medical treatment the patient will receive.

A medical power of attorney allows a patient to choose and appoint someone (a health care proxy) to make medical treatment decisions if the patient is unable to speak, communicate or make decisions.

What kind of hospice care can I expect in an at-home situation?

Hospice care involves a team of health professionals and volunteers who provide medical, psychological and spiritual support to terminally ill patients who are diagnosed as having less than six months to live. Working in tandem with families, hospice care is based primarily in the home allowing patients and their loved ones to remain together during the dying process. Hospice emphasizes palliative (calming) treatment, which includes pain management, daily caregiving needs and resolving emotional family issues.

What kind of hospice care can I expect at a long-term care facility?

Hospice can also provide its comprehensive care to patients in assisted-living facilities and nursing homes 223. This care includes pain management, symptom control and bereavement assistance. At times, a nursing home may be the best option if more skilled medical services are required, or if family members are unable to accommodate all the patient's needs. The hospice team serves to supplement the usual nursing home care.

What decisions might I need to make before I die?

Type of Care — **Organ Donation** — **Estate Planning**

Many important end-of-life decisions are better made when patients are able to communicate their wishes. These decisions may include:

Type of Care
- Choosing the type of end-of-life medical treatment you would want. This can require preparing an advance directive. 317

Organ Donation
- Organ donation and the types of organs, if any, that will be donated.

Estate Planning
- Estate planning, which can entail determining care for young children, legally appointing a person to make financial decisions, organizing records and writing a will. 319

Care Provider
- Choosing the best place to receive care or best-at-home provider. 223

Medicare-certified hospices are available for patients whose life expectancy is 6 months or less.

75% of all Americans approve of living wills. 317

The US Supreme Court reaffirmed the right of competent patients to refuse unwanted medical treatments and to receive adequate pain treatment at the end of life.

ACTION ITEMS Evaluating end-of-life care

1 Physical and emotional symptoms
Are physical and emotional symptoms such as pain, fatigue, depression, nausea and fear evaluated and treated?

What is the response time to serious symptoms and how does it vary based on the patient's setting (home, hospital, etc.)?

2 Support of function and autonomy
Is help provided to maintain the patient's functional activities such as eating and sleeping?

3 Aggressive care near death
Will the patient's wishes for avoiding or withdrawing aggressive end-of-life treatment be followed and respected?

Will the patient be allowed to die where they wish (home, hospital, etc.)?

4 Patient and family satisfaction
Will the healthcare providers be concerned with the satisfaction of the family when it comes to decision-making, outcomes and quality of life?

What kind of hospice care can I expect in a hospital?

The majority of patients with terminal illnesses will receive some of their care in a hospital. As many as 50% of these patients will die in the hospital. The types of palliative care programs developed by hospital and hospice partners include:

- A hospice team in the hospital to facilitate hospice admissions
- A hospice inpatient unit
- An inpatient palliative care unit and consultation service
- A Medicare Hospice Benefit contract
- A comfort suite for patients and their families
- Outpatient palliative care consultation

What kind of care can I expect at a hospice?

Choosing care in a hospice center is an option when patients have no family or friends available to help at home, or when patients develop acute or fluctuating medical needs that require intensive management. Most hospice centers do not offer long-term care, but assist patients and families in finding this service.

A hospice center provides the inclusive medical, psychological and spiritual care as well as a high staff-to-patient ratio, an on-call registered nurse, private rooms, kitchen facilities and meals, family rooms and 24-hour visiting privileges.

Two million people die in the US annually, and 80% of these deaths occur in hospitals, nursing homes or hospice centers.

Sources: Merck Health Library, mercksource.com; American Hospice Foundation, american-hospice.org; Hospice Association of America, hospice-america.org; partnershipforcaring.org; hospicenet.org; WebMD Health Encyclopedia, mywebmd.com; The Halquist Memorial Hospice Center, The Hospices of the National Capital Region, thehospices.org; American Academy of Family Physicians, aafp.org; Center to Advance Palliative Care; Hospice of Northwest Ohio, hospicenwo.org; The Visiting Nurse Association of Porter County, vnacounty.org.

Care Provider

"I wish I didn't have a brain tumor," claims Bernie Goldhirsch, founder of *Inc.* magazine. "But dealing with it has been the most exciting and dangerous journey of my life."

80% of hospice care takes place at home.

88% of adults would prefer to be cared for in their own home or a family member's home if they became terminally ill.

20% of Americans have completed advance directives. 317

Many hospitals and hospices provide grief support to survivors for up to 1 year following a death.

50 states and the District of Columbia have laws authorizing the use of some type of advance directives. 317

5 Global quality of life
Will the patient's support system (family, friends, clergy) be able to participate in the care of the patient?

Will additional support (i.e., counseling) be sought if needed?

6 Family burden 237
Will the patient's support system be assisted with the emotional, physical and financial challenges of direct caregiving?

7 Survival time
Will the patient and family be given realistic expectations on survival time?

8 Provider continuity and skill
Are relationships and plans made in one area of the program continued when the patient moves to another area (i.e., hospital to hospice)?

9 Bereavement
Will counseling or support group referrals be offered to the family following the patient's death?

*J*ust as there is no consensus about when conscious life begins, there is none about when it ends. Determining the precise time of death is, in fact, medically and scientifically impossible, says Atlanta cardiologist Michael Sabom. "It used to be thought that the point of death was a single moment in time," says Sabom. "It is now thought that death is a process, not a single moment." We need something to go by, though. So our society has come up with various legal and social definitions to give us a sense of finality. Here are the terms we're most familiar with:

Clinical Death Breathing and heartbeat have stopped. A person might still be able to be resuscitated with CPR or other means, depending on why the vital signs ceased and under what conditions.

Brain Death The lower brain, or brain stem, which controls automatic body functions, stops working. A person can be kept alive only with the help of life-support machines. The length of the period that the brain-stem must be inactive before a person is declared legally dead varies from jurisdiction to jurisdiction. Complicating the issue, the same person can be considered legally dead if about to become an organ donor, but legally alive if not.

Persistant Vegetative State The brain stem still functions, keeping the heart, lungs and digestive system working, but the sensing, thinking part of the brain has shut down. It may be possible to keep the body functioning for long periods with life-support systems.

Whole Brain Death Both lower and higher brain functions have ceased.

As if these definitions were not confusing enough, some religious leaders and experts in various disciplines questions whether consciousness or the "soul" has truly departed a body that meets any of the above criteria for death.

"When Do You Die?" by Anita Bartholomew reprinted with permission from the August 2003 Reader's Digest. © 2003, The Reader's Digest Association, Inc.

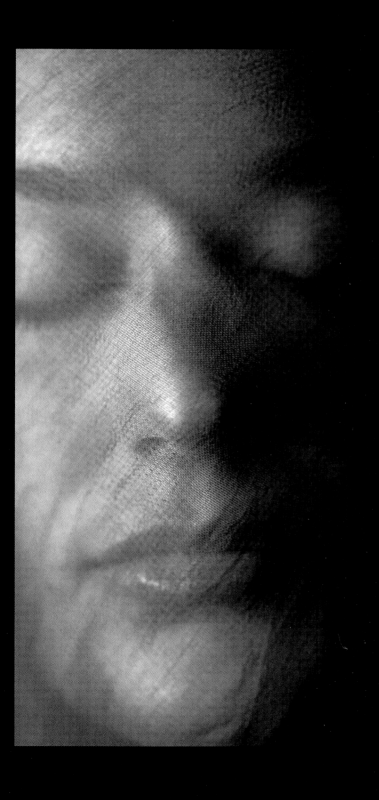

? What are the warning signs?

BRAIN CANCER

A brain tumor increases the mass inside the skull and may block the flow of cerebrospinal fluid. This pressure can cause:
- nausea
- vomiting
- headaches

More specific symptoms of brain cancer depend on exactly where the tumor is located within the brain.

Source: oncologychannel.com.

HEAD AND NECK CANCER

Common symptoms include:
- persistent pain in the throat
- pain or difficulty in swallowing
- persistent hoarseness or a change in voice
- bleeding in the mouth or throat
- pain in the ear

SKIN CANCER

These are some of the early signs:
- a firm red lump
- a small, pale, smooth, shiny or waxy lump
- a sore that begins bleeding or oozing
- a sore red spot that becomes scaly or crusty
- a sore that becomes itchy, tender or painful
- a spot that becomes red and/or swollen
- a mole that grows or changes its appearance

Use this simple ABCD of early skin cancer diagnosis:

A: look for **asymmetrical lesions:** the different halves of a mole do not look like each other.
B: look for **border irregularity:** the edges of the mole are indented or notched.
C: look for **color variation:** the mole is not the same color all over and may have patches of different colors.
D: look for a **diameter** greater than the size of a pencil eraser tip.

HEART DISEASE 75

Heart attacks can occur without warning, but the symptoms may have been there for some time. Common warning signs are:
- chest pain with exertion or activity
- shortness of breath
- swelling in the legs or feet
- high blood pressure
- high blood cholesterol

HEART ATTACK 77

- discomfort in the center of the chest for more than a few minutes
- pain in one or both arms, the back, neck, jaw or stomach
- shortness of breath (can occur before any chest discomfort)
- cold sweat, nausea or lightheadedness

MACULAR DEGENERATION

- blurred vision

LUNG CANCER

The main symptoms are:
- cough
- shortness of breath
- wheezing
- chest pain
- bloody, coughed-up sputum
- loss of appetite
- weight loss
- inflammation of the lungs (pneumonia)

STROKE 115

- sudden numbness or weakness of face, arm or leg, especially on one side of the body
- sudden confusion, trouble speaking or understanding
- sudden trouble seeing in one or both eyes
- sudden trouble walking, dizziness, loss of balance or coordination
- sudden severe headache with no known cause

CARDIAC ARREST

Cardiac arrest strikes immediately and without warning. Here are the signs:
- sudden loss of responsiveness
- no response to gentle shaking
- no normal breathing
- no signs of circulation
- no movement or coughing

ACTION ITEMS

When to go to the emergency room

Use good judgment in deciding when to use emergency medical services. Learn the signs of serious illness and trust your instincts. If you are alarmed by unusually severe symptoms, it is best to seek immediate care. If unsure, call your primary care physician and describe your symptoms so he can advise you on whether emergency treatment is necessary.

Here are some situations that warrant immediate care:

❶ Loss of consciousness

❷ Signs of heart attack that last two minutes or more

❸ Signs of a stroke 115

❹ Severe shortness of breath

❺ Bleeding that does not stop after 10 minutes of direct pressure.

❻ Sudden, severe pain

❼ Poisoning
(Note: If possible, call your local poison control center first and ask for immediate home treatment advice. Certain poisons should be vomited as soon as possible while others should be immediately diluted with water. Such preliminary home treatment could save your life.)

PANCREATIC CANCER

Diagnosis is often delayed because symptoms are non-specific. Jaundice (yellowing of the skin) is present in about half of cases, and patients may suffer weight loss, fatigue, discomfort in the abdomen, loss of appetite and glucose intolerance. The patient may not notice the gradual onset of these symptoms.

BLADDER CANCER

- blood in the urine
- frequent urination
- painful urination

Type I DIABETES

These symptoms occur suddenly and must receive immediate medical attention.

- frequent urination (in large quantities)
- excessive thirst
- extreme hunger
- rapid weight loss
- fatigue
- irritability
- nausea and vomiting
- high amounts of sugar in the blood and/or urine

Type II DIABETES 121

These symptoms occur gradually, but must still receive medical attention as soon as possible.

- blurred vision
- tingling or numbness in the legs, feet or fingers
- frequent infections of the skin
- recurring skin, gum or urinary tract infections
- itching skin or genitals
- drowsiness
- slow healing of cuts and bruises
- any symptoms listed under type I diabetes

There are clear warning signs for most major and life threatening health problems.

Learn what they are so that you will know when a trip to the emergency room might mean the difference between life and death.

CERVICAL CANCER

- abnormal vaginal bleeding
- abnormal vaginal discharge
- low back pain
- painful sexual intercourse
- painful urination

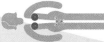

BREAST CANCER 93

- dimpling of the breast
- lump in the underarm or breast
- nipple discharge, pain or inversion
- skin irritation of the breast or nipple
- swelling

OVARIAN CANCER

- bloating
- abnormal pelvic discomfort or pressure
- nausea or loss of appetite
- changes in bowel function or urinary frequency
- back or leg pain
- malnourished or wasted appearance
- fatigue
- gastrointestinal symptoms (gas, stomach pain, indigestion)
- unusual vaginal bleeding

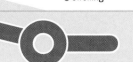

COLORECTAL CANCER 89

- feeling tired and weak
- jaundice
- pain or cramps in the abdomen
- difference in the usual bowel movements
- feeling of fullness in bowel after movement
- bleeding from rectum
- blood in stool
- reduced appetite

ARTHRITIS 107

- joints feel stiff and may be hard to move
- daily tasks such as climbing stairs or opening a jar may be hard to do
- pain and stiffness may be more severe during certain times of the day, or after doing certain tasks
- some types of arthritis cause swelling, or inflammation, and skin over the joint may appear red and hot to the touch

Is it a	COLD...	or FLU?
fever	rare	102°-104°
headache	rare	prominent
aches & pains	rare	usual, often severe
fatigue or weakness	slight	extreme
runny, stuffy nose	common	sometimes
sneezing	usual	sometimes
sore throat	common	sometimes
chest pain, cough	mild to moderate cough	common, can be severe

Source: missourifamilies.org.

8 A severe or worsening reaction to a medication, especially if breathing is difficult

9 A major injury such as a head trauma

10 Unexplained stupor, drowsiness or disorientation

11 Coughing up or vomiting blood

12 Severe or persistent vomiting

13 Suicidal or homicidal feelings 61

14 A broken bone when bone is showing or causes limb deformity

15 An insect sting accompanied by difficult breathing

16 Convulsions caused by fever

17 Fever over 101° in an infant under three months of age 143

18 Rectal bleeding not associated with a bowel movement

19 Profuse rectal bleeding (more than 1/2 cup) with a bowel movement

An allergy is a physical reaction to a substance in the environment. When a child comes into contact with one of these substances, known as an allergen, either by touching, breathing, or eating it, or having it injected, his body releases histamines to fight it.

Allergies

Chicken pox is an itchy rash that starts as small red bumps which quickly change into thin-walled water blisters on a pink base. The blisters then develop into clear fluid blips, which finally become dry brown crusts in about four days. Highly contagious through touch, sneezing, coughing or even breathing.

Chicken Pox

Asthma is a chronic condition in which a person's airways tend to become inflamed and fill with mucus when exposed to cigarette smoke, a known allergen, cold or exercise. The body reacts with coughing and wheezing.

Asthma

A cold is characterized by a stuffy or runny nose (thick, clear, white, yellow, or green mucus), a cough and sometimes a sore throat. Medicine will not cure the cold faster, but you can help your baby feel better and keep her from getting worse by giving her lots of rest and liquids (breast milk or formula only for babies under six months).

Cold
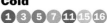

- **1 Fever** Rectal temperature more than 100.4° F
- **2 Diarrhea**
- **3 Cough**
- **4 Breathing problems/ wheezing**
- **5 Congestion/ stuffy nose**

- **10 Rash/ purple spots or sores**
- **11 Sore Throat**
- **12 Nausea/ vomiting**
- **13 Crying or fussiness**
- **14 Itchy/watery eyes**

Ear Infection

An ear infection can result when fluid and bacteria build up in the area behind your baby's eardrum. When the eustachian tube is blocked (common during colds, sinus infections, even allergy season), the fluid gets trapped in the middle ear and bacteria growth causes the eardrum to bulge. Symptoms include pus draining from the ear, baby tugging at her ear, fever and irritability.

Stomach Flu

A stomach flu caused by a virus is one of the most common causes of vomiting and diarrhea in a toddler. Avoid spreading germs by insisting that everyone in the house wash their hands thoroughly after changing diapers or using the bathroom.

Pneumonia

Pneumonia is an infection of the lungs that can be caused by bacteria and viruses. The infected child may develop pneumonia after two or three days of having a cold or sore throat. Symptoms may include fever and unusually rapid breathing. The most common type begins suddenly and can be prevented by immunization.

Gastric Reflux

Gastric reflux disease is characterized by frequent stomach eruptions and vomiting. Reflux is exactly what it looks and sounds like—frequent uprisings of stomach fluid—and it makes for a cranky baby who won't eat much and, in the worst cases, wheezes, coughs and gags.

ACTION ITEMS

When should I call the pediatrician?

You're the best judge of whether your baby is really ill, so call if you're worried, no matter what his temperature is. Besides, temperature isn't the only indication of whether his illness is serious. His age is a factor (fever is more serious in babies under three months), and so is his behavior (a high fever that doesn't stop him from playing and feeding normally may not be cause for alarm). Keep in mind that he'll feel hotter if he's been running around than if he's waking up from a nap.

With all this in mind, you should call the doctor if:

1 Your child is younger than three months and has a rectal temperature of 100.4° F (38° C) or higher.

2 Your child is three months or older and has a rectal temperature above 101° F (38.3° C).

3 You are worried—no matter what the time or temperature.

Coxsackie causes hand, foot and mouth syndrome and herpangina, with blister-like sores in mouth and throat and on feet and hands. Highly contagious, the virus spreads from mouth to mouth, feces to hand to mouth, or through sneezing or coughing, usually striking in the first two years of life.

Coxsackie

Croup is an infection in the upper respiratory tract that swells the trachea and larynx (windpipe and voice box). Children tend to develop a harsh, barking (like a seal) cough. Most cases of croup are caused by the parainfluenza virus (the adenovirus is another offender).

Croup

Respiratory Synctial Virus (RSV) is the most common cause of lower respiratory tract infections in children worldwide. It is the leading cause of pneumonia and bronchiolitis in infants.

RSV
 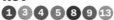

Use the chart at left to help determine what may be causing your child's symptoms. See a doctor for severe or persistant symptoms.

And, don't send your child off to school or childcare with a fever, a gastrointestinal illness, a rash linked to infection, pinkeye, strep throat or untreated head lice.

Source: Understanding Children, understandingchildren.com, TOP and Civitas.

Ear pain

7 Runny Nose Clear

8 Listlessness

9 Refuses food/liquid

15 Sneezing

16 Mucus Thick white, yellow or green

17 Fluid draining from ear White or yellow

18 Gas

Whooping Cough

Whooping cough (also known as pertussis) is a rare bacterial infection that inflames the airways. The pertussis bacteria set up shop in the windpipe, where they bring on a persistent, violent cough. The coughing spell can last for 20 to 30 seconds. Whooping cough is rare and very serious and can be prevented by immunization.

Eczema

Eczema is an itchy skin rash that can appear on a baby's skin when the child is as young as two months old. It generally shows up on the forehead, cheeks, or scalp and sometimes spreads to the arms or chest. The rash often causes the skin to appear dry, thickened and scaly.

Colic

Colic is a term used to describe persistent crying (usually in the afternoon or evening) in an otherwise healthy baby. If your baby is under five months old and cries for more than three hours a day, more than three days a week for more than three weeks, and there is no medical explanation for the distress, chances are he's colicky.

Any of the following symptoms could indicate a more serious problem when coupled with a fever and should be treated by a physician. Page your pediatrician, call 911 or go to the emergency room immediately if:

 Your baby has lost her appetite, has little energy or is noticeably pale; or you notice other changes in her behavior and appearance.

 Your baby has small, purple-red spots on his skin that don't turn white when you press on them or large purple blotches; both of these can signal meningitis, an infection of the brain.

3 Your baby has difficulty breathing even after you clear her nose with a bulb syringe.

4 Your baby seems delirious, glassy-eyed, or extremely cranky or irritable; these could signal a serious viral or bacterial illness.

Source: BabyCenter.com.

My wife talked me into going to this charity auction last year," said Dave, a 47-year-old accountant and volunteer firefighter from Denver. "It had about as much appeal to me as going to the dentist. But I'll tell you what, it saved my life."

One of the items up for bid was the yearlong services of a local GP. "I'm into health so it caught my eye. I figured why not have a doctor at my beck and call."

Dave won the bidding and met Dr. John Bowen, who was also attending the event. "What's the catch?" he asked the young doctor. "Just think of me as your own personal advocate. Call me whenever you need me," Dr. Bowen said handing Dave his card.

I'd been having trouble with diarrhea for the past several months and was headed to the hospital for some tests so I asked him to come along and help explain things to me.

Don't know what questions to ask? Check out
MerckSource. This Web site has a list of topics
(everything from diabetes to fibroids to yoga) and
provides you with a list of questions that go with
your topic choice.

www.mercksource.com

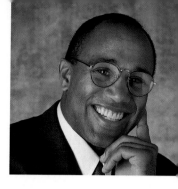

At the hospital, Dr. Bowen listened in on Dave's initial talk with his doctor. "Dave's always been healthy," said his doctor. "I'm sure it's nothing, but we'll run some tests."

"Here I am thinking this is no big deal and then Dr. Bowen starts asking questions about my symptoms that my other doctor hadn't asked me. The two of them started talking about possible causes and other tests. Suddenly, I started taking this much more seriously."

After testing, Dave was diagnosed with a slow-growing colon cancer.

"If Dr. Bowen hadn't been with me that day, I don't think the cancer would have been discovered in time," Dave said. "He saved my life. He's been with me through this whole process. I don't think I'll ever go to another doctor appointment without having my wife, a friend or somebody else with me."

Dave found that having a good healthcare advocate can make the difference between life and death.

Signs and symptoms of colon cancer:
  Rectal bleeding
  Stomach cramps or pain
  Change in bowel habits
  Tiny amounts of blood in stool
  Anemia
  Weight loss with no apparent cause
  Sometimes no symptoms at all
Source: Mayo Clinic Family Health Book.

Resources for advocates:
www.patientpowernetwork.org
www.agingresearch.org
www.acurion.com
www.drugpolicy.org
www.vh.org

8 questions to ask your doctor

If you're seeing a doctor for the first time, organize your personal health information and take it with you. Include details of your health history, test results, x-rays or scans, and immunization dates. You can keep this information in a notebook, on your computer, even online.

The Savard Health Record is a six-step system for keeping your own complete, accurate and continually updated medical chart. With your *Health Record* in hand at every office visit, you're helping your doctor give you the best care.

Source: *The Savard Health Record.*

About **50%**

of people with chronic illnesses feel that their doctor offers them choices, discusses pros and cons, and asks for their input on treatment on a consistent basis. The other half feel they aren't adequately involved in making decisions with their doctors.

Source: Robert Wood Johnson Foundation, FACCT – Foundation for Accountability, *A Portrait of the Chronically Ill in America*, 2002.

Nearly **95%**

of diagnosis is based on your medical history. The more your doctor knows about you the better. The control of that information is in your hands. After all, you're the source!

Source: Association for American Physicians and Surgeons, Inc.

Minutes spent with the doctor	
1-10	23%
11-15	36%
16-30	30.3%
31+	6.5%
0	4.2%

Source: National Center for Health Statistics, based on 880 million office visits, in 2001.

What's wrong and what caused it?

What are my treatment options? 199

Do I need tests and what are they? 158-191

Your doctor will keep your discussions confidential, unless you give permission to share the information. It's important to provide medical details even if they are embarrassing to you.

Do I need medication, and what kind?

What are the side effects of the medication?

What do I do next and when should I see you again?

If you don't feel comfortable talking with your doctor, you might want to consider making a change. 229 Good doctor/patient communication is vital to your health.

Can I ask you questions by email?

Can you email my test results?

Source: Association of American Physicians and Surgeons, *For Patient Power: The Patient's Handbook.*

ACTION ITEMS What to take to your doctor's visit

1 **A buddy**
For support and to help you remember details about the visit

2 **Questions**
A list of questions about your concerns

3 **Symptom list**
A detailed list of symptoms or problems

4 **Medical records**
Your personal health records

5 **Medications**
Either make a list of the medications and their dosages or bring the actual containers with you.

6 **A note pad**
Write down the answers to your questions, instructions the doctor gives you, explanation about your condition, how you should take your medications.

Source: Yale Medical Group.

What should I expect from my doctor?

Your doctor should communicate with you in a **clear and understandable** way. After every doctor visit, you should walk away with:

 An understanding of your **condition** and any tests or procedures that you might need.

Instructions for treating your condition.

 Instructions for prescribed **medications** and an understanding of potential side effects.

An estimate of how much your care will **cost.**

Understandable **answers** to all your questions. (If you don't understand your doctor's expla-nation, ask again and again until you do!)

Source: The Journal of the American Medical Association.

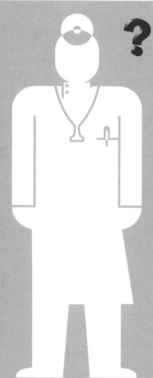

 ## What kind of doctor should I see? 225

The two largest groups of primary care doctors for adults are family physicians and internists. Some women see obstetricians/gynecologists for some of their primary care needs.

Physician assistants 232 , nurse practitioners 231 and certified nurse midwives are trained to deliver many aspects of primary care. Physician assistants must practice in partnership with doctors. Nurse practitioners and certified nurse midwives can work independently in some states, but not in others.

Specialists 15 concentrate on specific parts of the body, age groups or complex procedures that diagnose or treat certain conditions. Your doctor may refer you to a specialist or you may want to seek one out for a second opinion.

Sources: Agency for Healthcare Quality and Research, Journal of the American Medical Association.

How can I get the most out of a doctor's visit?

Be prepared and plan ahead. Write a list of questions to ask. Be very specific about all of your symptoms.

Remember to include equally important factors like stress or tension at work or at home.

Sources: *Understanding and Using the Health Care System,* Chapter 37; Memorial Sloan-Kettering Cancer Center; Psycho-Oncology Forum.

CONSUMER ALERT

Give information to your doctor. Don't wait to be asked! Tell your doctor about how you're feeling and what symptoms you have. Research says that patients who have good communication with their doctor tend to be more satisfied with their care and have better results.

Source: Agency for Healthcare Quality and Research.

Resources

American Medical Association
515 N. State Street
Chicago, IL 60610
312.464.5000
www.ama-assn.org

American Board of Medical Specialties Public Education Program
Verify a doctor's certification status.
800.776.2378
www.certifieddoctor.org

● **Guide to Clinical Preventive Services, 2nd edition**
Agency for Healthcare Research and Quality Office of Health Care Information
Executive Office Center
2101 East Jefferson Street, Suite 501
Rockville, MD 20852
301.594.1364
www.odphp.osophs.dhhs.gov/pubs/guidecps

Wellness check-ups

The information below is for typical wellness visits. Your child's doctor should be available whenever necessary. Call your pediatrician or bring your child in for a visit whenever you feel there is a problem.

Questions the doctor may ask

Are you having any problems with breastfeeding?

How is your baby sleeping?

When, how, and how often is your baby eating?

How is baby's elimination?

What are your baby's bowel movements like?

What is your baby's crying pattern like?

What sounds does your baby make?

Can your baby roll over one way or sit with support?

How are your baby's motor skills developing?

Does your baby seem ready for solid food?

What games does your baby like to play?

How does your baby react to strangers?

How many teeth does your baby have?

Is your baby standing? Walking?

Does your baby point at objects?

What does your baby say?

How are your baby's social skills developing?

Is your child showing any signs of toilet training readiness?

Are you cleaning your child's teeth and gums?

Has your child been saying "no" a lot or throwing temper tantrums?

Is your child talking a lot?

What new words is your child learning?

Does your child play well with others?

How does your child react when left at school or with someone else?

Immunizations

Hepatitis B

DTaP or DTP

Hib

Polio

Pneumococcal conjugate

MMR (measles, mumps, rubella)

Chicken pox

Developmental assessment

Height and weight

Vision and hearing

Head circumference

General development and behavior

Sleep, bedtime behavior and routines

Elimination, bowels, constipation

Feeding and nutrition

Skills, new and old

Health and hygiene

Umbilical cord, circumcision

Car seat and home safety

Cradle cap, baby acne, diaper rash

Return to work, child care, transitions

Ear infections, colds, flu, diarrhea, croup

Cuts, bumps and falls

Toilet training

ACTION ITEMS

Make doctor's visits less traumatic

 Don't get there early
Arrive at the doctor's office just in time for the appointment, not early. For that long wait in the tiny examining room, make sure you have a favorite toy and a snack or drink. Sing, cuddle and talk about all of the things in the room. Let your child touch anything she wants except the dreaded "medical waste can." You can even wash her hands in the sink. After the nurse gets the necessary information, try undressing while counting fingers and toes or doing the "head and shoulders, knees and toes" song.

 Treat the doctor's staff like friends
If you are friendly and comfortable with the staff in your doctor's office, it will help your child be more relaxed, too. For reinforcement at home, take a picture of your child with the doctor and nurse and take a look at it together every now and then. Before appointments, you can go over everyone's names and get your child excited to see them.

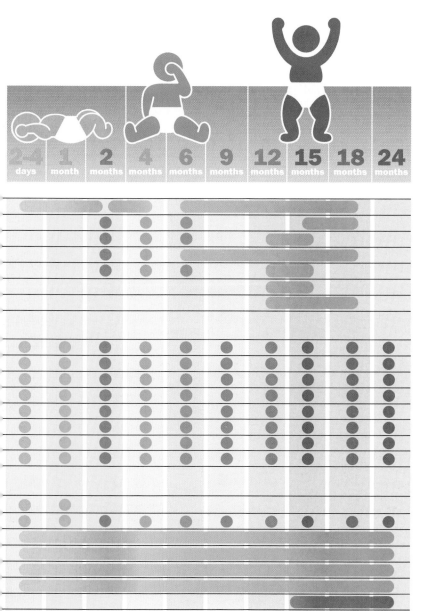

Choosing the right pediatrician is more important than you might think

The average new parent and baby visit the pediatrician's office 11 times in the first year for six routine well-baby visits and five other visits. Choose well, and the doctor you pick might treat your child all the way from her first cold to her pre-college physical.

Sources: Understanding Children, understandingchildren.com, TOP and Civitas; American Academy of Pediatrics; Centers for Disease Control and Prevention.

3 Make it a family affair
If you have more than one child, try to take them all with you to doctor and dentist appointments. That way, each child takes turns being "the patient" and they can see that the doctor's office is not necessarily a scary place.

4 Bring a toy
Take your baby's favorite toy with you to the doctor. While playing with the toy and sitting on your lap, your child will be preoccupied and comfortable—making it easier for you, your baby and your doctor.

5 Keep the same doctor
Try to keep the same doctor. That way your child can get to know the doctor and the surroundings.

Source: BabyCenter.com.

❓ What are major causes of a visit to the emergency room?

People complaining of **chest pains or discomfort that suggests a heart problem** account for 7 million visits to the emergency room a year. But when symptoms such as jaw pain, dizziness, sweating, nausea, mild chest and left arm pain appear, many people don't realize they are in serious trouble. A recent survey showed that of nearly 900 people seen in a hospital for chest pain, only 23% had used emergency medical service (EMS) transport to get there.

Sports-related injuries cause 3.7 million visits to emergency departments a year. Two-thirds (2.6 million) of the visits are by people age five to 24, and most are male. Basketball and cycling are the sports causing the most injuries, followed by football, baseball, roller and ice skating, skateboarding, gymnastics cheerleading, water and snow sports and playground injuries.

❓ What kind of care will I get in an emergency room?

Advances in medicine and new technology now gives emergency staffs the ability to turn off a heart attack in midstream by using clot dissolving medications or angioplasty (the use of a tiny balloon that is inflated to flatten the clot in a clogged blood vessel). By preserving heart muscle function, prompt treatment like this can reduce in-hospital deaths. A new test, the **cardiac sestambi scan**, can help emergency room doctors to more accurately rule out suspected heart attacks.

Source: WebMDHealth.

INSIDE AN AMBULANCE

Most emergency ambulances are fully equipped wih first aid and other specialized medical equipment. Paramedics are trained to carry out life-saving treatment on the scene of an accident, at a person's home and on the trip to the hospital.

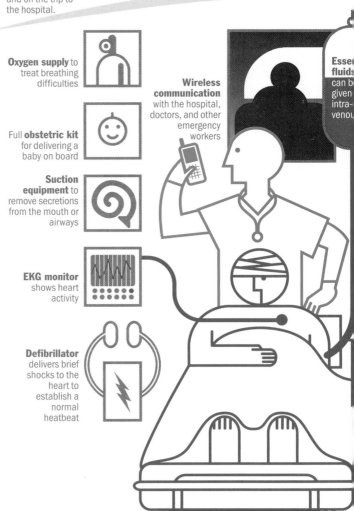

Oxygen supply to treat breathing difficulties

Full **obstetric kit** for delivering a baby on board

Suction equipment to remove secretions from the mouth or airways

EKG monitor shows heart activity

Defibrillator delivers brief shocks to the heart to establish a normal heatbeat

Wireless communication with the hospital, doctors, and other emergency workers

Esse fluids can b given intra- venou

Stretcher is secured into the ambulance

ACTION ITEMS Handling an emergency

Calling for help can be the most important thing you can do for yourself or someone else in an emergency. If you find yourself at the scene of an emergency:

1 Make sure that the scene is safe.

2 Call 911 immediately yourself or, if you are not alone, send someone else to call. Answer the technician's questions as clearly and concisely as possible. You will likely be asked for the following information:

- exact location of emergency
- your name
- nature of emergency
- condition of victims
- help being given at scene

The dispatcher may ask you to stay on the line until an ambulance arrives and most are trained to assist you with instructions for certain life-saving techniques like CPR.

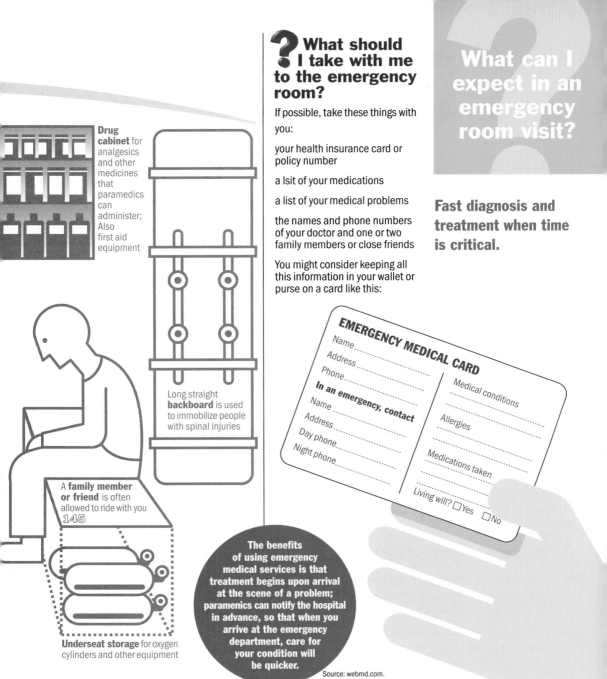

Drug cabinet for analgesics and other medicines that paramedics can administer; Also first aid equipment

Long straight **backboard** is used to immobilize people with spinal injuries

A **family member or friend** is often allowed to ride with you
145

Underseat storage for oxygen cylinders and other equipment

145

❓ What should I take with me to the emergency room?

If possible, take these things with you:

your health insurance card or policy number

a lsit of your medications

a list of your medical problems

the names and phone numbers of your doctor and one or two family members or close friends

You might consider keeping all this information in your wallet or purse on a card like this:

EMERGENCY MEDICAL CARD

Name..........

Address..........

Phone..........

In an emergency, contact

Name..........

Address..........

Day phone..........

Night phone..........

Medical conditions
....

Allergies
....

Medications taken
....

Living will? ☐ Yes ☐ No

The benefits of using emergency medical services is that treatment begins upon arrival at the scene of a problem; paramenics can notify the hospital in advance, so that when you arrive at the emergency department, care for your condition will be quicker.

Source: webmd.com.

❓ What can I expect in an emergency room visit?

Fast diagnosis and treatment when time is critical.

---

3 Care. Return to care for the victim until an ambulance arrives. If the victim is conscious, try to help him rest comfortably and keep him calm. Watch for changes in the victim's breathing and consciousness. If the victim is unconscious, is not breathing and has no pulse, administer CPR.

Adult CPR

❶ Find hand position on breastbone.

❷ Give 15 compressions.

❸ Give 2 slow breaths.

❹ Repeat compressions and breaths 3 times.

❺ Recheck pulse and breathing.

❻ Continue cycle until victim regains consciousness, help arrives or the scene becomes unsafe.

This is intended only as a supplement to information learned in a complete CPR training course. Contact you local Red Cross, American Heart Association or fire department for information on CPR certification.

Why does the medical profession try to rule in diseases, then try to rule them out? By ruling in a disease, diagnosticians are casting as wide a net as possible to be sure that no one who might have a disease is missed. However, once the wide net is cast, those healthy people who are caught in the net must be ruled out.

What is meant by "ruling in" and "ruling out?"

When women go for a mammogram, they go to **rule in** the possibility of breast cancer. If abnormalities show up only a fraction of them will actually be cancer. But those with abnormalities will then go for a biopsy to **rule out** cancer*. In general, **diagnostic sensitivity** refers to tests that rule in; these tests cast a wide net. **Diagnostic specificity** refers to tests that rule out; these tests are stringent in omitting healthy individuals.

*Mammograms have been criticized for casting too wide a net, resulting in unnecessary biopsies.

Differences between sensitive and specific tests	
Tests for ruling in disease:	**Tests for ruling out disease:**
are more sensitive	are more specific
cast a wide net	narrow the net
produce false positives	produce false negatives
are less invasive	are more invasive
are less risky	are more risky
cost less	cost more

What is a "pathognomic finding?"

The most useful tests are those that establish the presence of a disease. The results of these tests are called **pathognomonic findings.** A pathognomonic finding is when cancer cells are seen in a tissue biopsy: if there are cancer cells present, the patient has cancer.

What is meant by "false positive?"

False positive results are also known as errors of inclusion. This means that a test (usually a sensitive test) shows that you have a disease when you are actually healthy. When the test is positive but you do not have the disease, the result is called false positive.

What is meant by "false negative?"

False negative results are also known as errors of exclusion. This means that a test (usually a specific test) shows that you are healthy when you actually have the disease being tested for. When the test is negative, suggesting that no disease is present, but you do have the disease but you do not have the disease, the result is called false negative.

What are diagnoses of exclusion?

Some diseases are identified by **diagnoses of exclusion**—that is, there are presently no known tests to produce a final diagnosis. If a patient complains of very general problems, such as lethargy and overall fatigue, it's possible that the disease is chronic fatigue syndrome. But there is no specific test for that disease, so the doctor has to rule out other diseases (by using their specific tests) until there is nothing left to account for the symptoms.

ACTION ITEMS

Questions for your doctor

You've just gotten the news—good or bad. Before you celebrate, or jump off the nearest roof, sit down with your doctor and ask a few questions.

1. Why was this test ordered?

2. What are the results of the test?

3. What do the results of this test mean?

4. What results are considered "normal" for someone of my age and sex?

5. Do the results of this test fit my overall health profile?

6. Are the results of this test definitive?

7. Who interpreted the results of this test?

8. What other factors were considered when interpreting the results of this test?

9. How accurate is this test?

? What are reference ranges?

Some test results are compared to a set of average values, known as **reference ranges.** Different lab techniques often result in wide differences in their results (see the example on this page). So each lab publishes its own set of ranges that they have established for their own procedures. It's possible in some cases for computers to adjust the results to take into account other factors, such as your age, sex, general health, race and weight. But you should know that these ranges are no more than guidelines. **What a lab calls normal for you may not be normal for the next person.** In general, laboratories use their reference ranges to represent the middle 95% of tested people. This means that the remaining 5% of healthy patients will have values that are categorized as abnormal.

Medical tests have two fundamental purposes: to rule disease in and to rule disease out.

Two test results from the same blood

These examples showing the results of two different labs' analysis of blood samples taken on the same day show why **you should question the results of your tests.**

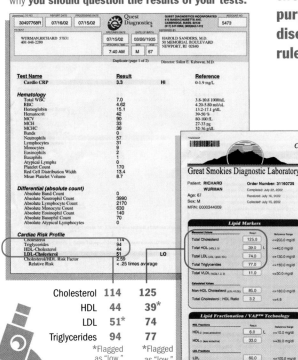

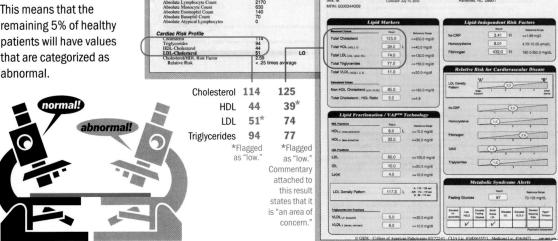

Cholesterol	114	125
HDL	44	39*
LDL	51*	74
Triglycerides	94	77

*Flagged as "low."   *Flagged as "low." Commentary attached to this result states that it is "an area of concern."

normal!   abnormal!

---

10 What is the chance of a false positive (or false negative) for this test?

11 Is there anything that could have caused inaccurate results (food, drugs, time of day)?

12 Why did you choose the lab that produced the results for this test?

13 Should this test be performed again to confirm these results?

14 Is there another test that can be done to confirm the results?

15 Should I get a second opinion?

16 Will you be recommending any additional tests?

Some say that in processing language, imaging results show that women use areas on both sides of the brain, while men are more likely to use only the left side.

Because of body size, male brains typically are **10%** larger than female brains.

Girls typically score slightly higher than boys on language and reading tests, while boys out-perform girls slightly in math. It is not known, however, the degree to which genes and socialization contribute to these differences.

Some gender differences may go back to the way our ancestors' brains developed where males were hunters (outdoors/visual/spatial) and women were gatherers (indoors/nurture).

FEMALES

pay attention longer in infancy.

have more acute sensory perception when they're infants.

tend to be somewhat more socially attuned.

tend to perform better verbally and be more emotionally aware.

MALES

tend to out-perform girls in visual-spatial integration.

tend to perform better on tasks like mental rotation of objects.

look at objects for shorter but more active periods as infants.

need more space to play, work.

The **brain** develops very early in embryonic life, earlier than limbs or internal organs.

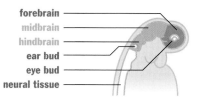

forebrain
midbrain
hindbrain
ear bud
eye bud
neural tissue

embryo at 4 weeks
In the tube of neural tissue at the back of the embryo, three areas (the primary vesicles) develop into the main parts of the brain.

actual size of a 4-week embryo

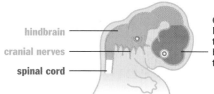

hindbrain
cranial nerves
spinal cord

embryo at 7 weeks
Nerves grow from the hindbrain, and bulges form on the forebrain.

actual size of a 7-week embryo

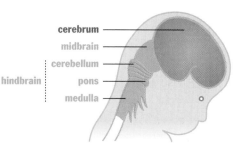

cerebrum
midbrain
cerebellum
hindbrain
pons
medulla

embryo at 11 weeks
One of the bulges on the forebrain becomes the cerebrum; this grows back over the midbrain towards the hindbrain, which has separated into three parts.

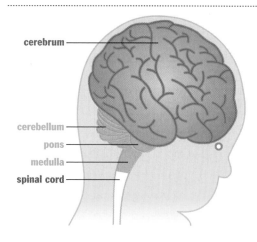

cerebrum
cerebellum
pons
medulla
spinal cord

birth
The cerebrum grows to be the largest part of the brain, and folds appear in the gray matter (the cerebral cortex) which covers it.

The pattern of folds is different in each human being.

By age three, the brain has reached 90% of its adult size, while the body is still only about 20% of full size.

ACTION ITEMS

Want to know more?

Right from Birth: Building Your Child's Foundation for Life

Craig and Sharon Ramey

Child development experts help parents understand the most important practices to enhance a baby's overall development and raise a confident, creative and happy child.

Brain Wonders

www.zerotothree.org

Learn about what happens in infant development at various stages from birth to 18 months. This website addresses areas of child development including brain growth, vision, hearing, touch, crying, breast feeding, emotional, cognitive/learning, coordination and social development.

Brain Connection

www.brainconnection.com

Brain Connection is a fascinating website that features high quality, easy-to-read information about brain development and how people learn. Special features include a research library, animations of brain function and an image gallery on topics including brain anatomy, vision and development.

Here's what's inside your child's **brain:**

the cerebrum
represents **70%** of the brain, and is divided into four lobes:

the occipital lobe
detects and interprets visual images and is active shortly after birth, but does not reach maturity until after preschool.

the parietal lobe
is active from the second or third month for space perception and some aspects of math.

the frontal lobe gradually becomes active at the end of the first year, at the same time as reasoning and speech develop. Skilled movements are controlled by neurons in this part of the brain, which is not fully mature until mid to late adolescence.

the temporal lobe deals with hearing, language and smell. This area also controls memory formation.

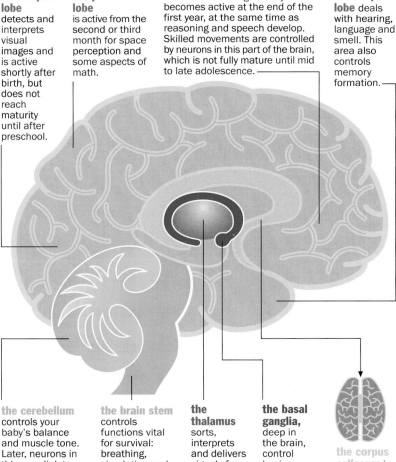

the cerebellum
controls your baby's balance and muscle tone. Later, neurons in this area link to other regions of the brain, coordinating smooth and precise movement, and speech.

the brain stem
controls functions vital for survival: breathing, circulation and heartbeat, and reflexes such as swallowing and vomiting. It is completely wired at birth.

the thalamus
sorts, interprets and delivers signals from the sensory systems to the appropriate parts of the cerebrum.

the basal ganglia,
deep in the brain, control basic voluntary movements such as walking.

the corpus callosum is a bundle of nerve fibers that connects the two hemispheres of the brain.

The human brain contains over 100 billion neurons (brain cells) at birth. Each neuron connects through electro-chemical structures (synapses) with thousands of others, creating the architecture that determines who we are.

Most pruning, or streamlining, after birth is the result of stimuli coming from the environment. So, the "wiring" of a baby's brain is a work in progress.

Sources: Understanding Children, understandingchildren.com, TOP and Civitas; Your Child from Birth to Three, Newsweek.

At birth, there are ten times as many neurons in the brain as there are stars in the Milky Way.

From Neurons to Neighborhoods
edited by Jack Shonkoff and Deborah Philips

This book stresses the importance of early child development and provides thought-provoking conclusions and recommendations on four main themes.

- Children are born wired for feelings and ready to learn.

- Early environment matters, and nurturing relationships are essential.

- Society is changing without addressing the needs of young children.

- Interactions among the early childhood disciplines of science, policy and practice are problematic and demand dramatic rethinking.

What's Going On in There? How the Brain and Mind Develop in the First Five Years of Life
Lise Eliot

Explains brain development and its implications for children's emerging motor, emotional, language and other cognitive skills.

Recent studies suggest that behavioral problems in children **2-3** years of age may occur if they sleep less than **11** hours at night. Children this age should sleep up to **13** hours at night.

Lack of sleep can cause behavioral problems such as acting out, behaving aggressively and hyperactively. **Conversely, children's behavioral problems have been said to contribute to a lack of sleep in children.**

Different children need various amounts of sleep. If a child does not look well rested, he probably needs more sleep.

Waking up at night, a problem that occurs in **33**% of children **2-4** years old, can also cause behavioral problems.

Researchers believe that regular amounts of sleep deprivation may have long-term effects on brain function.

Studies on rats show that sleep is necessary for survival, demonstrating that life expectancy decreases with sleep deprivation.

Sleep is a dynamic activity.

The five stages of sleep progress in a cycle from stage 1 to **REM** sleep, then the cycle starts over.

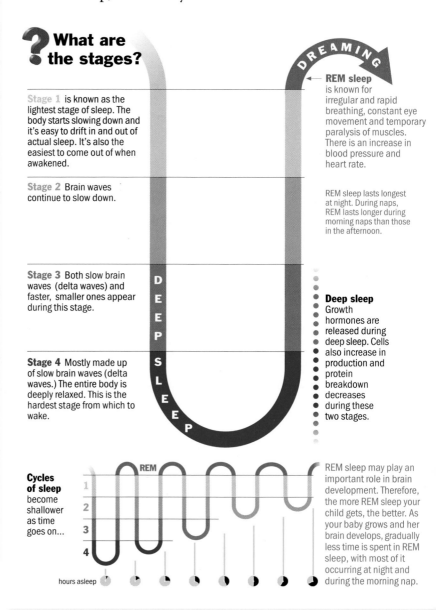

? What are the stages?

Stage 1 is known as the lightest stage of sleep. The body starts slowing down and it's easy to drift in and out of actual sleep. It's also the easiest to come out of when awakened.

Stage 2 Brain waves continue to slow down.

Stage 3 Both slow brain waves (delta waves) and faster, smaller ones appear during this stage.

Stage 4 Mostly made up of slow brain waves (delta waves.) The entire body is deeply relaxed. This is the hardest stage from which to wake.

DREAMING

REM sleep is known for irregular and rapid breathing, constant eye movement and temporary paralysis of muscles. There is an increase in blood pressure and heart rate.

REM sleep lasts longest at night. During naps, REM lasts longer during morning naps than those in the afternoon.

DEEP SLEEP

Deep sleep Growth hormones are released during deep sleep. Cells also increase in production and protein breakdown decreases during these two stages.

Cycles of sleep become shallower as time goes on...

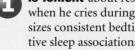

hours asleep

REM sleep may play an important role in brain development. Therefore, the more REM sleep your child gets, the better. As your baby grows and her brain develops, gradually less time is spent in REM sleep, with most of it occurring at night and during the morning nap.

ACTION ITEMS

Help your child get healthy sleep

What's the best way to help your child develop good sleep habits? There are many expert views about what role parents should play when it comes to helping their children develop good sleep habits. Ultimately, the choice is yours. If you like an approach that:

1 **is lenient** about responding to your baby when he cries during the night and emphasizes consistent bedtime routines and positive sleep associations, check out Dr. Jodi Mindell's book, *Sleeping Through the Night: How Infants, Toddlers and Their Parents Can Get a Good Night's Sleep.*

2 **advocates sticking firmly to routine** and letting your child cry at bedtime for extended intervals of time before you provide her with comfort, read Dr. Richard Ferber's book, *Solve Your Child's Sleep Problems.*

The brain is always active.

Since the 1950s, we've learned that our brains are very active during sleep. Neurotransmitters, or nerve-signaling chemicals in our brains, control whether we are asleep or awake. Neurons, which connect the brain to the spinal cord, produce other neurotransmitters which keep some parts of the brain active during sleep and while awake.

? What are dreams?

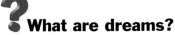

Infant **REM sleep** was first studied in 1953. However, scientists still do not fully understand the need for and purpose of dreams. **Sigmund Freud** believed that dreams are part of a human's unconscious desires.

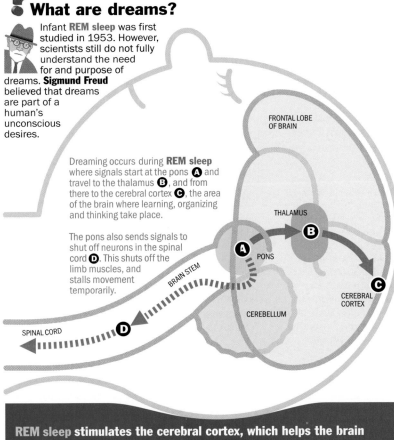

FRONTAL LOBE OF BRAIN

Dreaming occurs during **REM sleep** where signals start at the pons **A** and travel to the thalamus **B**, and from there to the cerebral cortex **C**, the area of the brain where learning, organizing and thinking take place.

The pons also sends signals to shut off neurons in the spinal cord **D**. This shuts off the limb muscles, and stalls movement temporarily.

THALAMUS

A PONS

B

C CEREBRAL CORTEX

BRAIN STEM

CEREBELLUM

D

SPINAL CORD

While sleeping, humans pass through 4 stages and REM (Rapid Eye Movement)—in repeating cycles throughout the night.

Sources: Understanding Children, understandingchildren.com, TOP and Civitas; NINDS, Brain Resources and Information Network; Healthy Sleep Habits, Happy Child, Marc Weissbluth, MD; Guide to Your Child's Sleep, American Academy of Pediatrics.

REM sleep stimulates the cerebral cortex, which helps the brain develop learning ability. Scientists believe that's why infants spend 50% of their time in **REM sleep**.

3 focuses on training your baby to go to sleep and comfort himself on his own by keeping nighttime feedings short, waking him if his daytime naps last more than a few hours and using your voice or a gentle pat to comfort him when he cries, try the American Academy of Pediatrics' book, *Guide to Your Child's Sleep*.

4 promotes the family bed and other ways of being there for your child to provide a comforting, relaxing sleep environment, look at Dr. William Sears' book, *Nighttime Parenting*.

5 emphasizes the prevention of sleep problems and teaches healthy sleep habits by synchronizing soothing techniques with your child's natural rhythms, read Dr. Marc Weissbluth's book, *Healthy Sleep Habits, Happy Child*.

AND REMEMBER, whichever approach you choose, be consistent.

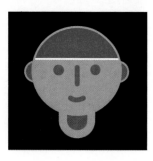

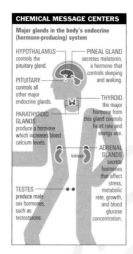

The brain is the major organ of the nervous system. It is composed of more than one hundred billion nerve cells, each of which is connected to thousands of others, which make it far more complex than any mere computer.

The average human brain weighs approximately three pounds. There is no correlation between normal variations in brain size and intelligence.

Hormone Testing

Blood and urine—collected in the usual manner—are tested for hormone levels.

Results

High or low levels of cortisol or other pituitary hormones may indicate malfunction of the pituitary or adrenal glands which often suggests a tumor in one of these glands. Abnormal levels of testosterone may indicate a problem with the pituitary gland which may be caused by tumors or a malfunctioning thyroid.

Spinal Tap/ Lumbar Puncture

An area in the lower back or back of the neck is anesthetized and sterilized. A needle is then inserted between two vertebrae to withdraw a sample of cerebrospinal fluid.

Results

The presence of certain types of cells in the fluid can indicate infection or leakage from the brain. Cerebrospinal fluid may be tested for the presence of Amyloid Beta Protein which can indicate Alzheimer's and other dementias, red blood cells which may indicate bleeding from an aneurysm or certain proteins that may indicate multiple sclerosis.

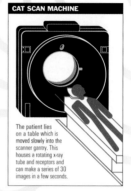

CAT SCAN MACHINE

The patient lies on a table which is moved slowly into the scanner gantry. This houses a rotating x-ray tube and receptors and can make a series of 30 images in a few seconds.

Computerized Axial Tomography (CAT or CT Scan)

The patient lies on a table which moves into a scanner while pictures are taken. Sometimes an iodine contrast dye is injected intravenously to help obtain clearer pictures.

Results

This type of scan provides sharp, two- and three-dimensional images of the brain and can be used to localize tumors, clots or other brain abnormalities which may show brain tumors, evidence of a stroke or treatable causes of dementia.

Carotid Ultrasound

A hand-held probe is passed over the neck and sound waves are converted to a picture.

Results

The technician or doctor can see and report immediately any abnormalities. Clots and arterial plaques, which can increase the risk of stroke, can be detected.

Electroencephalography (EEG, Brain Wave Test)

The patient lies down. Up to 30 electrodes are adhered to the scalp with conductive gel. A machine attached to the electrodes graphs brain activity over time. The patient may be asked to lie still, be shown bright lights, be sedated or asked to breathe heavily. This painless test lasts up to an hour.

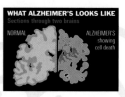

WHAT ALZHEIMER'S LOOKS LIKE
Sections through two brains
NORMAL   ALZHEIMER'S showing cell death

ACTION ITEMS

What to do if...

1 You are claustrophobic.
(MRI, CT) Ask your doctor if the facility doing the testing has an "open" MRI—a larger unit that is open on some sides. Otherwise, you may ask to be sedated during the procedure.

2 You are obese.
(MRI) Extremely overweight people may not fit in a standard MRI unit. Ask your facility if they have an "open" unit that will accommodate your size.

3 You have metallic implants.
(MRI) Because of the strong magnetic field created by an MRI scanner, you may not be able to have an MRI if you have an implanted metallic device like a pacemaker. Be sure to tell your doctor and the radiologist.

4 You are pregnant.
(MRI and Octreotide Scans) Be sure to tell your doctor if there is any chance you may be pregnant. Because these tests may be harmful to a fetus, pregnant women should not have MRI or Octreotide scans. CAT scans are rarely performed on pregnant women.

Results

Abnormal readings can indicate brain tumors, stroke, blood clots, epilepsy and seizures. The test is also used to establish whether a person is brain-dead. A variation of this test, called an Evoked Potential Study, provides external stimulus to the brain during the EEG to measure response.

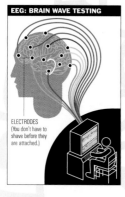

EEG: BRAIN WAVE TESTING

ELECTRODES
(You don't have to shave before they are attached.)

Electromyography

The patient lies on a table, and electrodes are adhered with gel to the nerve pathway or muscles to be tested. A meter measures electrical current as the patient tenses and relaxes certain muscles. This test can be uncomfortable.

Results

This test examines the function of nerves in the body by investigating the electrical pathways between the brain and the muscles it controls.

The results can indicate nerve and brain disease such as multiple sclerosis, myopathy, diabetes, polio and Lou Gehrig's Disease.

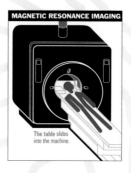

MAGNETIC RESONANCE IMAGING

The table slides into the machine.

Magnetic Resonance Imaging (MRI)

The patient lies on a table, which slides into the machine. The patient lies still as the imager thumps and moves around for 30 to 90 minutes. In some cases, just before the test begins, a safe contrast dye may be injected in a vein to provide greater clarity.

Results

The images produced can help diagnose tumors, aneurysms, multiple sclerosis, infection. blood clots and hemorrhages.

Octreotide Scan

A radioactive substance is injected into a vein. This substance is absorbed in greater concentrations by different types of tissue. A gamma camera is used to take pictures of the entire body and show the different tissues in clear contrast.

Results

This nuclear test is used to find and monitor brain tumors.

Positron Emission Tomography Scan (PET)

This test begins with the inhalation or injection of a radioactive element. The patient lies on a table which slides into a large scanning device. Recent use of caffeine, alcohol, tobacco or other drugs may affect test results.

Results

This imaging test combines techniques from the nuclear scan and biochemical assessment, and is used to search for tumors or evidence of heart attack and strokes.

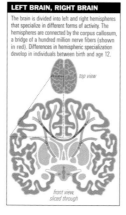

LEFT BRAIN, RIGHT BRAIN

The brain is divided into left and right hemispheres that specialize in different forms of activity. The hemispheres are connected by the corpus callosum, a bridge of a hundred million nerve fibers (shown in red). Differences in hemispheric specialization develop in individuals between birth and age 12.

top view

front view, sliced through

Today's technology provides procedures for both structural and functional analysis of the brain.

Structural analysis helps find problems with the anatomy of the brain—like tumors, hemorrhages, blood clots and lesions. Functional analysis measures and locates brain activity which helps diagnose problems like epileptic seizures.

Sources: Diagnostic Tests for Men, Diagnostic Tests for Women.

TIP

Treatment within three hours of a stroke can make the difference between permanent disability or death and the return to normal function.

5 You are allergic to iodine or shellfish.
(CAT) Be sure to tell your doctor and the technician of any allergies before testing. Iodine-based contrast dye can cause a severe allergic reaction in those allergic to iodine or shellfish. If a problem is suspected, you may be given an antihistamine-steroid mixture to reduce your risk of a reaction.

6 You cannot assume a curled position.
(Spinal Tap) If you are unable to lie in the required position, an alternate procedure, called a cisternal puncture, may be performed. In this case, the cerebrospinal fluid would be drawn from between vertebrate in the neck.

7 You have increased intracranial pressure.
(Spinal Tap) A higher-than-normal intracranial pressure may exclude you from having this test. If you are aware you have this condition, be sure to tell your doctor.

8 You have widespread skin infection.
(Electromyography) Because the needle electrodes used for this test can pass infection from the skin to the muscles, you may not be able to have this procedure.

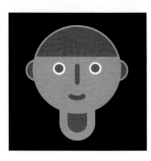

The poet who said that "the eyes are the windows of the soul" was only half right. They are the windows to the workings of the body, too.

Almost half of Americans over age 65 will develop at least one of three chronic eye diseases: glaucoma, macular degeneration and diabetic retinopathy.

Muscle Integrity Evaluation

The patient is asked to perform simple motions with the eye—back and forth, up and down.

Results

If the patient has a problem moving the eye, or a discrepancy between one eye and the other, it could indicate muscle or nerve damage or deterioration.

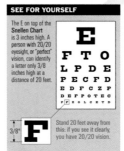

SEE FOR YOURSELF

The E on top of the Snellen Chart is 3 inches high. A person with 20/20 eyesight, or "perfect" vision, can identify a letter only 3/8 inches high at a distance of 20 feet.

E
F T O
L P D E
P E C F D
E D F C Z P
D E F P O T E C

3/8" **F** Stand 20 feet away from this: if you see it clearly, you have 20/20 vision.

Visual Acuity

The patient is asked to read a Snellen Eye Chart set 20 feet away until the letters are no longer clear. The test is done one eye at a time, and first done without glasses, then with them, if the patient wears them. To test near vision, a Jaeger card, placed at a closer distance, is used in a similar manner.

Results

Visual acuity is expressed as a fraction, the top portion of which is always 20, indicating the 20-foot distance from the patient to the Snellen chart. The bottom portion of the fraction compares the patient's eyesight against the norm. Someone with 20/60 vision sees at 20 feet what those with perfect vision can see at 60 feet.

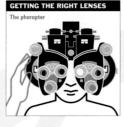

GETTING THE RIGHT LENSES

The phoropter

Phorometry

The patient looks at a Snellen Chart, and later a Jaeger card, through a goggle-like instrument called a phoropter. Different lenses are placed between the eye and the chart and the patient is asked which lens makes the letters appear clearer.

Results

This test helps the doctor determine the strength of glasses or contact lenses to prescribe.

Visual Field Test (Perimetry)

The patient rests his head in a chin rest, facing a bowl-shaped instrument. A series of lights go on and off and the patient is asked to respond to what is seen.

Results

The absence or reduction of sensitivity in one or more areas of the visual field may indicate one or more disorders, including glaucoma.

Intraocular Pressure Determination (Tonometry)

Following anesthetic drops, the eyeball is touched gently with a pen-like tube. A variation on this procedure is "air puff" tonometry, which requires no direct contact.

Results

This test measures the internal pressure of the eye, and should be performed with each eye examination. Since high pressure can indicate glaucoma, this test can be extremely important as a preventive measure.

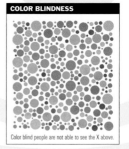

COLOR BLINDNESS

Color blind people are not able to see the X above.

Color Defectiveness Determination

The test involves looking at a series of color patterns within which are numbers and letters which are obvious to normal eyes, but not to those that are color defective.

ACTION ITEMS
Be good to your eyes

1 **Use UV protection.**
Wearing sunglasses when you're outdoors is one of the biggest favors you can do for your eyes. Make sure that the ones you choose have proper UV protection. Ask your eyecare professional if you have any questions.

2 **Limit alcohol and caffeine.**
Both alcohol and caffeine act as diuretics in your body. And, this dryness is likely to affect your eyes as well. Try to avoid, or at least limit, your intake of alcoholic and caffeinated beverages.

3 **Stay away from smoke.**
If you're a smoker and are looking for one more reason to quit, here it is: Smoking is not good for your eyes. Non-smokers should also avoid secondhand smoke and other smoky environments, which can be drying to the eyes.

4 **Shield your eyes from the wind.**
If you spend a lot of time outdoors, consider investing in goggles or glasses with side shields to protect your eyes from the wind. Try a store that specializes in outdoor recreation or ask your eyecare professional.

Results

This test measures the ability to discern differences among various colors. Several types of color defectiveness exist that make two different colors appear the same.

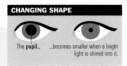

The pupil... ...becomes smaller when a bright light is shined into it.

Pupillary Reflex Response

A bright light is shined into the patient's eye.

Results

This test measures how fast the pupil closes. Any abnormality can be an indication of nerve damage or damage to the cornea or iris.

Dry Eye Test (Schirmer Tear Test)

A sterile strip of filter paper is gently inserted under the patient's lower eyelids. After five minutes, the strips are removed and the length of the moistened area is measured in millimeters.

Results

This test assesses the functioning of the lacrimal glands in the eye.

Slit Lamp Exam (Biomicroscopy)

The patient rests his chin on a stand and looks straight ahead while the doctor moves a special lamp around and looks into the eye.

Results

The doctor can examine the surface, cornea and lens for infection, inflammation or damage.

A-Scan (Ocular Biometry)

A clear plastic cup connected to a transducer is moved over the surface of the eyeball.

Results

Using computer technology, the shape, thickness and power of the eye's natural lens is determined, so that a plastic replica can be made for cataract surgery.

Retinal Examination (Direct Ophthalmoscopy or Fundoscopy)

Using a small beam light and magnifying lens (an ophthalmoscope), the doctor examines the inside and rear of the eye.

Results

The doctor can get an idea of the patient's general health, find evidence of high blood pressure or diabetes, check the retina for damage and identify "floaters," retinal detachment, macular degeneration and other problems.

Corneal Topography and Corneal Pachymetry

During a pre-surgery exam, sophisticated equipment is used to take measurements of the cornea's thickness and map the curvature of the eye's surface.

Results

These tests are used to determine the patient's eligibility for laser vision correction and to diagnose corneal disease. If topography reveals an irregular-shaped cornea or pachymetry finds a too-thin cornea, you may be rejected for laser surgery.

Most tests for the eyes are simple, painless and noninvasive.

A few of the tests for macular degeneration or optic nerve damage may require hospital-based x-ray or scanning technology, but most eye diagnostics are conducted by eyecare professionals during regular office visits

Sources: Diagnostic Tests for Men, Diagnostic Tests for Women.

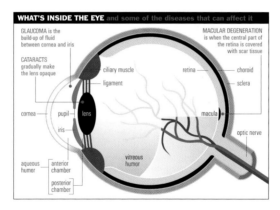

WHAT'S INSIDE THE EYE and some of the diseases that can affect it

GLAUCOMA is the build-up of fluid between cornea and iris

CATARACTS gradually make the lens opaque

MACULAR DEGENERATION is when the central part of the retina is covered with scar tissue

ciliary muscle — retina — choroid
ligament — sclera
cornea — pupil — lens
iris — macula
optic nerve
vitreous humor
aqueous humor — anterior chamber
posterior chamber

5 **Take breaks from the computer.**
Extended periods of computer work can be especially drying to the eyes because you tend to blink less. Try to take a short break at least once an hour. Rest your eyes, or try focusing on something far away.

6 **Give your eyes a rest from contacts.**
Follow your eyecare professional's advice when it comes to daily- or extended-wear contacts. Wearing eyeglasses periodically and using rewetting drops regularly can go a long way to protect your eyes from the strain of dryness.

7 **Use a humidifier.**
Keep some moisture in the air during the winter months by using a humidifier. Dry air caused by indoor heat can be terribly drying to your eyes.

8 **Pay attention to your medications.**
If you've been having dry eyes, your medications could be to blame. Over-the-counter antihistamines are particularly drying. Ask your doctor or pharmacist about your prescription medications, too. They may be able to recommend an alternate medication that won't bother your eyes.

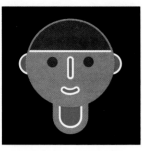

The ear, nose and throat (ENT) specialty is called Otorhinolarynology—"oto" for ear, "rhino" for nose and "laryn" for the voice box area of the throat.

The human sense of smell usually functions in tandem with the sense of taste. Because the nose is 10,000 times more sensitive, you lose nearly 90% of taste sensations when your nose is blocked.

EARS

Audiometry

The patient is asked to listen to various sounds and indicate when and in which ear a tone is heard.

Results

Abnormal results may point to damage from trauma or deterioration.

Auditory Brainstem Response

Electrodes placed on the patient's head measure electrical impulses while the patient is exposed to a series of tones and clicks played through headphones.

Results

This test measures the brain's response to sound and can measure hearing loss or indicate tumors.

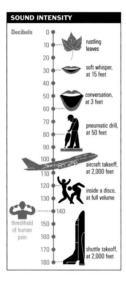

HEARING THINGS

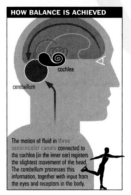

tympanic membrane (eardrum) — auditory nerve — malleus (hammer) — incus (anvil) — stapes (stirrup) — cochlea — sound waves — ear flap

Sound waves cause the eardrum to vibrate. Three tiny bones amplify the vibrations, which pass to fluid in the cochlea. Movement in the fluid sets off nerve impulses and these travel to the brain via the auditory nerve

Electronystagmogram (Caloric Study, ENG)

The patient is asked to follow a series of light flashes along a wall. After that, water, first cold, then warm, is poured into the ears to stimulate

HOW BALANCE IS ACHIEVED

cochlea — cerebellum

The motion of fluid in three semicircular canals connected to the cochlea (in the inner ear) registers the slightest movement of the head. The cerebellum processes this information, together with input from the eyes and receptors in the body.

involuntary eye movement. (This part of the test may cause nausea and vomiting.) Electrical charges caused by eye movement are picked up by electrodes placed near the eyes and recorded for analysis.

Results

Any abnormalities in movement of the eyes or the electrical impulses can be traced to hearing

loss, vertigo or nerve damage, possibly due to brain damage, inflammation or cancer.

Tympanogram

The patient wears headphones equipped with a rubber plug, which fits into the ear and up against the eardrum. Pressure is exerted on the plug to test the elasticity of the membrane.

Results

Abnormal results may indicate infection, trapped fluid or a perforation.

HOW WE SMELL

We can detect more than 10,000 different smells; all of them are derived from seven primary odors.

olfactory bulb

Odor molecules stimulate tiny hairs attached to the olfactory bulb, above the roof of the nasal cavity. From there the signal goes to the brain.

NOSE

Aspiration and Excisional Biopsies

After a local anesthetic is administered, tissue or

SOUND INTENSITY

Decibels	
0	
10	rustling leaves
20	
30	soft whisper, at 15 feet
40	
50	conversation, at 3 feet
60	
70	pneumatic drill, at 50 feet
80	
90	
100	
110	aircraft takeoff, at 2,000 feet
120	
130	inside a disco, at full volume
140	
150	threshhold of human pain
160	
170	shuttle takeoff, at 2,000 feet
180	

ACTION ITEMS

What to do if...

1 You have ringing in the ear.
(Audiography) Discuss your tinnitus (ringing in the ear) with your doctor. This condition may interfere with your hearing test.

2 You are regularly exposed to load noises.
(Audiography) You should schedule your test for a time when you can avoid loud noises for at least 16 hours.

3 You have a pacemaker.
(Electronystagmogram) Be sure to tell your doctor or the technician if you wear a pacemaker and an ENG has been ordered. The equipment may interfere with the pacemaker's function.

4 You have a perforated eardrum.
(Electronystagmogram) Because of the risk of infection, an ENG should not be performed on a patient with a perforated eardrum.

fluid is removed from the sinus area with a needle or scalpel and sent for analysis.

Results

Tests performed on sinus tissue can reveal infection, tumors and other problems.

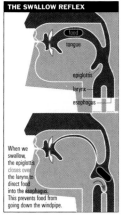

THE SWALLOW REFLEX

food
tongue
epiglottis
larynx
esophagus

When we swallow, the epiglottis closes over the larynx to direct food into the esophagus. This prevents food from going down the windpipe.

THROAT

Laryngoscopy

Before the test begins, the mouth and throat are anesthetized with a spray. A laryngoscope—a flexible, tubular instrument with a light source and biopsy equipment— is inserted into the throat either through the nose or mouth. This is slightly uncomfortable and often produces the urge to gag.

Results

The visualization equipment of the scope can show doctors or technicians infections or tumors of the throat and allow a general internal inspection. Other instruments on the scope allow for fluid or tissue collection from the throat area. These samples can be analyzed in a lab for infection and cancerous cells.

Throat Culture

A cotton swab is inserted deep into the throat to collect potentially infected mucus and saliva which is then rubbed onto a culture plate.

Results

The presense of bacteria indicates infection.

Excisional Throat Biopsy

While the patient is under general anesthesia, a small tissue sample is removed from the throat with surgical tools.

Results

The biopsy of the throat can analyze infected tissue, or, more likely, tumors or other growths.

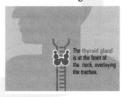

The thyroid gland is at the front of the neck, overlaying the trachea.

Thyroid Stimulating Hormone (TSH) Blood Test

Blood is drawn from a vein in the arm and sent to a laboratory to be analyzed.

Results

The presence and quantity of TSH and another hormone, thyroxine, can indicate the beginnings of hypo and hyperthyroidism at levels undetectable in other types of exams.

Radioactive Iodine Uptake (RAI)

Iodine is administered either orally or intravenously. Radioactive pictures of the thyroid area are taken over a period of several hours.

Results

Since iodine is a chemical absorbed almost exclusively by the thyroid, the pictures measure absorption over time. Too much or too little indicates that the thyroid is under- or overactive.

Thyroid Radioisotope Scan

After ingesting a radioactive substance, the patient lies down on an x-ray table, neck stretched out by a brace. The scanner passes over the patient multiple times and takes pictures of the thyroid area.

Results

The test is used to evaluate nodules (lumps) in the thyroid and may indicate the likelihood of the nodule being benign or malignant.

The ears, nose and throat offer opportunities for doctors to obtain indications of general health in addition to information about a specific organ.

As with other senses, many disorders of the ears and nose are age-related and should be tested more frequently as we get older.

Sources: Diagnostic Tests for Men, Diagnostic Tests for Women.

TIP

Only 10% of those who could be helped by hearing aids actually wear them even though very small models are now available.

5 **You are allergic to iodine or shellfish.**
(Radioactive Iodine Uptake) Before testing, be sure to tell your doctor and the technitian if you are allergic to iodine or shellfish. Iodine can cause a severe allergic reaction.

6 **You take hormone supplements.**
(Thyroid Tests) Hormone supplements and other medications can effect the results of many thyroid tests. Be sure your doctor is aware of all the medications (herbs, too) that you take.

7 **You've recently had a nuclear scan**
(Thyroid Tests) If you have been injected with a radioactive substance for another test, be sure to tell your doctor or technician.

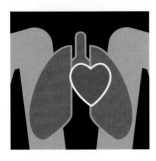

The heart is the muscular pump that beats continuously from before you are born to your last day of life. During an average lifetime, the heart contracts more than 2.5 billion times.

A new blood test that measures the levels of the enzyme myeloperoxidase may soon help doctors predict future heart attacks and more quickly treat emergency room patients.

Electrocardiogram (EKG or ECG)

The patient disrobes from the waist up and lies down. Electrodes are attached to the chest, wrists and ankles with gel. The test lasts about 15 minutes as the electrodes take amplified readings of the heart's electrical activity.

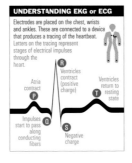

UNDERSTANDING EKG or ECG

Electrodes are placed on the chest, wrists and ankles. These are connected to a device that produces a tracing of the heartbeat. Letters on the tracing represent stages of electrical impulses through the heart.

Atria contract — P
Ventricles contract (positive charge) — R
Ventricles return to resting state — T
Impulses start to pass along conducting fibers — Q
Negative charge — S

Results

The result, a 12-line graph, can reveal the presence of abnormal rhythms, heart inflammation and heart disease. Although it gives no indication as to whether a heart attack is imminent, it is useful to compare electrocardiograms done at different times on the same patient, because it can identify warning signs. Several variations of this test exist. One, a Holter Monitor, measures the heart for an entire day, watching for changes which occur during varied activities.

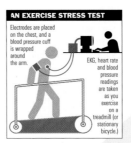

AN EXERCISE STRESS TEST

Electrodes are placed on the chest, and a blood pressure cuff is wrapped around the arm.

EKG, heart rate and blood pressure readings are taken as you exercise on a treadmill (or stationary bicycle.)

Another is called an exercise stress test. During this test, the patient exercises on a treadmill instead of lying down to show the response of the heart to physical exercise.

Chest X-Ray

The patient undresses from the waist up. The x-ray camera is aimed at the chest. Frontal and side views are usually taken.

Results

Abnormal heart size or shape and lung congestion may be visible indicating heart failure.

Echocardiogram

The patient undresses from the waist up and lies down on a table. Gel is spread on the chest to help transmit sound waves. The transducer, a pen-like instrument used in all ultrasounds, is passed over the chest to take readings.

Results

From the images converted from the bounced sound waves, the doctor can determine the internal size of the heart chamber, the thickness of the chamber walls, whether there is excess fluid building up around the heart, contractile power of the heart muscle, and whether the four valves of the heart are narrowed, inflamed or leaking.

Coronary Angiography with Cardiac Catheterization

The patient, who has fasted and taken a sedative, is monitored by an EKG during the test. After a local anesthetic is injected, a thin catheter is inserted into a vein or artery of the body, usually in the upper leg or groin. The catheter is guided through the body into the heart and dye is injected. As the dye spreads x-rays are taken.

Results

The doctor can clearly see clogged arteries or malfunctioning heart tissue. Findings may help the doctor make decisions about bypass surgery, angioplasty, revascularization procedures or drug therapy.

Nuclear Heart Scans: Thallium, Stress-Thallium, Technetium

One of several nuclear isotopes is injected into the body. Shortly after, a gamma camera is used to photograph the heart.

ACTION ITEMS

What to do if...

 You have arrhythmias.
(EKG) If you have certain arrhythmias, a standard EKG may not produce useful data. Instead, a signal-averaged EKG—that averages results over a 15-20 minute period—may be used.

2 **You take heart medication.**
(EKG) Remind your doctor which heart medications you're taking. They may affect your results from an EKG.

 You are pregnant.
(Chest X-Ray) Be sure to tell your doctor if there is any chance you may be pregnant. X-rays are generally not recommended for women who may be pregnant. If you must have this procedure, a lead apron should be draped over the belly during exposure. (Angiogram, CT, Nuclear Heart Scan)Be sure to tell your doctor if there is any chance you may be pregnant. Because these tests may be harmful to a fetus, pregnant women should not have nuclear heart scans.

Results

The test can help detect heart tissue damage from a heart attack. The doctor can also see if some areas of the heart are not getting sufficient oxygen or are not pumping properly.

Electron Beam Computed Tomography (EBCT) or Ultrafast CT

The patient lies on a large tray which slides into an ultrafast electron beam scanner. The patient lies still during the 20-30 minute test.

Results

This test measures the amount of calcium in coronary arteries, which some experts believe may predict heart disease.

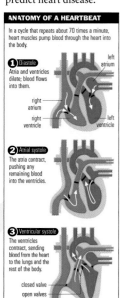

ANATOMY OF A HEARTBEAT

In a cycle that repeats about 70 times a minute, heart muscles pump blood through the heart into the body.

1 Diastole
Atria and ventricles dilate; blood flows into them.

left atrium
right atrium
right ventricle
left ventricle

2 Atrial systole
The atria contract, pushing any remaining blood into the ventricles.

3 Ventricular systole
The ventricles contract, sending blood from the heart to the lungs and the rest of the body.

closed valve
open valves

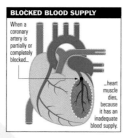

BLOCKED BLOOD SUPPLY

When a coronary artery is partially or completely blocked...

...heart muscle dies, because it has an inadequate blood supply.

Blood Tests for Lipids/Cholesterol, Triglycerides, HDL, LDL

Blood is drawn after the patient has been fasting, and is sent to a lab for analysis.

Results

These blood tests measure lipids (fat) in the blood and can help evaluate risk of heart disease, clogged arteries, diabetes and pancreatitis (in the case of triglycerides). Cholesterol is a fatty compound which is produced in the body and is necessary in small quantities, but can build up and clog arteries. Triglycerides are the most dominant lipid in the body, and have some correlation to heart disease. HDL (High Density Lipoprotein)decreases the risk of heart disease. LDL (Low Density Lipoprotein) is the opposite, increasing the risk.

Apolipoproteins Blood Test

Blood is taken from a vein and sent to a lab for analysis.

Results

High levels of lipoprotein can indicative a risk of coronary artery disease and other illnesses.

Blood Test for Heart Enzyme, CPK, CK, SGOT, LDH

Blood is drawn from a vein and sent to a lab for analysis.

Results

Elevated levels of these enzymes can indicate damage from a heart attack.

Blood Test for Vitamin B1

After the patient has fasted, blood is drawn from a vein and sent to a lab for analysis.

Results

A low level of B1, usually due to poor diet, can lead to muscle weakness and heart failure.

Hematocrit Blood Test

Blood is drawn from a vein or collected from a finger prick and separated in a centrifuge. The percentage of red blood cells is measured.

Results

A low reading can indicate anemia, while an abnormally high reading can mean poor oxygenation of the blood, which can occur from certain congenital heart diseases or emphysema.

Heart tests may be ordered by your primary care physician, or you may be referred to a cardiologist— a physician who specializes in diseases of the heart.

More is known about gender differences involving the heart than any other organ, yet such differentiation is not always recognized in medical diagnostic testing.

Sources: Diagnostic Tests for Men, Diagnostic Tests for Women.

TIP

Men who smoke ten cigarettes or more per day have an 80% higher risk of dying from heart disease.

 You are obese.
(Chest X-Ray) Images from x-rays performed on extremely overweight people may be difficult to read.
(Echocardiogram) If you are obese and need an echocardiogram, an esophageal echocardiogram may be performed instead. In this variation, the readings are taken through a tube fed down the esophagus.

 You are allergic to iodine or shellfish.
(Angiogram) Be sure to tell your doctor and the technician of any allergies before testing. Iodine-based contrast dye can cause a severe allergic reaction in those allergic to iodine or shellfish.

 You are claustrophobic.
(MRI, CT) Ask your doctor if the facility doing the testing has an "open" MRI—a larger unit that is open on some sides. Otherwise, you may ask to be sedated during the procedure.

Source: American Cancer Society.

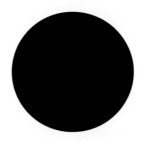

average size of breast tumor
at diagnosis in early 1980's
when only 13% of women were
getting regular mammograms

*average size of breast tumor
at diagnosis in late 1990's
when 60% of women were
getting regular mammograms*

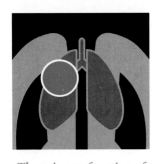

The primary function of the female breast is to provide milk for nursing infants. each contains 15 to 20 lobes of milk-secreting glands that are embedded in fatty tissue. During pregnancy, estrogen and progesterone stimulate these glands and cause the nipple to enlarge for feeding.

Breast cancer may occur in men as well as women, but is much more common in women.

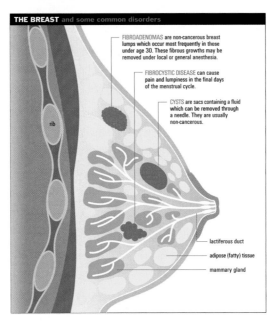

THE BREAST and some common disorders

FIBROADENOMAS are non-cancerous breast lumps which occur most frequently in those under age 30. These fibrous growths may be removed under local or general anesthesia.

FIBROCYSTIC DISEASE can cause pain and lumpiness in the final days of the menstrual cycle.

CYSTS are sacs containing a fluid which can be removed through a needle. They are usually non-cancerous.

rib

lactiferous duct
adipose (fatty) tissue
mammary gland

Mammogram

This important test is an x-ray of breast tissue. Mammography can detect a lump up to two years before it can be felt by manual examination. The test may be done lying down, sitting or standing. The breasts are x-rayed, one at a time. The woman places one breast between two plates which compact the breast and spread it out. The x-ray machine, attached to the plate, then takes a picture. The procedure is repeated with the other breast. This procedure is, at best, uncomfortable and embarrassing. At worst, it can be painful. Communicate to your doctor or technician your level of discomfort and request reasonable adjustments.

Results

The pictures of the breast show fat and duct tissue in the breast. Tumors as well as duct tissue will stand out from the breast tissue. If a tumor is suspected from a mammogram, a biopsy will likely be performed.

Thermography

This is an alternative technique for diagnosing breast cancer, not requiring x-ray radiation. It measures heat in the breast using an infrared camera. However, it is not as precise as a mammogram. Like in a mammogram, the woman places each breast in turn between two plates, spreading each out. The infrared camera then photographs the breast. This camera is sensitive to heat.

Results

Areas which are hotter than others receive more than normal blood flow. Therefore, if an area shows up "hot" on the infrared camera, it can be suspected to be tumorous, and a biopsy can be ordered.

Tumor Marker Blood Tests, Cancer Antigen (CA) Blood Tests

A number of blood tests have been discovered which can detect cancers in specific parts of the body, as in the breast, and can also be used to monitor the spread of cancers and the effectiveness of treatment. Blood is drawn from a vein and sent to a lab for analysis.

Results

Though these tests can be used to detect and monitor cancer, particularly breast and ovarian cancer, they also pick up on benign tumors and, sometimes, cirrhosis of the liver. Though they may be improved as genetic technology advances, currently only the first wave of tests are available.

ACTION ITEMS

What to do if...

1 **You are under the age of 50.**
(Mammogram) Consult with your doctor. There is some controversy about the usefulness of mammograms in younger women. Because younger women have more dense glandular tissue, which makes spotting tumors more difficult, there is a higher likelihood of a false-positive test result. This can lead to unnecessary biopsies. Ultrasound testing is often a preferred method of breast testing in younger women who have found a lump.

2 **You are pregnant.**
(Mammogram) Be sure to tell your doctor if there is any chance you may be pregnant. Because this test may cause harm to a fetus, pregnant women should not have mammograms.

3 **You have a family history of breast cancer.**
Talk to your doctor if you are concerned about your risk for breast cancer because of family history or other factors. You may want to begin regular mammograms at an earlier age than is usually recommended.

TEST YOURSELF (once a month, 2 or 3 days after the end of your period)

❶

IN THE SHOWER, raise your left arm. With the fingers of the right hand, carefully examine the left breast. In a circular pattern, starting from the outer top, press firmly enough to feel the tissue inside the breast. Complete one full circle, then move toward the center and circle again. Continue until you reach the nipple.

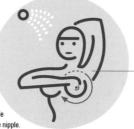

Check the area above the breast, including the armpit, for lumps.

Repeat the examination on your right breast.

❷

IN FRONT OF A MIRROR, place your hands at your sides and check your breasts for any changes in color, shape, or size. Also look for any dimpling or scaling of the skin.

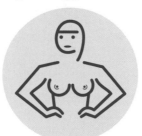

❸
STILL IN FRONT OF THE MIRROR, place your hands on your hips. Press your shoulders and elbows forward to flex the chest muscles.

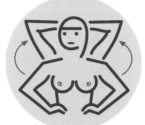

Then raise your hands and clasp them behind your head. Check for everything in step 2.

❹

LIE DOWN, and place a pillow under your left shoulder. Raise your left arm above your head. Using the circular method from step 1, examine your left breast.

Repeat the process for your right breast.

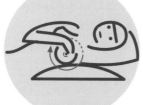

FINALLY, gently squeeze each nipple to check for discharge. Report any changes to your doctor.

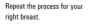 **A Clinical Breast Examination (CBE)** is essentially the same procedure as the self-exam, except it is performed more thoroughly by a doctor, who has more expertise, and who may use the CBE as an opportunity to educate patients in techniques for their self-exams.

How are the breasts evaluated?

Early detection is the key to isolating and stopping breast cancer.

Although most breast cancers are self-detected, a mammogram is one of the best ways for women to protect themselves against breast cancer.

Sources: Diagnostic Tests for Men, Diagnostic Tests for Women.

TIP

Although a painful, soft lump is less likely to be cancerous, all lumps should be brought to the attention of your doctor.

---

❹ **You want more information.**
Contact one of these organizations for more information on preventing, diagnosing and treating breast cancer.

Y-Me National Organization for Breast Cancer Information and Support
800.221.2141

National Alliance of Breast Cancer Organizations
212.719.0154

Breast Implant Information Line
Food and Drug Administration
800.532.4440

The Mayo Clinic Breast Cancer Decision-making Guidelines
www.mayohealth.org/mayo/9907/htm/breastcan.htm

The Breast Cancer Information Clearinghouse
www.nysernet.org/breast/Default.html

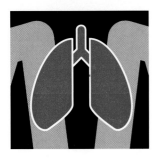

The lungs are the main organ of the respiratory system. They supply the body with oxygen and eliminate carbon dioxide.

Lung disease is the number three cause of death in the United States, responsible for one in every seven deaths.

Arterial blood gases

Blood is taken from an artery—usually found deeper in the arm than veins.—and then sent to a lab for analysis.

Results

This test measures levels of oxygen, carbon dioxide and acid in the blood in order to determine lung function. Abnormal levels of the various gases may indicate the lungs are failing to bring oxygen in and expel CO2 properly, suggesting lung disease. Lung disease and heart disease often go hand-in-hand.

Carboxyhemoglobin

Blood is drawn from a vein and sent to a lab for analysis.

Results

If more than 5% of hemoglobin is found to have carbon monoxide, it is likely that some external factor is contributing the gas to the body. Acute carbon monoxide exposure is often deadly. And, long-term exposure at low levels, which can occur at factories or in some homes, can cause serious medical problems.

Pulmonary Function Test (PFT or Spirometry)

This test simply involves breathing down a tube into a machine which measures lung capacity and strength. The patient is given a mouthpiece attached to a machine and is instructed to breathe into it normally, inhale or exhale deeply, or perform similar tasks.

Results

The results of this test are measured on an instrument called a spirogram. Examples of these measures include how much air is taken in with one breath, how fast it can be expelled and how much is left after letting the breath out. Results can be used to diagnose diseases such as asthma and emphysema, or to see how these diseases are affecting breathing ability.

Bronchogram

This test requires a considerable amount of patient preparation, including fasting and taking both a sedative and a medication to decrease mucus production. The mouth is also anesthetized or "numbed" with a spray or swab, and anesthetic drops are placed deeper into the throat. A plastic tube called a catheter is inserted through the mouth into the lungs. Contrast material (which shows up on an x-ray) is injected into the lungs through the catheter, where the progress of breathing dis-

tributes it throughout the lungs. X-rays are then taken of the lungs.

Results

The contrast material outlines the airway tubes, and shows up on an x-ray. The appearance of the x-rays can help make a diagnosis. Although this x-ray is not needed frequently, it is designed to get a clearer picture of the lungs than a normal chest x-ray can provide.

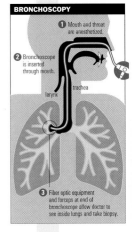

Bronchoscopy

As with the bronchogram, the mouth and throat are anesthetized. The patient takes a sedative and is given other medication to decrease secretions. The bronchoscope, a flexible tube, is inserted through the mouth, down the windpipe and into the bronchial tubes. At the end is fiber optic visual-

ACTION ITEMS
What to do if...

1 **You have a bleeding disorder.**
(Arterial Blood Gas) Because blood is drawn from an artery, people with severe bleeding disorders should not have this test. (Thoracentesis) Pleural fluid collection may be dangerous for patients with bleeding disorders.

2 **You have unstable asthma.**
(Pulmonary Function Test) These types of inhalation studies can trigger asthmatic episodes. Although bronchodilators are kept nearby, if your asthma is unstable, this test may not be safe for you.

3 **You take anticoagulants.**
(Bronchoscopy) Because they may cause bleeding, patients are often asked to discontinue the use of anticoagulants or nonsteroidal antiinflammatory drugs before having a bronchoscopy. Always be sure to tell your doctor about all the medications you take, including herbs and supplements. (Mediastinoscopy) Your doctor will ask you to stop taking anticoagulants for some time before having mediastinoscopy. Always make sure your doctor is aware of the medications you take.

ization and biopsy equipment. A biopsy can be obtained with forceps that actually cut a piece of tissue, or with a brush that gathers cells for collection.

Results

This test allows the doctor to look directly into the lungs and observe closely any tumors, clots or foreign objects. Biopsies can be performed on the tissue and blood and fluid samples can also be taken.

Mediastinoscopy

The patient is put to sleep in an operating room, and an incision is made in the notch at the top of the ribcage. An endoscope is inserted and can withdraw fluid, allow visualizations or obtain tissue samples from the lymph nodes between the lungs.

Results

Doctors may suspect cancer of the lymph nodes or lungs, which can be detected with a biopsy. Other diseases of the lung, such as tuberculosis, can also be diagnosed through this procedure.

Sputum culture

The patient coughs up sputum into a cup, which is taken to a lab for analysis. A mist which promotes coughing may be administered.

Results

An analysis of sputum can help diagnose pneumonia and bronchitis and, most importantly, tuberculosis.

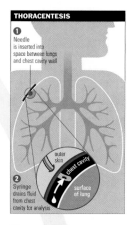

THORACENTESIS

❶ Needle is inserted into space between lungs and chest cavity wall

outer skin

chest cavity

❷ Syringe drains fluid from chest cavity for analysis

surface of lung

Thoracentesis

A small area of the chest is injected with a local anesthetic. Then, a needle is inserted and is positioned into the space where fluid has collected. Fluid is removed with a syringe for analysis. If needed, a larger amount can be drained if it is causing discomfort or intruding on normal body functions such as breathing.

Results

The analysis from the lab reports on the content of the fluid. This can include protein, glucose, bacteria and cancerous cells. Fluid around the lungs can indicate lung cancer and pneumonia, as well as other chest abnormalities or infections.

Lung scan

There are two types of this nuclear scan, which tests for blood clots in the lung, abnormal oxygen absorption and lung function. In the first, a radioactive substance is injected into a vein and spreads to the lungs. A "gamma camera" then takes pictures of the lungs. In the second, the patient inhales a gas containing radioisotopes into the lungs and pictures are then taken. Both types, together called a "ventilation-perfusion" lung scan, are often performed when a blood clot is suspected.

Results

The images show which parts of the lung are effectively exchanging air.

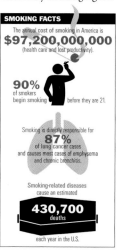

SMOKING FACTS

The annual cost of smoking in America is
$97,200,000,000
(health care and lost productivity).

90% of smokers begin smoking before they are 21.

Smoking is directly responsible for
87% of lung cancer cases and causes most cases of emphysema and chronic bronchitis.

Smoking-related diseases cause an estimated
430,700 deaths
each year in the U.S.

Lung disorders may range from acute infections like bronchitis to chronic conditions like asthma to life-threatening diseases like lung cancer.

Although some common diagnostic tests may be ordered by your physician, more severe or chronic cases may be handled by a pulmonologist—a doctor with several years of specialized training in diseases of the lungs.

Sources: Diagnostic Tests for Men, Diagnostic Tests for Women.

TIP

Cigarette smoking is the main cause of lung cancer. At least 9 in 10 lung cancer deaths are attributed to smoking.

4 **You've been taking antibiotics.**
(Sputum Culture) Let your doctor know if you've been taking antibiotics recently. It may affect the accuracy of your culture.

5 **You are pregnant.**
(Lung Scan) Be sure to tell your doctor if there is any chance you may be pregnant. Because these tests may be harmful to a fetus, pregnant women should not have this type of test.

6 **You've had another type of nuclear scan recently.**
(Lung Scan) The results of your lung scan could be inaccurate if you've had other nuclear testing beforehand.

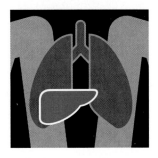

The liver manufactures and regulates chemicals, converts glucose, breaks down fats and proteins, produces blood-clotting enzymes, produces bile, and filters drugs and alcohol.

The normal human liver is the size of a football and weighs between 2.5 and 3.3 pounds.

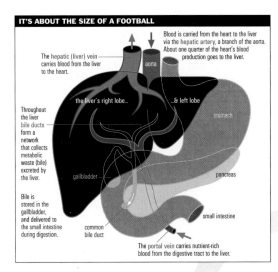

IT'S ABOUT THE SIZE OF A FOOTBALL

Blood is carried from the heart to the liver via the hepatic artery, a branch of the aorta. About one quarter of the heart's blood production goes to the liver.

The hepatic (liver) vein carries blood from the liver to the heart.

aorta

the liver's right lobe...

...& left lobe

stomach

Throughout the liver bile ducts form a network that collects metabolic waste (bile) excreted by the liver.

gallbladder

pancreas

Bile is stored in the gallbladder, and delivered to the small intestine during digestion.

small intestine

common bile duct

The portal vein carries nutrient-rich blood from the digestive tract to the liver.

Endoscopic Retrograde Cholangiopancreatography (ERCP)

The patient fasts for 12 hours before the test to clear the intestine. The mouth and throat are anesthetized and a sedative may be given. An endoscope is then guided through the mouth into the stomach and small intestine. The endoscope injects dye into the bile ducts. X-rays are then taken of the liver area. Other endoscopic procedures may be performed, including the removal of stones.

Results

The x-rays of the liver area should be very clear because of the dye injected. Bile duct infections and blockages should be visible. Because the scope allows detailed inspection of this area of the body, other problems or blockages may be revealed. The material removed from the biopsy can be tested for cancers or infections.

Abdominal Ultrasound

The patient disrobes from the waist up and lies down on an examination table. A gel is put on the abdomen to help transmit sound waves. The technician then moves an ultrasound transducer over the parts of the abdomen that are important to the doctor.

Results

Like other ultrasound results, these appear on a screen that can be studied by the doctor. This test reads gallstones and kidney stones especially well.

It can detect inflammations and also differentiate between solid and fluid-filled masses, useful for examining suspected tumors. It is helpful in identifying masses outside the liver or gallbladder that are compressing these organs.

Computed Tomography of the Biliary Tract and Liver (Liver CT Scan)

The patient lies down on an x-ray table positioned in the opening of a scanner gantry. A contrast medium is given orally (after fasting) or intravenously. The patient is asked to remain as still as possible during the scanning process which can take as long as an hour.

Results

The size, shape and function of the liver can be observed, as well as cysts, tumors and abscesses .

Percutaneous Liver Biopsy

Under local anesthesia, a special hypodermic needle is inserted through the chest wall into the liver, and a sample of tissue is drawn out by aspiration. Under certain circumstances, the needle may require guidance to a particular place in the liver, in which case, CT scanning or ultrasound may be performed simultaneously with the biopsy.

ACTION ITEMS

What to do if...

1 **You are pregnant.**
(ERCP, Computed Tomography) Be sure to tell your doctor if there is any chance you may be pregnant. Because ionizing radiation may be harmful to a fetus, pregnant women should not have these tests.

2 **You are allergic to iodine or shellfish.**
(ERCP, Computed Tomography) Iodine-based contrast dye can cause a severe allergic reaction in those allergic to iodine or shellfish. Be sure to tell your doctor and the technitian of any allergies before testing.

3 **You are obese.**
(Abdominal Ultrasound) Since fat may interfere with sound wave transmission, this type of ultrasound may not produce clear results for obese patients.
(Percutaneous Liver Biopsy) It may be difficult to obtain a proper tissue sample in extremely obese patients using this biopsy method. In extreme cases the biopsy may be taken using a laparoscope—a tube inserted through a small incision in the abdomen.

Results

The specimen of tissue must be transported to the laboratory for analysis immediately. Examination of the tissue may reveal signs of cirrhosis, hepatitis or infection such as tuberculosis. Tissue analysis may also identify cancerous or non-cancerous tumors.

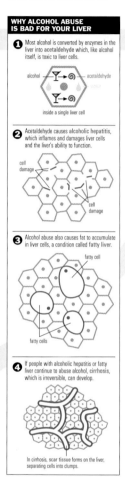

WHY ALCOHOL ABUSE IS BAD FOR YOUR LIVER

❶ Most alcohol is converted by enzymes in the liver into acetaldehyde which, like alcohol itself, is toxic to liver cells.

alcohol ⟶ acetaldehyde

inside a single liver cell

❷ Acetaldehyde causes alcoholic hepatitis, which inflames and damages liver cells and the liver's ability to function.

cell damage

cell damage

❸ Alcohol abuse also causes fat to accumulate in liver cells, a condition called fatty liver.

fatty cell

fatty cells

❹ If people with alcoholic hepatitis or fatty liver continue to abuse alcohol, cirrhosis, which is irreversible, can develop.

In cirrhosis, scar tissue forms on the liver, separating cells into clumps.

Alanine Aminotransferase Blood Test (ALT) or Serum Glutamic-Pyruvic Transminase Blood Test (SGPT) or Alkaline Phosphatase (ALP)

Blood is drawn from a vein and sent to a lab for analysis.

Results

An elevated level of ALT in the blood is a sign of liver inflammation from things like hepatitis or alcohol abuse.

Alpha-fetoprotein Blood Test (AFP)

Blood is drawn from a vein and sent to a lab for analysis.

Results

Elevated AFP in the blood may indicate cirrhosis, chronic active hepatitis or cancer, in particular, testicular cancer.

Alkaline Phosphatase Blood Test (ALP)

Blood is taken from a vein and sent to a lab for analysis.

Results

Elevated levels of this compound in the bloodstream may indicate cirrhosis, obstruction of the bile duct or a liver tumor.

Bilirubin Blood Test

Blood is drawn and sent to a lab for analysis.

Results

Excessive red blood cell destruction from disease leads to elevated bilirubin, as can blocked bile ducts caused by cancer, gallstones or scarring.

Protein, Albumin, Serum Protein, Globulin and Serum Electrophoresis Blood Tests

Blood is drawn from a vein and sent to a lab for analysis.

Results

Low albumin is a sign of liver or kidney disease. Decreased levels of the other proteins are signs of malnutrition, starvation, liver disease or cancer.

Hepatitis Blood Test

Blood is drawn from a vein and sent to a lab for analysis.

Results

Results may indicate the presence of the hepatitis virus or antibodies, the latter of which may be present due to vaccination.

Ammonia Level Blood and Urine Test

Blood and urine samples are taken and sent to a lab for analysis.

Results

Ammonia is always present in blood and urine, but in high quantities can indicate severe liver

CT scans can detect cirrhosis, cysts and tumors. Blood tests can help detect hepatitis and other liver problems. The liver can also be biopsied and examined to diagnose cancer.

Cirrhosis is used to describe a multitude of chronic diseases that cause scarring of the liver. After alcoholic liver disease, viral hepatitis is the second most common liver disorder.

Sources: Diagnostic Tests for Men, Diagnostic Tests for Women.

TIP

Liver disease due to excessive alcohol consumption outnumbers all other types of liver disorders by five to one.

❹ **You are dehydrated.**
(Abdominal Ultrasound) If you are dehydrated, it may be difficult to distinguish between different types of tissues during an abdominal ultrasound.
(Computed Tomography) Because the contrast dye used for this test can cause renal failure in patients with chronic dehydration, liver function testing prior to a CT scan may necessary.

❺ **You have a lung infection.**
(Percutaneous Liver Biopsy) Infection near the biopsy site may preclude you from having this procedure as it may spread the infection.

❻ **You take anticoagulants.**
(Percutaneous Liver Biopsy) Because they may cause bleeding, patients are asked to discontinue the use of anticoagulants, aspirin or nonsteroidal antiinflammatory drugs before having this procedure. Always be sure to tell your doctor about all the medications you take, including herbs and supplements.

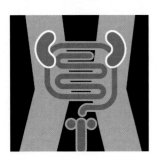

The kidneys, ureter, bladder and urethra comprise the urinary tract. Kidneys remove liquid waste from the blood in the form of urine, keep a stable balance of salts in the blood, regulate blood pressure and produce erythroprotein, a hormone that aids in the production of red blood cells.

Human kidneys are about four inches long and filter approximately 40 gallons of blood daily.

Blood Urea Nitrogen (BUN), Creatinine, Creatinine Clearance

Blood and urine samples are taken over the course of a day.

Results

Too little BUN may be an indication of liver problems or of malnutrition. Too much urea nitrogen or creatinine in the blood can indicate kidney failure. The creatinine clearance test rates the kidney's function by its ability to remove this waste.

Urinalysis

Urine collected in a sterile container is sent to a lab for analysis.

Results

Cloudiness, blood or an abnormal number of particles dissolved in the urine can alert doctors to kidney problems. Glucose can indicate diabetes or other kidney problems. Ketones indicate diabetes or starvation. Nitrite is a good indication of infection. Protein usually means the kidney filters have been damaged.

Urine Culture

Urine collected in a sterile container is sent to a lab for analysis.

Results

Bacteria in the urine is a sign of a urinary tract infection.

Sodium Test

Blood is taken from a vein and sent to a lab for analysis.

Results

Excess sodium building up in the body may be an indicator of kidney failure or malfunction.

Calcium Test

Blood is taken from a vein and sent to a lab for analysis.

Results

Chronically low calcium levels can indicate kidney failure.

Potassium Test

Blood is taken from a vein and sent to a lab for analysis.

Results

Abnormal levels of potassium in the blood can indicate kidney failure.

24 Hour Urine (Steroids, calcium and protein)

Urine collected from an entire day in one sterile container is sent to a lab for analysis.

Results

Too much calcium can predict future kidney stones or damaged hormone regulation. Uric acid is found in the urine of patients with gout and leukemia, and can contribute to kidney stones as well. Excessive amounts of steroids can indicate disease in the

organs where they are produced.

Electrolytes

Blood is drawn from a vein and sent to a lab for analysis.

Results

Abnormal electrolyte levels can indicate dehydration or kidney malfunction.

Magnesium

Blood is taken from a vein and sent to a lab for analysis.

Results

Magnesium in the blood is usually a sign of overconsumption, but can also point to kidney failure or liver disease.

Phosphorus

Blood is taken from a vein and sent to a lab for analysis.

Results

High phosphorus levels can mean future kidney failure.

Urine Amino Acid Screen

Urine collected in a sterile container is sent to a lab for analysis.

Results

High amounts of amino acids can indicate kidney disease.

Abdominal X-ray

The patient dons a hospital gown and two x-ray

ACTION ITEMS

What to do if...

1 **You are pregnant.**
(Abdominal X-Ray, Cystography, Cystoscopy, Cystometry, Pyelography, Renal Angiogram, Renal Scan) Be sure to tell your doctor if there is any chance you may be pregnant. Because ionizing radiation may be harmful to a fetus, pregnant women should not have these tests.

2 **You've had other recent contrast xrays.**
(Cystography, Cystoscopy, Cystometry, Pyelography, Renal Angiogram) Contrast dye or barium in your system from a recent diagnostic test can affect the accuracy of your cystography or pyelography results.

3 **You are allergic to iodine or shellfish.**
(Cystography, Cystoscopy, Cystometry, Pyelography, Renal Angiogram) Be sure to tell your doctor and the technician of any allergies before testing. Iodine-based contrast dye can cause a severe allergic reaction in those allergic to iodine or shellfish.

4 **You are dehydrated.**
(Pyelography, Renal Angiogram) Because the contrast dye used for this test can adversely affect kidney function and cause renal failure, this test may not be appropriate for patients with chronic dehydration, diabetes or decreased kidney function.

THE URINARY TRACT

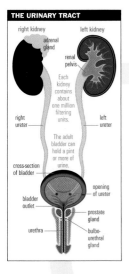

right kidney
left kidney
adrenal gland
renal pelvis

Each kidney contains about one million filtering units.

right ureter
left ureter

The adult bladder can hold a pint or more of urine.

cross-section of bladder

bladder outlet

opening of ureter

prostate gland

urethra

bulbo-urethral gland

pictures are taken, one lying down and one standing.

Results

This simple x-ray can show intestinal blockages, tears, tumors and deposits such as kidney stones and gallstones.

Cystography, Cystourethrogram

A catheter is inserted via the urethra into the bladder. The bladder is drained, dye is injected and x-rays are taken.

Results

Results can indicate bladder malfunctions or tumors.

Pyelogram

A dye is injected intravenously. After it has spread through the blood to the kidneys, x-rays are taken before and after the patient empties their bladder.

Results

Size, shape and abnormalities are evident. Cancer of the kidney can be seen, as can infections and kidney stones. If the dye does not spread properly this indicates bad blood flow and possible kidney failure.

Renal Angiogram

A local anesthetic is injected into the skin near the femoral artery. A catheter is then inserted into this artery and maneuvered up into the body next to the kidney. A contrast dye is injected directly into the kidney area, and x-rays are taken.

Results

This test can help diagnose kidney failure, kidney stones, tumors, cancer and blood vessel blockages.

Cystoscopy

The urethra is anesthetized with an injection and an endoscope is inserted through the urethra into the bladder.

Results

This test can visually detect problems, like tumors or other growths, in the prostate, the kidney and especially the bladder. Samples taken during the procedure can be analyzed for cancer and infection.

Cystometry

Different fluids are inserted and drained out of the bladder through a catheter. The patient describes any unusual sensations. The bladder is then filled completely with liquid, measuring the bladder's size and pressure. The fluid may be drained from the bladder and replaced with carbon dioxide for further measurements.

Results

This test measures bladder pressure, sensitivity and other functions. Abnormalities usually lead to further testing.

Renin Assay, Plasma

Blood is taken from a vein and sent to a lab for analysis.

Results

The presense of this kidney-produced enzyme in the blood is an indication of blood vessel blockage or kidney failure.

Renogram, Renal Scan

A radioisotope is injected into a vein, and spreads to the kidneys. Pictures of the kidney area are taken with a gamma camera.

Results

This test can show kidney failure, hypertension, tumors, cysts and non-function.

Kidney stones, one of the most common disorders of the urinary tract, are usually detected through urinalysis and confirmed with an x-ray technique-called pyelography.

Kidney stones occur more frequently in men than women and are extremely painful. They develop from crystals, usually made largely of calcium, which form in the urine.

Sources: Diagnostic Tests for Men, Diagnostic Tests for Women.

TIP

Kidney disease can occur from taking large quantities of pain killers over many years.

 You have a urinary tract infection.
(Cystography, Cystoscopy, Cystometry) Because these tests may exacerbate your condition, it is often recommended that they are postponed or cancelled if you have any infection of the urinary tract.

 You've recently had pyelography.
(Renal Scan) You should wait at least 24 hours after pyelography before having a renogram.

 You take antihypertensive medication.
(Renal Scan) Patients are usually asked to discontinue the use of antihypertensive drugs before having this procedure. Always be sure to tell your doctor about all the medications you take, including herbs and supplements.

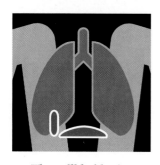

The gallbladder is a small pear-shaped sac located under the liver which stores and distributes bile.

The pancreas is a carrot-shaped gland that lies behind the stomach secreting digestive enzymes and hormones, insulin and glucagon, into the body.

About 1 million people are diagnosed with gallstones every year.

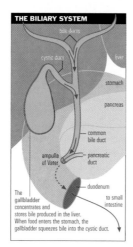

THE BILIARY SYSTEM

bile ducts
cystic duct
liver
stomach
pancreas
common bile duct
ampulla of Vater
pancreatic duct
duodenum
to small intestine

The gallbladder concentrates and stores bile produced in the liver. When food enters the stomach, the gallbladder squeezes bile into the cystic duct.

GALLBLADDER

Endoscopic Retrograde Cholangiopancreatography
172

Oral Cholecystogram

If an ultrasound is unable to make a clear diagnosis of pain source in the gall-bladder, this test may be ordered. The oral chole-cystogram utilizes a contrast dye to highlight the gallbladder. In this test, the patient swallows a capsule containing a contrast dye the evening before the test. The dye is digested and makes its way into the bile the liver produces. X-rays are then taken about 12 hours later when the bile has been stored in the gall-bladder.

Results

The dye makes the gall-bladder stand out on the x-rays. Blockages, inflammations, gallstones, and, rarely, tumors, should all be visible. Cholescintigraphy differs because the radionuclide contrast dye is injected in a vein.

Percutaneous Transhepatic Cholangiography (PTC)

The patient is placed on an x-ray table and the abdominal wall or lower chest wall is anesthetized. Using televised fluoro-scopic monitoring, a needle is passed through the abdominal wall and into the liver. A biliary branch is located and punctured. When bile is flowing freely into the needle, radiographic dye is injected. The dye passes into the biliary tract. X-rays are then taken. If an obstruction is found, a catheter or stent is left temporarily in the biliary tract to establish drainage and decompression. The patient may feel some discomfort when the needle is introduced, even though the area is anesthetized. This procedure will take approximately one hour. The patient may feel abdominal pain for several hours after the test, and will normally remain under observation for that period. Open cholangiograms may be performed during a sur-gical operation where dye is injected directed into the biliary tracts to make sure that there is no obstruction in this area.

Results

The dye should make the gallbladder stand out. Blockages, inflammations and stones will be visible.

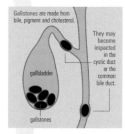

Gallstones are made from bile, pigment and cholesterol.

They may become impacted in the cystic duct or the common bile duct.

gallbladder

gallstones

PANCREAS

Amylase

Blood is drawn from a vein and sent to a lab for analysis.

Results

If the pancreas or salivary organs are inflamed or damaged, amylase leaks into the bloodstream. Increased presence of this enzyme in the blood indicates these conditions.

C-peptide

Blood is drawn from a vein and sent to a lab for analysis.

Results

This test is primarily used to monitor insulin in the body, although too much of this enzyme can be a sign of kidney failure. This

ACTION ITEMS

What to do if...

1 **You are pregnant.**
(Oral Cholecystogram, Percutaneous Transhepatic Cholangiography) Be sure to tell your doctor if there is any chance you may be pregnant. Because ionizing radiation may be harmful to a fetus, pregnant women should not have these tests.

2 **You are allergic to iodine or shellfish.**
(Oral Cholecystogram, Percutaneous Transhepatic Cholangiography) Be sure to tell your doctor and the technician of any allergies before testing. Iodine-based contrast dye can cause a severe reaction in those allergic to iodine or shellfish.

3 **You want more information.**
Contact one of these organizations for more information on preventing, diagnosing and treating diseases of the gallbladder and pancreas.

National Digestive Diseases Information Clearinghouse
2 Information Way
Bethesda, MD 20892-3570
www.nddk.nih.gov

American Gastrointestinal Association
www.gastro.org/gallstones.html

American Society for Gastrointestinal Endoscopy
www.asge.org

enzyme is in the bloodstream in proportion to insulin, but stays in the body longer, making it a more accurate measure.

Glucose

This blood test measures glucose levels in the body. A variation of the test, called the glucose tolerance test, is ordered on known diabetics. A known (usually large) quantity of glucose is given to the patient to eat, and blood tests are done over time to see how the patient reacts. Blood is drawn from a vein and sent to a lab for analysis. The glucose tolerance test takes both blood and urine samples at half-hour intervals after the meal is eaten.

Results

Too little glucose, hypoglycemia, is a sign of starvation or an overdose of insulin. Symptoms include dizziness and light-headedness. Too much glucose, hyperglycemia, is a strong indication of diabetes.

Hemoglobin A1C (Glycohemoglobin)

Blood is drawn from a vein and sent to a lab for analysis. This test is usually ordered in those who have already had a glucose test which requires further investigation or to follow the effectiveness of

a diabetic patient's treatment. It monitors the average level of hemoglobin AlC over the ninety days a red blood cell lives.

Results

If high hemoglobin A1C is found as well as high glucose, these factors are a strong indication of diabetes. This test is also used to monitor how well diabetics are controlling their sugar levels with insulin therapy. Glucose combines with hemoglobin, a component of blood, to form hemoglobin A1C. This is a long-term measure of glucose which does not fluctuate with meals, as normal glucose would.

Ketones

Blood is drawn from a vein and urine is collected in a sterile container. Both are sent to a lab for analysis.

Results

Ketones, chemical compounds in the blood, exist in high quantities when the body has to burn fat reserves because it is unable to use carbohydrates. Both diabetics and people who are dehydrat-

THE TOP 4 WARNING SIGNS OF DIABETES

- Frequent urination.
- Excessive thirst and hunger.
- Family members with diabetes; it often runs in families.
- Sugar binges; diabetes can be detected with blood and urine tests for glucose.

ed or suffering from starvation may exhibit high ketone levels. Ketosis, the accumulation of excessive amounts of ketones in the body, is usually a medical emergency.

Lipase

Blood is drawn from a vein and sent to a lab for analysis.

Results

Elevated levels of this digestive enzyme in the blood occurs when the pancreas is infected or blocked by cysts. This test is less sensitive than the test for amylase, but will detect pancreatic inflammation for a longer period of time after the infection occurs.

Sweat Test

An area of skin is cleaned and dried. A drug which induces sweat is dropped onto the skin. An electrode is placed on top of the skin, and another on a nearby patch of skin. Low voltage current running between them allows the drug to seep in and sweating begins. The skin is cleaned and dried again, and a piece of absorbent paper is placed on the skin. It absorbs sweat for up to an hour.

Results

The sweat can be tested for the presence of minerals which indicate cystic fibrosis.

Gallbladder testing is usually conducted by your primary care physician. Because the pancreas is part of both the digestive and endocrine systems, pancreatic tests may also be overseen by either a gastroenterologist or an encronologist.

Gallstones are the most common problem with the gallbladder. By far the most common pancreatic disorder is diabetes mellitus.

Sources: Diagnostic Tests for Men, Diagnostic Tests for Women.

TIP

Obesity, crash dieting and prolonged fasting are all major risk factors for gallstone formation.

The National Pancreas Foundation
PO Box 600590
Newtonville, MA 02460
877.NPF.FUND or 877.673.3863
www.pancreasfoundation.org

Pancreas.org
www.pancreas.org

American Diabetes Association
149 Madison Avenue
New York, NY 10016
800.342.2383
www.diabetes.org

National Institute of Diabetes and Digestive Diseases
Diabetes Prevention Program
www.preventdiabetes.com

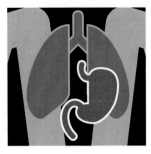

The upper gastrointestinal tract (upper GI) includes the esophagus, stomach and small intestine.

The average adult stomach holds 1.5 quarts (or three pints). The small intestine is about 21 feet long.

Fecal Occult Blood Test

A small sample of stool is obtained by the patient either at home or in the doctor's office for analysis in the laboratory.

Results

This test examines the patient's stool for the presence of hidden (or occult) blood. If the test indicates that there is blood present in the stool, it does not necessarily indicate cancer. A number of non-cancerous bleeding conditions, such as hemorrhoids or ulcers, may exist.

Gastrin Blood Test

Blood is drawn from a vein and sent to a lab for analysis. Sometimes injections of substances which stimulate gastrin production are given before the blood sample is taken. This helps determine the cause of high gastrin levels.

Results

Excessive gastrin, a hormone which stimulates acid secretion, may indicate tumors (usually in the pancreas). This test is useful in patients with ulcer disease.

Upper GI Series or Barium Swallow

The patient first drinks about four ounces of chalky barium liquid, which is often flavored to make it more palatable. The barium coats the esophagus, stomach and small intestine. X-rays are taken as it does so and after it has had time to settle. These can be taken both sitting up and lying down. It spreads into the stomach for x-ray in about half an hour, but can take four hours to spread to the small intestine. The barium may cause constipation. Although the "barium cocktail" is distasteful to most patients, it is a safe and important diagnostic tool.

Results

Tumors and ulcers should stand out in the esophagus and stomach due to the outlining effect of the barium. If tumors are detected in a barium swallow procedure, a biopsy is usually required for further analysis. The extent of damage from reflux, the bubbling of

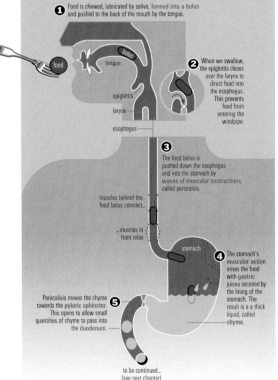

A BITE'S PROGRESS: PART ONE

① Food is chewed, lubricated by saliva, formed into a bolus and pushed to the back of the mouth by the tongue.

food
bolus
tongue

② When we swallow, the epiglottis closes over the larynx to direct food into the esophagus. This prevents food from entering the windpipe.

epiglottis
larynx
esophagus

③ The food bolus is pushed down the esophagus and into the stomach by waves of muscular contractions, called peristalsis.

muscles behind the food bolus contract...
...muscles in front relax
stomach

④ The stomach's muscular action mixes the food with gastric juices secreted by the lining of the stomach. The result is a a thick liquid, called chyme.

⑤ Peristalsis moves the chyme towards the pyloric sphincter. This opens to allow small quantities of chyme to pass into the duodenum.

to be continued...
(see next chapter)

ACTION ITEMS

What to do if...

1 **You regularly take vitamin C supplements.**
(Fecal Occult Blood Test) Ingesting vitamin C supplements or an abundance of food containing vitamin C before giving a stool sample for this test can result in a false-negative result.

2 **You have difficulty swallowing.**
(Upper GI Series) Because of the risk of aspirating barium into the lungs, this test may not be appropriate for patients with impaired swallowing reflex.

3 **You may be pregnant**
(Upper GI Series) Be sure to tell your doctor if there is any chance you may be pregnant. Because ionizing radiation may be harmful to a fetus, pregnant women should not have this test.
(Gastric Analysis) Because of the stimulating hormone injected, this test is not recommended for women who may be pregnant.

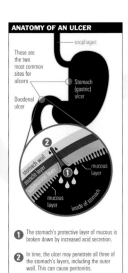

ANATOMY OF AN ULCER

esophagus

These are the two most common sites for ulcers

Stomach (gastric) ulcer

Duodenal ulcer

stomach wall
muscia layer
submucosa
mucous layer

mucous layer

inside of stomach

1 The stomach's protective layer of mucous is broken down by increased acid secretion.

2 In time, the ulcer may penetrate all three of the stomach's layers, including the outer wall. This can cause peritonitis.

stomach juices up into the esophagus, can be seen as well. In particular, tumors and ulcers become more apparent on x-rays using barium.

Esophagogastroduodenoscopy (EGD) or Gastroscopy or Upper GI Endoscopy

The patient usually fasts for several hours beforehand to empty the stomach. The throat is anesthetized with a spray, and a sedative is given so the patient relaxes. A flexible endoscope is inserted through the mouth, down the esophagus and into the stomach and duodenum (first part of the small intestine). The interior of these organs can be examined and tests can be performed using the endoscope.

Results

Ulcers are the most common problem discovered during this test. Inflammation or cancers of the stomach and of the esophagus can be seen, and biopsied. This is an excellent method of finding the cause of bleeding in this part of the body.

Gastric Analysis

The test begins with the patient fasting up to eight hours before the test, to ensure that the stomach will be completely empty. A narrow, flexible tube is inserted through the nose and down into the stomach. Every fifteen minutes for one hour, the doctor or technician withdraws a sample of stomach juice from the tube. Then the patient is injected with a chemical that will cause the stomach to produce acid. Generally, four more samples are collected every 15 minutes.

Results

The samples are analyzed and compared for their acid content. If the injected chemical has no effect on acid production in the stomach, this may indicate gastritis, gastric ulcer or cancer. Increased acid in the stomach is associated with ulcers, tumors and endocrine disease.

Heliobacter Pylori Tests

The heliobacter pylori bacteria—a microbe recognized as contributing to gastric diseases such as duodenal ulcers, gastritis and gastric carcinomais—is sometimes found in the mucus layer that lines the stomach and can be can be detected by several methods: a cultured specimen, a gastric mucosal biopsy, a blood test or a breath test. A biopsy or mucus specimen for culturing may be obtained by an esophagogastro-duodenoscopy (EGD), as described above. The specimen should be transported to the lab within 30 minutes of collection. Analysis of blood drawn from a vein, however, is an equally accurate and simpler procedure. The breath test requires the patient to swallow a dose of radioactive C or nonradioactive C urea.

Results

A biopsy or culture will be tested for heliobacter pylori or for antibodies. Similarly, blood can be analyzed for the presence of these antibodies. The breath test is based on the ability of helicobacter pylori to break down urea into carbon dioxide and ammonia. The CO_2 concentration will reveal the presence of the microbe.

Problems with the stomach, esophagus and small intestine are frequently diagnosed and treated by a gastroenterologist.

The most common serious stomach ailment is the peptic ulcer—a breakdown in the stomach lining (gastric ulcer) or first part of the small intestine (duodenal ulcer) resulting from stress, injury or infection. Esophagitis is the inflamation of the esophagus—commonly causing the symptom of heartburn

Sources: Diagnostic Tests for Men, Diagnostic Tests for Women.

TIP

Smoking, drinking alcohol and caffeine and taking aspirin and other NSAIDs can irritate an ulcer.

 You might have an upper GI perforation
(Upper GI Series) If your doctor suspects that you have a perforation in your upper GI tract, you may be given a water-soluble contrast dye instead of barium to minimize the risk of inflammation.
(EGD) An esophagogastroduodenoscopy may worsen an upper GI perforation.

 You've recently had an upper GI series.
(EGD) Because barium in your system will make it difficult for the doctor to make a clear inspection, it is recommended that you schedule your EGD at least two days after having a barium swallow.

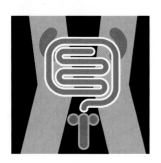

The lower gastrointestinal tract (lower GI) is comprised of the cecum, colon, rectum and anal canal. The largest section, the colon, is a segmented tube approximately four-and-a-half feet long. Its primary function is to absorb water before waste leaves the body.

Approximately 130,000 Americans were diagnosed with colon cancer in 1998. More than 55,000 were diagnosed too late for effective treatment and died. Unfortunately, only 20% of American adults are regularly tested for colorectal cancer.

Routine Stool Lab Tests (Occult Blood, Stool and Rectal Cultures)

This is one of the most common and most important tests of the lower gastrointestinal tract. A stool sample provided by the patient is studied for overall appearance and then may also be evaluated for fat content, in order to diagnose potential problems in the intestinal tract. Cultures can be conducted on stool samples to detect certain harmful bacteria, which can then be treated. Stool is also examined for parasites and blood. The presence of blood may be the first sign of a tumor, and is therefore an important diagnostic indicator. The patient should avoid red meat for two days prior to this test to avoid false-positive results.

Results

Abnormalities in the consistency, content, odor and color of stool may reflect disease anywhere along the path food travels from top to bottom. Stool naturally contains a lot of bacteria. Some, however, are indications of abnormalities or poisons in the intestine, and these can be identified in the test. Blood in the stool, usually not evident to the naked eye, can be an indication of cancer, colitis, ulcer formation, hemorrhoids or inflammation. Stool is also examined for parasites or eggs. If blood is in the stool, further diagnostic tests may be recommended.

Proctosigmoidoscopy or Sigmoidoscopy

The patient is given oral laxatives or an enema just before the test to clear the colon. The patient then lies on an examination table, knees up to chest, as the doctor inserts a lubricated proctosigmoidoscope into the rectum. Polyps or tissue samples may be removed during the exam.

Results

The doctor may detect polyps, colitis or cancer. Biopsy material may be analyzed by a lab.

Colonoscopy

The patient restricts eating the day before and takes a heavy laxative that night. Sometimes enemas are also needed to clear the colon. During the test, the patient lies on his side on an examination table with knees drawn up. The doctor lubricates and inserts a colonoscope

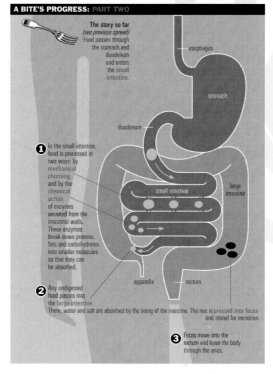

A BITE'S PROGRESS: PART TWO

The story so far *(see previous spread)* Food passes through the stomach and duodenum and enters the small intestine.

esophagus

stomach

duodenum

1 In the small intestine, food is processed in two ways: by mechanical churning, and by the chemical action of enzymes secreted from the intestinal walls. These enzymes break down proteins, fats and carbohydrates into smaller molecules so that they can be absorbed.

small intestine

large intestine

2 Any undigested food passes into the large intestine. There, water and salt are absorbed by the lining of the intestine. The rest is pressed into feces and stored for excretion.

appendix

rectum

3 Feces move into the rectum and leave the body through the anus.

ACTION ITEMS

What to do if...

1 **You regularly take vitamin C supplements.**
(Occult Blood Test) Ingesting vitamin C supplements or an abundance of food containing vitamin C before giving a stool sample for this test can result in a false-negative result.

2 **You've recently had a barium test.**
(Sigmoidoscopy, Colonoscopy, Barium Enema, CT Colonoscopy) Because barium in your system will make it difficult for the doctor to make a clear inspection, it is recommended that you schedule these tests at least one week after having a barium test.

3 **You have painful hemorrhoids.**
(Sigmoidoscopy, Colonoscopy) Anorectal conditions like hemmorrhoids or fissures may preclude you from having this test.

4 **You have a suspected colon perforation.**
(Colonoscopy) Because of the danger of causing additional damage, colonoscopy should not be performed on patients with suspected colon perforations.
(Barium Enema) If your doctor suspects that you have a perforation in your lower GI tract, you may be given a water-soluble contrast dye instead.

LOOKING INSIDE THE COLON

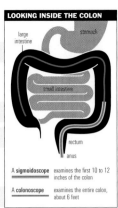

large intestine

stomach

small intestine

rectum

anus

A **sigmoidoscope** examines the first 10 to 12 inches of the colon

A **colonoscope** examines the entire colon, about 6 feet

---

into the rectum. Air is sometimes passed through the scope to inflate the bowel, allowing the scope to penetrate further. A sedative is often given to relax the patient both physically and mentally before the test.

Results

As the scope is removed, the doctor can see any abnormalities inside the colon, including tumors, polyps, colitis and diverticular disease. Fluid samples or biopsy material gathered by the colonoscope may be analyzed.

Barium Enema or Air Contrast Enema

The patient's colon is first cleared out, either with a laxative or by fasting or, if needed, with enemas. After a plain x-ray of the colon is taken first, the barium enema is inserted into the patient's rectum. A balloon on the enema

---

inflates to hold it inside the rectum, and barium begins to flow into the colon. As it is distributed through the colon, additional x-ray pictures are taken. In an air contrast enema, air is introduced, causing the barium to coat the colon thinly for clearer pictures.

Results

The barium makes polyps, tumors and diverticular disease much more visible than in a normal x-ray.

CT Colonoscopy

Following a cleansing enema or fasting, air is inserted into the patient's colon. A helical CT scanner passes over the patient gathering images.

Results

The images from the CT scan reveal all polyps that are larger than one centimeter in size and most other smaller polyps. Until clinical studies are completed, this procedure should not be considered a standard of care.

Laparoscopy

The lower abdomen is cleaned and sterilized, and general anesthesia is administered. A small incision is made in the skin and the laparoscope slipped inside. The scope is then used to observe and test the internal organs.

Results

From this perspective, doctors can detect cancers and liver disease. Any fluid or tissue collected may be analyzed.

Carcinoembryonic Antigen Blood Test (CEA)

Blood is drawn from a vein and sent to a lab for analysis.

Results

Although this is helpful in following known cases of colon cancer, it is not a good screening test. Seventy percent of patients with colon cancer have an elevated level of this antigen in their blood. The antigen may also elevated in cases of cancers elsewhere in the body and in the blood of smokers.

Rectal Digital Examination

The doctor wears sterile latex gloves, and, using one finger, he probes and touches the anal area and the entrance to the rectum.

Results

The doctor may discover the presence of hemorrhoidal tissues, scarring, polyps or growths. In this important test for men, the doctor may be able to detect enlargement or hardening of the prostate gland.

How is the lower GI evaluated?

Screening, looking for disease before symptoms are present, not only can find colorectal cancer at an early curable stage, it can also prevent it by locating and allowing the removal of polyps that might become cancer.

Although being screened before symptoms occur is better, colorectal cancer can also be found early if you report any symptoms to your doctor right away.

Sources: Diagnostic Tests for Men, Diagnostic Tests for Women, cancer.org.

TIP

Eating a high-fiber, low-fat diet, maintaining a healthy body weight and being physically active will reduce your risk of colon cancer.

 You have an extremely dilated colon. (Colonoscopy, Barium Enema) These tests are not appropriate for patients with a condition called megacolon, where the colon is extremely dilated.

 You take anticoagulants. (Colonoscopy, Laparoscopy) Because they may cause bleeding, patients are often asked to discontinue the use of anticoagulants or nonsteroidal antiinflammatory drugs before having a colonoscopy or laparoscopy. Always tell your doctor about all the medications you take, including herbs and supplements.

 You have suspected internal bleeding. (Laparoscopy) Because blood in your abdomen can make inspection difficult, it is usually recommended to postpone laparoscopy if internal bleeding is suspected.

 You may be pregnant. (Laparoscopy) Be sure to tell your doctor if there is any chance you may be pregnant. Because ionizing radiation may be harmful to a fetus, pregnant women should not have this test.

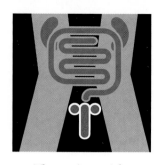

The penis, testicles and surrounding organs make up the male genitalia. The testicles produce sperm and the male hormone testosterone.

Proteonics, a technique that studies proteins in blood and other tissues, may soon replace the PSA test, which produces false-positive results about 25-30% of the time, as a screening tool for protate cancer.

Prostate cancer is the second most common cause of death from cancer in men of all ages, killing over 40,000 men each year.

Prostate Specific Antigen (PSA)

Blood is drawn and sent to a lab for analysis.

Results

Men with prostate cancer have elevated PSA levels in their blood. Those who have already been diagnosed with prostate cancer may undergo regular PSA testing to monitor the progress of the disease and/or the effectiveness of therapy. It is important to note that elevated PSA levels are not necessarily indicative of prostate cancer. BPH (benign prostatic hypertrophy) and prostatitis (an infection of the prostate) will also generate elevated PSA levels in the blood.

Scrotal/Prostate Ultrasound

These types of ultrasound are useful in detecting disorders of the prostate and testicles, and can identify even non-palpable cancers. The patient is first given an enema. For a prostate ultrasound, the doctor examines the rectum and inserts the ultrasound probe. The probe gives off sound waves into the prostate. The sound waves which are bounced back appear on the screen, giving a picture of the area. For a testicular ultrasound, a jelly is spread on the scrotum and the testicles are visualized.

Results

Prostate ultrasound is a great aid in the specific diagnosis of prostate cancer. Testicular ultrasound detects tumors of the testicles.

Testicular Self-exam

Because testicular cancer often produces no symptoms, many doctors recommend monthly self-exams. The best time to examine your testicles is during or right after a warm bath or shower. The heat causes the skin of the scrotum to soften and relax. And, soapy skin may make it even easier to feel any lumps underneath. Examine each testicle separately with both hands by rolling the testicle between the thumbs and fingers. You'll feel a cord-like structure (the epididymis which stores and transports sperm) on the top and back of the testicle. Gently separate this tube from the testicle with your fingers to examine the testicle itself. Feel for any swelling, lumps or any change in the size, shape or consistency of the testes.

Results

Although most are not cancer, any lumps or other symptoms should be checked by a physician.

Infertility Testing/ Semen Analysis

Many semen tests are available to study male fertility. All require a sample that the patient provides at a testing facility.

Results

Semen analysis is the first test done for male infertility. It can reveal abnormal sperm, low sperm count and "lazy" sperm, which lack the ability to swim effectively. In addition, a blockage may be preventing sperm from leaving the body. Blockages are sometimes due to STDs such as gonorrhea. As many as one in six couples may have fertility problems. The top cause of male infertility is failure to produce enough healthy sperm.

AIDS Blood Serology

Blood is drawn from a vein and sent to a lab for analysis. Home HIV tests are now available, but no test is yet 100 percent conclusive.

Results

This blood test detects the HIV antibodies which lead to the AIDS virus. A positive test means that the patient has the human immunodeficiency virus, which can develop into full-blown AIDS. A number of different tests exist for the disease,

---

ACTION ITEMS

Choosing prostate cancer treatment

If you have been diagnosed with prostate cancer, you may be overwhelmed with an array of treatment options. Your course of action will, to some extent, be influenced by the character of your cancer. Your decisions should also reflect your personal priorities after weighing each potential benefit and possible harm for the treatment options available. Your age and health should also be considered. Treatment decisions are complicated by shortcomings in both prognosis and treatment. Although your Gleason score and PSA level provide good guidelines, there is still no way to know for sure how rapidly your prostate cancer will progress.

Many questions will need answers.

1 Is your cancer truly confined to the prostate gland, or has it spread to nearby- or even distant parts of your body?

2 Does your cancer appear to be aggressive or slow-growing?

3 What is your general health status? Are you healthy enough for surgery?

4 Are you young enough so that even a slow-growing cancer might someday pose a threat?

and testing positive with one test does not necessarily mean that HIV/AIDS is present. Positive results from one type of test are confirmed with an alternative diagnostic technique. If one test is positive and another negative, the patient should retest in three to six months. AIDS is the most serious sexually-transmitted disease. It acts by suppressing the immune system, magnifying the impact of otherwise mild, treatable illnesses. Those at most risk are sexually active homosexual and bisexual men, women with multiple partners, intravenous drug users, persons receiving blood tainted with HIV (the virus that causes AIDS), and infants exposed to the disease while in utero.

Herpes Test

Though diagnosed largely by sight, a fluid sample can be taken and tested, identifying this STD for monitoring. A swab is used to remove fluid from a suspected herpes lesion and examined under a microscope and cultured. Blood can also be taken from a vein and sent to a lab for analysis.

Results

If the infection grows in the culture, the patient is infected. Herpes is a viral infection that can become chronic. There is no known cure, although medications to treat the symptoms are quite effective. Herpes simplex virus (HSV) has two types. Type 1 produces cold sores and fever blisters, generally in the mouth area. HSV Type 2 is a sexually transmitted viral infection whose first manifestation is usually sores. Genital herpes is characterized by reddish, tender, fluid-filled vesicles. Sores can also appear on and in the mouth, or on other parts of the body. The lesions usually turn up about a week after sex with an infected person, and take 10 to 21 days to heal. Even after the vesicles subside, the person remains infected, and outbreaks of the sores may flare up again in the future. Although forty percent of those affected never have a second attack, recurrences most often take place when the body is run down. Herpes is extremely contagious when the sores are present.

Chlamydia/Gonorrhea Blood Tests

A culture is usually taken by swabbing the urethra, collecting some of the infected material present. Blood may also be drawn from a vein and sent to a lab for analysis.

Results

In the case of gonorrhea, the infection may be visible under a microscope. However, the most reliable test is a culture test in which urethral discharge is cultivated to see if it will grow the bacteria of these infections. If either grows, the patient is infected. Chlamydia is the most frequently occurring STD in the US. The infection begins with unusual discharge from the penis, and often causes pain in urination. Eventually it can cause infertility in both sexes. About 35% of those who have chlamydia also have gonorrhea, a similar infection, both causing cloudy discharge or painful urination, as well as an urge to urinate often. Gonorrhea can also lead to infertility. It primarily infects the genitals, but can spread as well. It can be transmitted through oral, anal and vaginal sex.

Syphilis Blood Test

Blood is drawn from a vein and sent to a lab for analysis.

Results

The presence of the antibodies produced in response to treponema pallidum, the spiral-shaped bacterium that causes syphilis, indicate the infection.

If men in general are resistant to medical testing (and they are), they are especially resistant to the testing of their reproductive system.

Early identification of prostate cancer is now possible by annual screening of men over 50. (Those with increased risk should begin screening at an earlier age.) This screening involves a digital rectal exam and a PSA (prostate specific antegen) blood test.

Sources: Diagnostic Tests for Men, Diagnostic Tests for Women.

TIP

Impotence is rarely psychological. The most common causes are vascular problems, nerve damage, low testosterone and drug side effects

5 Are you willing to risk serious, lifelong side effects to possibly reduce your chances of a cancer death?

6 How important is it for you, in your work or recreation, to maintain bladder or bowel control?

7 How important is it to be able to have erections?

8 Would you find it too worrisome to live with an untreated cancer, too stressful to face frequent monitoring?

Once you receive your doctor's opinion about what treatments you need, it may be helpful to get more advice before you make up your mind. Getting another doctor's advice is normal medical practice, and your doctor can help you with this effort. Many health insurance companies require and will pay for other opinions.

You may also consider contacting a prostate cancer support group in your area. Talking with other men who have experienced the various procedures available may help you to understand better the treatment options described by your doctor.

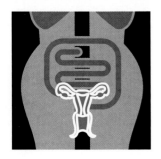

The female reproductive system is literally the cradle of human life. Pregnancy and childbirth have a powerful impact on the female reproductive system, including physical and hormonal changes.

Women who have had abnormal Pap results or who have certain STDs (HPV) should consider having Pap tests every year.

The "Pap" test is named after George Papanicolaou who invented it in 1928.

Pelvic Examination

The woman lies on her back with her knees bent or is seated in a gynecological examination chair. The doctor first inspects the external genitals for abnormalities. The doctor inserts two gloved fingers into the vagina to feel the size and position of the uterus and ovaries and to detect any pelvic swelling or growth. With a speculum in place, the doctor visually inspects the vagina and cervix.

Results

This simple physical examination provides the doctor with an overview of the health of a woman's reproductive system, and is often the basis for the consideration of further testing.

Pap Test or Pap Smear

While the patient is positioned for a gynecological

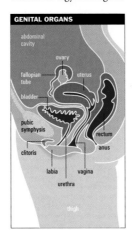

GENITAL ORGANS

abdominal cavity
ovary
fallopian tube
uterus
bladder
pubic symphysis
rectum
anus
clitoris
labia
vagina
urethra
thigh

exam, the doctor inserts a speculum and takes a sample from the mouth of the cervix with a swab or spatula. A slide is prepared and sent to a lab for analysis.

Results

This test, a part of most gynecological annual exams, can detect cervical cancer earlier than any other method. Although the Pap smear gives about a 75-90 percent chance of detecting precancerous cell changes, most abnormalities are not cancerous, and include herpes, other infections and irritation of the cervix.

Colposcopy

With the patient lying with her feet in stirrups, a speculum is inserted into the vagina. After swabbing the vagina and cervix to stain abnormal areas, a colposcope is placed at the vaginal opening. The doctor looks through the scope, focusing on the cervix. The doctor may also remove tissue for biopsy.

Results

A colposcopy almost always follows a repeated abnormal Pap smear. Cancer of the cervix can be detected with this test.

Pregnancy Tests

Pregnancy tests are readily available, but none are 100 percent accurate. In a

hospital or doctor's office, blood or urine is collected for analysis.

Results

The presence of certain hormones indicate that an egg has been fertilized. If the test is negative and menstruation has not occurred a week later, the test should be repeated.

Abdominal/Pelvic Ultrasound (Sonogram)

The patient's abdomen is coated with a gel and an ultrasound transducer is moved back and forth over the abdomen.

Results

The images from this test allow doctors to see the tissues of the uterus and ovaries. Tumors, cysts or the accumulation of fluid are often visible. In pregnant women, ultrasound is a noninvasive method to evaluate fetal health, and can identify number, position, sex and stage of development.

Vaginal Ultrasonography

The patient lies on her back with knees bent and wide apart. A probe, covered with a water soluble gel and a protective sheath is inserted into the vagina to obtain images.

Results

Problems such as ectopic pregnancy, blighted ovum, tubo-ovarian

---

ACTION ITEMS

Screening for cervical cancer

In 2002, about 4,100 women in the US died from cervical cancer. This number reflects a 70% decline from the mid-20th century, when the Pap test was first introduced as a screening tool. Cervical cancer screening is important to detect significant abnormal cell changes that may arise before cancer develops. The National Cancer Institute (NCI) supports these new guidelines on cervical cancer screening released by the US Preventive Services Task Force.

1 Cervical cancer screening should begin about three years after a woman begins having sexual intercourse, but no later than age 21.

2 Experts recommend waiting approximately three years following the initiation of sexual activity because transient HPV infections and cervical cell changes that are not significant are common and it takes years for a significant abnormality or cancer to develop. Cervical cancer is extremely rare in women under the age of 25.

3 Women should have a Pap test at least once every three years.

4 Women 65 to 70 years of age who have had at least three normal Pap tests and no abnormal Pap tests in the last 10 years may decide, upon consultation with their healthcare provider, to stop cervical cancer screening.

abscesses, fetal abnormalities and uterine bleeding can be diagnosed and evaluated.

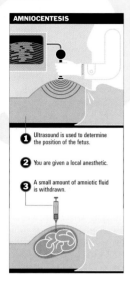

AMNIOCENTESIS

1 Ultrasound is used to determine the position of the fetus.

2 You are given a local anesthetic.

3 A small amount of amniotic fluid is withdrawn.

Amniocentesis

A long hollow needle is inserted through the abdomen into the uterus, and used to withdraw amniotic fluid. The procedure is usually done with a local anesthetic, generally in the fourteenth to sixteenth week of pregnancy. An ultrasound is usually performed beforehand to locate the fetus and minimize the chance that the needle will damage the baby or the placenta.

Results

A more precise age of the fetus can be determined, as well as the sex. Some serious defects and disorders, including Down's Syndrome, hemophilia, cystic fibrosis and spina bifida may also be revealed.

Chorionic Villus Sampling

After determining the position of the fetus through ultrasound, a needle is inserted either through the vagina or the abdomen into the uterus to take cells from the chorionic villus, a sac in the uterus.

Results

The cells taken in the sample are analyzed for genetic defects. The sex of the fetus can also be determined.

Oncoscint Scan

A radioactive dye is injected into the patient 48 to 72 hours prior to the test. After the dye has spread to the uterus, nuclear pictures are taken.

Results

If tumors are present, it is likely the dye with concentrate on these areas, making them stand out in the pictures. Although the test is not always reliable, it is used to diagnose cancers.

Alpha-fetoprotein Blood Test (AFP)

Blood is drawn and sent to a lab for analysis.

Results

Although this test is only 90% accurate, elevated Alpha-feto protein levels can be a strong indication of fetal abnormalities. AFP levels are also raised in multiple pregnancies and miscarriages. Further tests, including amniocentesis and ultrasound are usually recommended for clarification. Unusually low AFP levels may indicate Down's syndrome.

Chlamydia and Gonorrhea Blood Tests
183

Herpes Test
183

AIDS Blood Serology
182

Syphilis Blood Test
183

Hysterosalpingogram

A dye is injected into the cervix through a tube and x-rays are taken.

Results

This type of x-ray is used to visualize the uterus and detect abnormal tissue masses and blockages of the fallopian tubes, one of the most common causes of infertility.

Laparoscopy
181 This procedure can help diagnose endometriosis.

Tests of the reproductive organs are necessary for routine preventive health, as well as for detection of problems associated with pregnancy or menopause.

The greatest health risks for the female reproductive system are sexually transmitted diseases (STDs) and cancer. Women should have annual gynecological exams, including a Pap test.

Sources: Diagnostic Tests for Men, Diagnostic Tests for Women.

TIP

Don't forget that annual gynecological visit! Since the introduction of the Pap test, deaths from cervical cancer have dropped 70%.

5 Women who have had a total hysterectomy (removal of the uterus and cervix) do not need to undergo cervical cancer screening, unless the surgery was done as a treatment for cervical precancer or cancer.

6 Women should seek expert medical advice about when they should begin screening, how often they should be screened and when they can discontinue cervical screenings, especially if they are at higher than average risk of cervical cancer due to factors such as HIV infection.

Source: National Institutes of Health.

For more information on cervical cancer and cervical cancer screening, please contact:

The National Cancer Institute
800.4.CANCER
www.cancer.gov

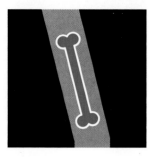

The human skeleton is comprised of over 200 bones which provide a rigid framework for the surrounding muscles and protect the essential organs in the skull and chest cavity.

Women middle-aged and older can cut their risk of hip fractures by 40% by walking four or more hours a week.

50% of women and 20% of men over the age of 65 will sustain bone fractures due to osteoporosis.

ALL ABOUT THE SPINE

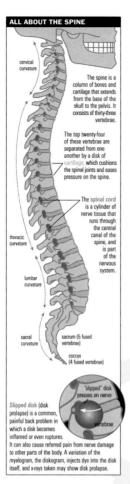

cervical curvature

The spine is a column of bones and cartilage that extends from the base of the skull to the pelvis. It consists of thirty-three vertebrae.

The top twenty-four of these vertebrae are separated from one another by a disk of cartilage, which cushions the spinal joints and eases pressure on the spine.

thoracic curvature

The spinal cord is a cylinder of nerve tissue that runs through the central canal of the spine, and is part of the nervous system.

lumbar curvature

sacral curvature

sacrum (5 fused vertebrae)

coccyx (4 fused vertebrae)

"slipped" disk presses on nerve

vertebrae

Slipped disk (disk prolapse) is a common, painful back problem in which a disk becomes inflamed or even ruptures. It can also cause referred pain from nerve damage to other parts of the body. A variation of the myelogram, the diskogram, injects dye into the disk itself, and x-rays taken may show disk prolapse.

Bone Densitometry

This is a safe and painless technique which utilizes x-rays to measure the absorption of photon radiation to determine bone density.

Results:

The images are used to determine bone mass, which is compared to standard mass for the patient's age, weight and gender. This test is used to screen for, diagnose and monitor osteoporosis.

X-ray and Magnetic Resonance Imaging Tests

These tests are frequently used to diagnose fractures of bones and arthritis. 107

Blood Test for Calcium

Blood is drawn from a vein and sent to a lab for analysis.

Results

Calcium is the most common mineral in the human body. It helps muscles contract, the heart beat, blood clotting and nerve impulses. Too much calcium in the blood may mean that calcium is being lost from bones. This may be an indication of hormone imbalance, cancer or kidney problems. There are two causes for calcium loss from bones: leaching and poor absorption from the gastrointestinal system.

Bone Marrow Aspiration

In this procedure, a small portion of bone marrow, where blood cells are manufactured, is removed for analysis. Marrow may be extracted from the hip or breast bone. The skin in the area is cleaned and sterilized, and a local anaesthetic is injected into both the skin and bone area. A long hollow needle is then inserted through the skin and into the bone itself, puncturing it. The bone marrow layer is reached, and bone marrow is extracted and analyzed. Despite the anaesthetic, this test may be painful. After the procedure the patient may be bruised and tender.

Results

The marrow is tested for the types and numbers of red and white blood cells to determine the presence of anemia and other blood diseases, such as leukemia and cancer. The ability of the marrow to create new blood cells can be determined as well. The marrow can be cultured or even cloned for future use.

BONE FACTS

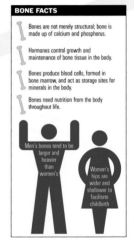

Bones are not merely structural; bone is made up of calcium and phosphorus.

Hormones control growth and maintenance of bone tissue in the body.

Bones produce blood cells, formed in bone marrow, and act as storage sites for minerals in the body.

Bones need nutrition from the body throughout life.

Men's bones tend to be larger and heavier than women's

Women's hips are wider and shallower to facilitate childbirth

---

ACTION ITEMS

What to do if...

1 **You are pregnant.**
(Bone Densitometry, Nuclear Bone Scan, Myelogram) Be sure to tell your doctor if there is any chance you may be pregnant. These tests may be harmful to a fetus, and are not appropriate for pregnant women.

2 **You regularly take calcium supplements.**
(Bone Densitometry) You should not take calcium supplements during the 24 hours prior to this test.

3 **You've recently had a barium test.**
(Bone Densitometry) Because barium in your system can affect the results, it is recommended that you schedule your test at least 10 days after having any barium test.

4 **You take anticoagulants.**
(Bone Marrow Aspiration) Because they may cause bleeding, patients are usually asked to discontinue the use of anticoagulants and nonsteroidal antiinflammatory drugs before having a bone marrow aspiration. Always tell your doctor about all the medications you take, including herbs and supplements.

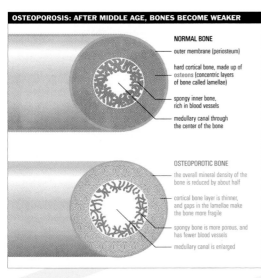

OSTEOPOROSIS: AFTER MIDDLE AGE, BONES BECOME WEAKER

NORMAL BONE
- outer membrane (periosteum)
- hard cortical bone, made up of osteons (concentric layers of bone called lamellae)
- spongy inner bone, rich in blood vessels
- medullary canal through the center of the bone

OSTEOPOROTIC BONE
- the overall mineral density of the bone is reduced by about half
- cortical bone layer is thinner, and gaps in the lamellae make the bone more fragile
- spongy bone is more porous, and has fewer blood vessels
- medullary canal is enlarged

Nuclear Bone Scan

Because some areas of abnormal bone do not show up well on x-rays, a nuclear scan may be ordered to better differentiate between normal and abnormal bone formation. A radioactive substance is injected into a vein. After approximately three hours, the patient lies still on a table for up to an hour as a nuclear camera takes pictures.

Results

The camera converts the images into a picture which looks like a skeleton. Abnormal areas, indicating weak, decayed, or cancerous bone, will show up as "hot spots" on the pictures. Bone scans also provide valuable information for those with unexplained bone pain, and may reveal otherwise undetected fractures and infections.

Myelogram

For this specialized x-ray, dye is injected into the spinal canal (the cerebrospinal fluid that surrounds the spine). The patient must lie face down on an x-ray table. A local anesthetic is put into the back with a needle. A larger needle is inserted into the space between the vertebrae, and into the spinal canal, and a small amount of dye is injected. With the needle still in place, the patient and the table may be tilted to allow the dye to spread throughout the spinal cord. After x-rays are taken, the needle is usually used to remove the dye. Sometimes cerebrospinal fluid is removed for analysis as well.

Results

Many disorders can affect the spine and spinal cord, including degeneration and rupture of disks, infections in the spinal fluid and arthritis of the vertebrae. The x-rays contribute to diagnosis of spinal cord abnormalities and tumors in the area as well. This examination has potentially serious aftereffects. The needle insertion, or spinal tap, may produce persistent leakage of cerebrospinal fluid, resulting in severe headache. The patient is often asked to remain in a reclining position for up to 12 hours after the test to avoid this problem. Depending on the material introduced, the patient may also be at risk for seizures after the test.

Vitamin D Blood Test

Blood is drawn from a vein and sent to a lab for analysis.

Results

Vitamin D is essential to the body because it helps calcium be absorbed by the body into bone and other tissue. It is present in dairy products and most products heavy in animal fats. A deficiency in the blood may point to a nutritional deficiency.

Broken bones due to trauma are a regular occurrence in childhood, but the most common bone disease in adults is osteoporosis.

Early detection is the most preventive measure. Low bone density can be easily and painlessly detected by x-ray, ultrasound and densitometry.

Sources: Diagnostic Tests for Men, Diagnostic Tests for Women, Journal of the American Medical Association.

TIP

Reduce your risk of osteoporosis: Add calcium and vitamin D to your diet, do weight-bearing exercise, don't smoke and limit caffeine and alcohol.

 You have impaired kidney function.
(Nuclear Bone Scan) Because poor kidney function may inhibit the absorption of the radioactive substance, this test may not have good results in patients with kidney disease.

 You are allergic to iodine or shellfish.
(Mylogram) Be sure to tell your doctor and the technician of any allergies before testing. Iodine-based contrast dye can cause a severe allergic reaction in those allergic to iodine or shellfish. If a problem is suspected, you may be given an antihistamine-steroid mixture to reduce your risk of a reaction.

 You have increased intracranial pressure.
(Mylogram) The spinal tap necessary for this test is not recommended for patients with elevated intracranial pressure.

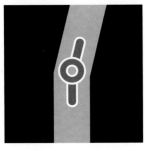

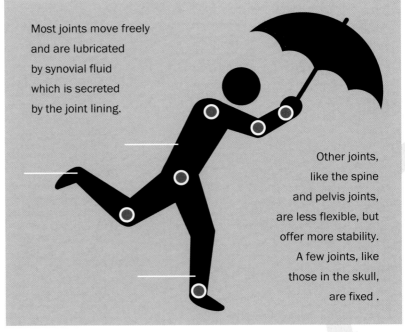

Most joints move freely and are lubricated by synovial fluid which is secreted by the joint lining.

Other joints, like the spine and pelvis joints, are less flexible, but offer more stability. A few joints, like those in the skull, are fixed .

Joints are defined as the junction of two or more bones.

They contain ligaments (tissue which connects bones), tendons (tissue that connects muscle to bone), cartilage (tissue that protects bones from rubbing each other directly) and membranes (that line the entire joint surface).

Osteoarthritis affects more than 21 million Americans and is the leading cause of disability in the US.

Arthroscopy

In this test a specialized arthroscope allows the physician to see directly inside the joint, including all the bones and connective tissue. A local anesthetic is injected into the joint to be examined. Depending on the joint, a general anesthetic may be administered as well. A buttonhole-sized incision is made in the skin, and the arthroscope is inserted through the hole into the joint area. The doctor then uses the scope to examine the joint visually. Arthroscopy may be accompanied by arthroscopic surgery.

Specialized surgical tools designed to repair torn tissue or remove fluid or loose fragments may be inserted through the same hole as the arthroscope. This type of surgery is preferable to an open surgical procedure (arthrotomy) because of its precision and because it opens up only a small hole in the skin. Because of the use of anesthesia, patients will be asked to refrain from food or water after midnight the day before the arthroscopy is performed.

Results

This test allows the doctor to see the bones

and connective tissues in a joint, and to view their functions directly. The patient may experience discomfort and swelling after the test is completed and should limit physical activity for several days. Physicians generally recommend that the patient not drive after the test.

Arthrocentesis (Joint Aspiration)

Synovial fluid lubricates the joints of the body. If a joint is painful or swollen, the doctor may perform an arthrocentesis to remove excessive synovial fluid or to examine

ACTION ITEMS

What to do if...

1 **You have fibrous ankylosis.**
(Arthroscopy) If you have fibrous ankylosis, which causes stiffening of the joints in a fixed position, arthroscopy may not be appropriate for you.

2 **You have local skin or wound infection.**
(Arthroscopy, Arthrocentisis) To avoid the risk of spreading infection, arthroscopy and arthrocentisis should not be performed on people with infection near the affected joint.

3 **You are allergic to iodine or shellfish.**
(Arthrogram) Be sure to tell your doctor and the technician of any allergies before testing. Iodine-based contrast dye can cause a severe allergic reaction in those allergic to iodine or shellfish. If a problem is suspected, you may be given an antihistamine-steroid mixture to reduce your risk of a reaction.

4 **You are claustrophobic.**
(MRI) Ask your doctor if the facility doing the testing has an "open" MRI—a larger unit that is open on some sides. Otherwise, you may ask to be sedated during the procedure.

the fluid. After the skin over the joint is cleaned and sterilized, a local anesthetic is injected. The doctor then inserts a needle into the joint cavity to withdraw synovial fluid. Despite the anesthetic, patients may experience mild discomfort when the needle is inserted. Depending upon the reason for the arthrocentesis, the synovial fluid may be examined after removal.

Results

An elevated white blood cell count is a good indicator for inflammation. Other studies that may be ordered include analysis of uric acid crystals (if gout is suspected) or a microscopic examination or culture (if infection is suspected).

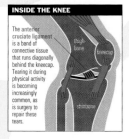

INSIDE THE KNEE

The anterior cruciate ligament is a band of connective tissue that runs diagonally behind the kneecap. Tearing it during physical activity is becoming increasingly common, as is surgery to repair these tears.

Arthrogram

Regular x-rays of joints have limited ability to differentiate between types of joint tissue. In this test dye is injected into the joints, which makes it possible to distinguish the soft tissue structures within the joints. It is

most often performed on the knee. The joint to be examined is cleaned and sterilized. A needle is inserted into the joint, and dye is injected. The patient moves the joint around to distribute the dye. X-rays are taken of the joint from different angles.

Results

These x-rays can show tears and loose pieces of tissue or bone, as well as the functioning of the joint. Arthroscopy is usually more accurate than an arthrogram and is often preferred to this test.

Uric Acid Blood Test

Blood is drawn from a vein and sent to a lab for analysis.

Results

Elevated uric acid levels predispose patients to attacks of gout—the painful swelling of the joints due to excessive accumulation of uric acid.

Magnetic Resonance Imaging (MRI)

The patient lies on a table, which slides into a machine. 257 The patient lies still as the imager thumps and moves around for 30 to 90 minutes. In some cases, just before the test begins, a safe contrast dye may be injected in a vein

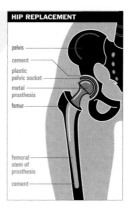

HIP REPLACEMENT

pelvis
cement
plastic pelvic socket
metal prosthesis
femur
femoral stem of prosthesis
cement

to provide greater clarity.

Results

The images produced can help diagnose joint problems, especially in the knee and shoulder.

Erythrocyte Sedimentation Rate (ESR Blood Test)

Blood is drawn from a vein and sent to a lab for analysis. When the blood is allowed to stand in a special tube, red blood cells settle at varying rates.

Results

This test measures how much a sample of red blood cells settle in an hour. An increased rate of settling often is a good indicator of the presence of an inflammatory condition (e.g., arthritis), while a slow or normal rate is usually present in healthy individuals. Results help diagnose diseases such as arthritis and cancer.

Joint problems, such as arthritis, are usually treated by a rheumatologist— a specialist in arthritis and other afflictions of the joints.

Arthritis is not a single disorder, but the name of a collection of joint diseases—the most common being osteoarthritis 107— which have a number of causes. In addition to arthritis, other common joint disorders include tears of joint tissue, such as the rotator cuff or other tendons.

Sources: Diagnostic Tests for Men, Diagnostic Tests for Women.

TIP

Numbness, tingling or shooting pain in the hands and arm can be signs of carpal tunnel syndrome and is often caused by overuse of the hand and wrist.

5 **You are obese.**
(MRI) Extremely overweight people may not fit in a standard MRI unit. Ask your facility if they have an "open" unit that will accomodate your size.

6 **You have metallic implants.**
(MRI) Because of the strong magnetic field created by an MRI scanner, you will not be able to have an MRI if you have an implanted metallic device like a pacemaker.

7 **You are pregnant.**
(MRI) Be sure to tell your doctor if there is any chance you may be pregnant. Because these tests may be harmful to a fetus, pregnant women should not have MRIs.

A river that flows through 60,000 miles of veins and arteries, blood's main function is as a transport system, carrying oxygen and nutrients to all organs and tissues of the body. Blood also has a major role in fighting infection.

The average adult man has about 10 pints of blood in his body.

Blood Pressure

A cuff is wrapped around the patient's arm and is pumped full of air, obstructing circulation in the arm. While the cuff is loosened, a stethoscope is used on the arm to detect the return of circulation and the pressure is noted. The pressure is noted again as the sound of the blood against the artery markedly diminishes and then disappears.

Results

Blood pressure readings are conventionally given as a fraction. The top number, called systolic pressure, refers to the pressure right after the heart has contracted, at its peak. The bottom number, called diastolic pressure, measures pressure when the heart is relaxed. Although previous thinking was that people with pressures under 140/90 were not at risk, new guidelines suggest that pressures higher than 120/80 can mean trouble.

Doppler Ultrasound of the Extremities

The patient lies on an examination table. A water-soluble gel that enhances sound wave transmission is applied to the area being tested. A transducer attached to an ultrasound machine is rubbed over the area.

Results

Blood flow in the limb is evaluated. Results may show clots, trauma or other problems. This test can also be used to monitor the progression of certain diseases.

Complete Blood Count (CBC), Red Blood Cell or White Blood Cell

Blood is drawn from a vein and sent to a lab for analysis.

Results

This routine group of blood tests analyzes red blood cells, hemoglobin levels, the hematocrit (percentage of red blood cells), white blood cells and platelets. Too few red blood cells and a low hematocrit mean anemia is present from causes such as infection, iron deficiency, internal bleeding or cancer. A high white-cell count can indicate infection, inflammation and, occasionally, cancer. A lack of platelets can affect the clotting ability of the blood, or be a sign of leukemia.

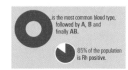

...is the most common blood type, followed by **A**, **B** and finally **AB**.

85% of the population is Rh positive.

Blood Typing

Blood is drawn from a vein and sent to a lab for analysis.

Results

There are a total of eight major blood types: A, B, AB, and O, each Rh positive or negative. This test is done before most surgical procedures and transfusions to determine the patient's blood type and to help prevent serious reactions.

Alcohol

Blood is drawn from a vein and sent to a lab for analysis.

Results

This test measures alcohol as a percentage of blood content. Anything over 0.05% impairs normal hand-eye coordination.

Blood Culture or Wound Culture

Blood is drawn or pus is obtained and sent to a lab for analysis.

Results

The sample is cultured in a lab, and if any growth results, it indicates an infection.

Blood Albumin and Globulin

Blood is drawn from a vein and sent to a lab for analysis.

Results

Too much globulin in the blood may indicate inflammatory diseases or certain forms of cancer. Too little albumin is

ACTION ITEMS

Dealing with anemia

Iron deficiency anemia occurs when the iron supply in the blood is decreased. Iron carries oxygen to all the blood cells in the body. If the red blood cells do not have enough oxygen, the cells cannot function properly. Here are some tips for recognizing and treating anemia.

Notify your physician if you have any of the symptoms listed, or if you are being treated for anemia and experience nausea, vomiting, fever, severe diarrhea or constipation.

1 Know the signs of anemia.

Fatigue
Weakness
Paleness
Tongue inflammation
Fainting
Shortness of breath
Elevated heart rate
Decreased appetite
Abdominal pain
Cravings for ice, paint or dirt
Frequent infections

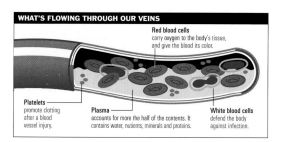

WHAT'S FLOWING THROUGH OUR VEINS

Red blood cells
carry oxygen to the body's tissue, and give the blood its color.

Platelets
promote clotting after a blood vessel injury.

Plasma
accounts for more the half of the contents. It contains water, nutrients, minerals and proteins.

White blood cells
defend the body against infection.

often due to kidney disease or poor nutrition.

Coombs' Test

Blood is drawn from a vein and sent to a lab for analysis.

Results

Certain antibodies in the blood, which can attack red blood cells, may point to an incompatible blood transfusion or certain types of anemia.

Infectious Disease Antibody

Blood is drawn from a vein and sent to a lab for analysis.

Results

Almost any kind of infection makes the body produce specific antibodies, which can be measured and used to diagnose illness or indicate a prior vaccination.

Iron, TIBC, Ferritin

Blood is drawn from a vein and sent to a lab for analysis.

Results

Iron-deficiency anemia is the most common diag-

nosis from this test. High iron levels result in a condition called hemochromatosis.

Hormone Testing

158

Lead

Blood is drawn from a vein and sent to a lab for analysis.

Results

High levels of lead, due to environmental exposure, can be quite toxic.

Prothrombin Time, Partial Thromboplastin Time, Bleeding Time

Blood is drawn from a vein and sent to a lab for analysis.

Results

These tests are used to see how well blood clots, and are given before some surgical procedures.

Reticulocyte Count

Blood is drawn from a vein and sent to a lab for analysis.

Results

This test measures the ability of bone marrow to

produce red blood cells. It also assists in the detection of some types of anemia and measures the effectiveness of certain vitamins and minerals to stimulate red blood cell production. Low reticulocyte counts generally indicate a failure of the bone marrow to respond normally because of a problem (e.g., iron deficiency, blood diseases such as leukemia and cancer).

Arterial Blood Gases

170

Carboxyhemoglobin

170

Erythrocyte Sedimentation Rate

189

Lipids/Cholesterol,

165

Triglycerides, HDL, LDL

165

Apolipoproteins

165

Heart Enzyme, CPK, CK, SGOT or LDH

165

Vitamin B1

165

Hematocrit

165

There are more tests of blood than there are of any other body component, and blood testing can reveal more about the body than just blood disorders.

There are three main types of blood tests: hematological (which look at components of the blood itself), biochemical (which look at chemicals in the blood) and microbiological (which examine the blood for bacteria, viruses and other small organisms).

Sources: Diagnostic Tests for Men, Diagnostic Tests for Women.

TIP

Toddlers are most at risk for chronic lead poisoning—a cause of brain, nerve and red blood cell damage, mostly from eating old, peeling paint.

 Consume adequate amounts of protein and iron through a well-balanced diet that includes meat, beans and leafy green vegetables. The foods below are especially good choices:

Iron-fortified breakfast cereal
Beef liver
Bran
Spinach
Kidney beans
Prune juice

 Limit milk.
Iron-deficient adults should limit milk to one pint a day, because milk can interfere with iron absorption.

 Follow your doctor's instructions.
If your health care provider recommends iron supplements, take them as instructed.

What are the risks of Down syndrome?

The risk of Down syndrome, a chromosomal disorder that causes mental retardation, increases dramatically with the mother's age. (Age is not sole risk factor.)

Mother's age:	Risk of Down syndrome is 1 in:
20	1,667
25	1,250
30	952
31	909
32	769
33	625
34	500
35	385
36	294
37	227
38	175
39	137
40	106
41	82
42	64
43	50
44	38
45	30
46	23
47	18
48	14
49	11

Screening vs. Diagnosis

Screening tests: Reveal only the possibility of problems with baby; often a good "starting point"

Diagnostic tests: Determine the existence of problem with a higher degree of certainty

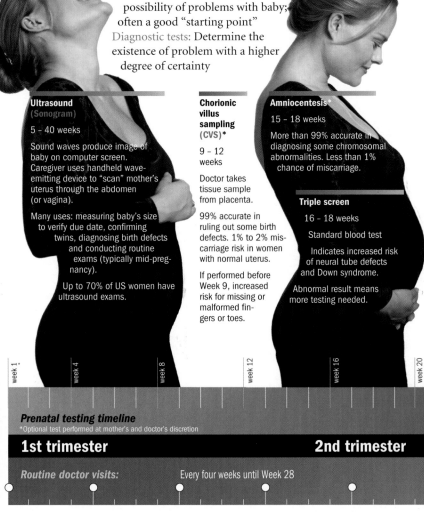

Ultrasound (Sonogram)

5 – 40 weeks

Sound waves produce image of baby on computer screen. Caregiver uses handheld wave-emitting device to "scan" mother's uterus through the abdomen (or vagina).

Many uses: measuring baby's size to verify due date, confirming twins, diagnosing birth defects and conducting routine exams (typically mid-pregnancy).

Up to 70% of US women have ultrasound exams.

Chorionic villus sampling (CVS)*

9 – 12 weeks

Doctor takes tissue sample from placenta.

99% accurate in ruling out some birth defects. 1% to 2% miscarriage risk in women with normal uterus.

If performed before Week 9, increased risk for missing or malformed fingers or toes.

Amniocentesis*

15 – 18 weeks

More than 99% accurate in diagnosing some chromosomal abnormalities. Less than 1% chance of miscarriage.

Triple screen

16 – 18 weeks

Standard blood test

Indicates increased risk of neural tube defects and Down syndrome.

Abnormal result means more testing needed.

week 1 | week 4 | week 8 | week 12 | week 16 | week 20

Prenatal testing timeline
*Optional test performed at mother's and doctor's discretion

1st trimester   **2nd trimester**

Routine doctor visits: Every four weeks until Week 28

Routine doctor visits: ■ First visit: Complete history and physical; due date estimated. Tests may include: Blood and Rh typing, anemia, rubella, Tay-Sachs disease, sickle-cell anemia, drug use, sexually transmitted diseases. ■ Every visit: Urine tests for diabetes and pregnancy-induced high blood pressure (preeclampsia). ■ Month 3 visit and thereafter: Baby's heartbeat monitored.

ACTION ITEMS

Choosing your health care provider

Start by asking friends, nurses or childbirth educators for their recommendations.

If you are not pleased with your current gynecologist (or other provider of well-woman care), this is the time to change. Do not feel a sense of obligation to a health care provider with whom you are not completely satisfied.

Determine your options. If you have special medical conditions (e.g., diabetes), you may need a professional who delivers in a hospital setting. If your history is less complicated, you may want to consider additional options, such as a certified nurse-midwife who works in a birthing center.

Phone screening: Questions for the office staff

- Where did the healthcare provider train? What are her credentials?
- How many other providers are in this practice?
- How likely will it be that the one I've chosen will attend my delivery?
- At which facilities (hospitals, birthing centers) does she deliver?
- What are the fees for all prenatal visits and delivery? When are payments due?
- Could I briefly interview (at no cost) the person I've chosen?
- How long are the routine office visits? How long of a wait (if any) should I expect when I have a scheduled visit?

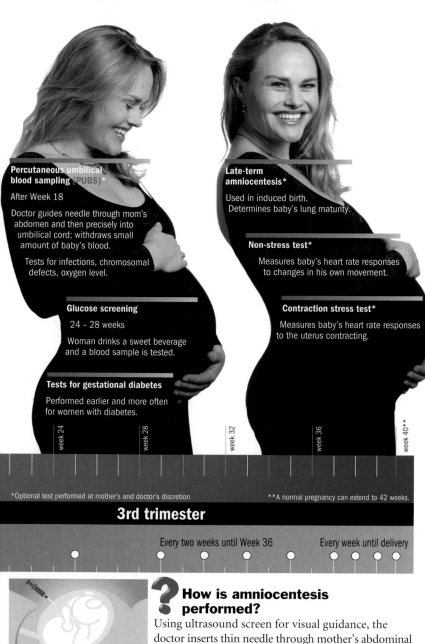

Percutaneous umbilical blood sampling (PUBS)*

After Week 18

Doctor guides needle through mom's abdomen and then precisely into umbilical cord; withdraws small amount of baby's blood.

Tests for infections, chromosomal defects, oxygen level.

Glucose screening

24 – 28 weeks

Woman drinks a sweet beverage and a blood sample is tested.

Tests for gestational diabetes

Performed earlier and more often for women with diabetes.

Late-term amniocentesis*

Used in induced birth. Determines baby's lung maturity.

Non-stress test*

Measures baby's heart rate responses to changes in his own movement.

Contraction stress test*

Measures baby's heart rate responses to the uterus contracting.

week 24   week 28   week 32   week 36   week 40**

*Optional test performed at mother's and doctor's discretion   **A normal pregnancy can extend to 42 weeks.

3rd trimester

Every two weeks until Week 36   Every week until delivery

? How is amniocentesis performed?

Using ultrasound screen for visual guidance, the doctor inserts thin needle through mother's abdominal wall and extracts a few teaspoons of amniotic fluid. Mother feels slight cramping or no pain at all.

Today a pregnant woman can learn a tremendous amount about the health of her baby.

Most tests ultimately reassure parents.

In some cases, less-than-conclusive results place parents in the position of having to make some very difficult decisions. And in still other cases, results give parents the option of having their baby undergo a surgery, blood transfusion or other treatment while still in the womb. A word of reassurance: the vast majority of babies are born healthy.

Source: Understanding Children, understandingchildren.com, TOP and Civitas.

Getting to know you: Questions for the healthcare provider

- How can I reach you in case of emergency? Can I call even if I have less urgent questions?
- Which type of childbirth classes do you recommend?
- Will you be the person attending my delivery? If not, who would be there in your place?
- How much time do you usually spend with a woman during labor?
- What advice do you give your patients about managing labor pain? How do you feel about epidurals and other medications?
- What percentage of your deliveries are cesarean sections?

Money matters: Questions for your insurance company

- What is the coverage for prenatal care?
- Can I choose whichever healthcare provider and facility I want? If not, what are my choices?
- Will I have to pay a deductible when I go to the hospital to deliver?
- How long of a hospital stay is covered for a normal delivery?
- Am I covered for any treatments or emergency care I might need during my pregnancy?
- Are there any treatments that are not covered?
- Am I covered for childbirth education classes?
- Will my baby's costs after delivery be covered? For how long?

❓ What's a full body scan?

A full body scan is an **early detection program for disease** that is non-invasive. Instead of waiting for symptoms of heart disease or cancer to appear, some doctors offer specialized scanning to detect tumors or blocked vessels before they become a medical problem.

The scans are done with an **electron beam computed tomography scanner**, often called a CT scanner. The procedure takes about 15 minutes.

How it works: a conventional x-ray shows front, rear or side views of the body. You see only the outside of the organs. A CT scan takes **axial views** of the body—**dozens of thin slices** through it—which can then be viewed separately, or reassembled by computers into three-dimensional, high-definition images of whole organs (soft tissue and blood vessels as well as bones). Since the images are digital, they can be sent to experts anywhere in the world for immediate analysis or a second opinion.

❓ How much does it cost?

Heart scans costs about $500; heart and lungs is about $850; **a full body scan can be anywhere from $1,000 to $1,500.** But there could

be additional costs: since no tests can be 100% reliable if the scan picks up unknown problems (which may be nothing at all) you may need surgery or other invasive procedures to rule out disease.

❓ What diseases & other problems might show up in the scans?

Usually, a "full body scan" covers areas from the shoulders to the pelvis; by examining the images produced, radiologists can detect evidence or early signs of these problems:

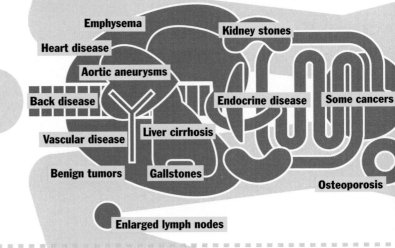

Emphysema
Heart disease
Aortic aneurysms
Back disease
Vascular disease
Liver cirrhosis
Benign tumors
Gallstones
Kidney stones
Endocrine disease
Some cancers
Osteoporosis
Enlarged lymph nodes

Area covered by a full body scan

Sources: FDA; HealthView; seniorsite.com, johnshopkinsafter50.com.

ACTION ITEMS Considering a full body scan

Consider these points when when deciding whether to have a full body scan.

1 Your attitude toward healthcare
Will you follow up with regular medical care even if you get a "clean bill of health?"

2 Your doctor's advice
Are you foregoing tests recommended by your doctor? *A full body scan can't detect problems like abnormal heart rhythm, high blood pressure, high PSA levels, high glucose levels and infection.*

3 Your age
How old are you? *The younger you are, the less likely a problem will be detected.*

4 Your health
Do you currently have any symptoms that warrant testing?

5 Your risk factors
Do you have risk factors that warrant this type of procedure even if no symptoms are present?

❓ Why is the procedure controversial?

Because the long-term benefits and risks have not been researched. The Food and Drug Administration has approved CT x-ray scanning only as a diagnostic tool to be used when symptoms exist, or when there is reason for the test. No studies have been done to support screening people without symptoms. Also the dose of radiation from a CT procedure can be 500 times larger than the dose from a conventional chest X-ray, according to FDA radiation physicists.

❓ Does a body scan replace other screening tests?

No. Even when the quality of a full body scan is good, it is not a substitute for other tests. These include: mammography for breast cancer, pap smear for cervical cancer, bone densitometry for osteoporosis, blood tests for prostate-specific antigen (prostate cancer), glucose for diabetes and cholesterol for heart disease. **However, scanning has been shown to be good in detecting pancreatic cancer,** the symptoms of which are often too far advanced by the time they are discovered by conventional diagnosis. And while the colonoscopy is currently thought to be the best way to detect colorectal cancer, **virtual colonoscopies** are seen to be a promising and valuable tool for body scanning.

Is it worthwhile to pay for a full body scan?

Probably not, if you are young and healthy with no symptoms or a family history suggesting disease.

❓ What does not show up in the scans?

The term full body scan misleads some people into thinking that everything that could be wrong with their body will appear. But scans cannot show high blood pressure, high cholesterol levels, infection or abnormal heart rhythm.

Pregnant women should not have a full body scan.

❓ Is a full body scan covered by insurance?

Probably not, especially if you are in good health. But if you had some symptoms in your abdomen, and your doctor wanted to see a scan of just that area, your insurance company might pay for that, but not for a full body scan.

THE CT SCANNING MACHINE
158

The patient lies on a table which is moved slowly into the donut-shaped scanner gantry. This houses a rotating x-ray tube and receptors. The machine makes a series of images—"slices" through the body—which can be viewed on computer monitors.

---

6 Radiation exposure
Are you willing to expose yourself to the levels of radiation produced by a full body scan?

7 The facility
Is the facility administering the test affiliated with a major hospital or other respected health facility?

8 The staff
Is the person performing the test a board-certified radiologist with experience reading CT scans?

9 The equipment
Does the testing facility have a state-of-the-art multi-detector CT (MDCT) that can reconstruct the data in 3-D images?

10 The follow up
Will the test include a comprehensive evaluation that's reported to your doctor?

11 Cost
Can you afford the test? Some will tell you you can't afford not to get tested. *Full body scans are only rarely covered by insurance.*

US News & World Report annually ranks "America's Best Hospitals." 247 Beginning with 6,003 facilities, the hospitals are narrowed to 203 different medical centers in 17 specialties from cancer to urology.
Source: US News & World Report.

At 86, Yan had lived a long and independent life—supporting himself as a bookkeeper into his mid-70s. He was a tough, independent, clear-headed man. He lived in the Boston area, surrounded by fine medical schools and hospitals, and greatly respected his white-coated doctors, well-known experts in their fields.

For over a decade Yan fought a rare blood disorder, constantly fine-tuning his medications and managing his lifestyle 201 to avoid problems. Now, his kidneys were acting up and his doctors said he needed a new heart valve and probably a bypass, too.

At nearly 90, he knew there weren't a great many years left to him. His three grandchildren were his greatest joy in life. His granddaughter was nearly a high school graduate and would soon head to college. Yan's twin grandsons would follow their sister the following year. For Yan, nothing meant more

Eating a healthy diet, exercising, taking your medicine exactly as prescribed and following the advice of your health care providers is good lifestyle management. You reduce your risks for disease and improve your chances for better health.
Source: American Heart Association.

There are alternative treatments for bypass surgery, though they aren't right for everyone. Medication is a non-surgical treatment as is balloon or laser angioplasty. Your doctor can help you decide on the best choice for you.
Source: American Heart Association.

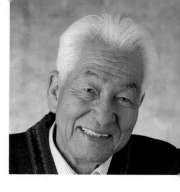

Yan may have lived longer had he known all the options.

than seeing all three of them graduate and start off in the world as adults.

Surgery, his family knew, would have some risks, but could prolong his life by two or three years. His surgeon assured them everything would be okay.

A family friend gently warned Yan's children that this looked like a fairly risky operation. Statistics suggested that as someone his age, with his health problems, he faced a 20 to 30 percent chance of death from the difficult surgery, and a high chance of other complications—like stroke 115—if he survived. His children responded, "He wants the surgery and he trusts his doctors." They didn't talk with Yan or his doctor about the chances of a bad outcome.

The surgery went well, but soon after Yan slipped into a coma. Three weeks later he died never knowing he had a choice.

Heart attack, stroke and kidney damage are severe complications from surgery. Though rare, they most often occur in patients with preexisting conditions.
Source: Mayo Clinic Family Health Book.

Informed consent lets you fully participate in your health care decisions. It means that a doctor talks to you about risks and benefits of all possible treatments before deciding on which one to use. And it means the doctor makes sure that that you understand the information presented to you.
Source: Ethics in Medicine, University of Washington School of Medicine.

For most disorders, an early, clear diagnosis, followed by the proper treatment, will give you the best chance of a successful outcome.

If you start your treatment late, there may be more risks involved and a longer recovery time afterwards. Before recommending a course of treatment your doctor should take into account your age and medical history. You may be advised to stop smoking or to lose weight.

What are the options?

Most treatment falls into one of these four categories:

**lifestyle
drugs
surgery
therapy**

It's likely that a combination of these will be used in most cases; for instance, surgery is often followed by a course of physical rehabilitation therapy.

You'll begin by discussing the case with your doctor.

For **minor illnesses,** this might be a short discussion. But for a **chronic 219 or more serious disorder**, you may have a choice between surgery and drugs, or different forms of surgery. You'll discuss the possible side effects and risks involved. Nothing will happen until you give your consent.

In the past, most people accepted the doctor's offer of treatment with little question. Today, given our access to the Internet 325, we are better equipped to ask questions and to be more involved in decisions about treatment.

Source: American College of Physicians
Complete Home Medical Guide.

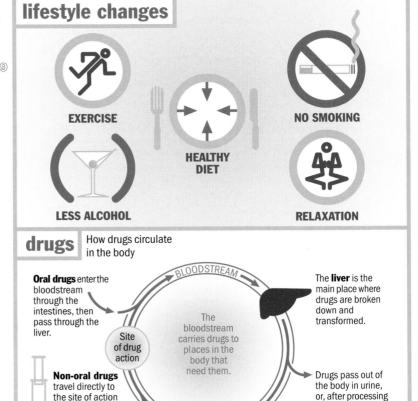

lifestyle changes

EXERCISE

HEALTHY DIET

LESS ALCOHOL

NO SMOKING

RELAXATION

drugs How drugs circulate in the body

BLOODSTREAM

Oral drugs enter the bloodstream through the intestines, then pass through the liver.

Site of drug action

The bloodstream carries drugs to places in the body that need them.

The **liver** is the main place where drugs are broken down and transformed.

Non-oral drugs travel directly to the site of action without passing through the liver.

Drugs pass out of the body in urine, or, after processing in the liver, are carried in bile to the intestines, then excreted in feces.

ACTION ITEMS
Questions to ask your doctor

1 What are all the treatment options available for my condition?

2 What are the benefits of this treatment and what will it do for me?

3 What are the negative and positive side effects of each treatment?

4 What is your success rate with this treatment? How long have you used it on your patients?

5 How do people my age and with similar symptoms respond to this treatment?

6 Does this treatment require a hospital stay? If so, for how long? Which hospital are you affiliated with? And what's the hospital's track record for this procedure?

7 How long will it take me to recover from this treatment?

8 Where can I read about the latest research about this treatment?

surgery 205

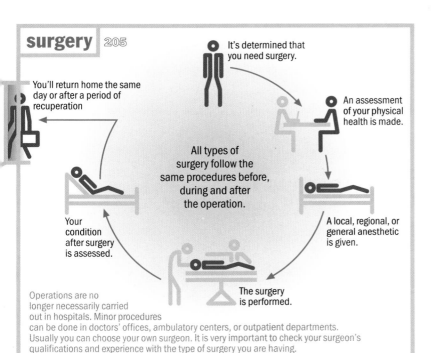

It's determined that you need surgery.

An assessment of your physical health is made.

A local, regional, or general anesthetic is given.

The surgery is performed.

Your condition after surgery is assessed.

You'll return home the same day or after a period of recuperation

All types of surgery follow the same procedures before, during and after the operation.

Operations are no longer necessarily carried out in hospitals. Minor procedures can be done in doctors' offices, ambulatory centers, or outpatient departments. Usually you can choose your own surgeon. It is very important to check your surgeon's qualifications and experience with the type of surgery you are having.

therapy

A range of therapies are available to treat illness and its aftermath.

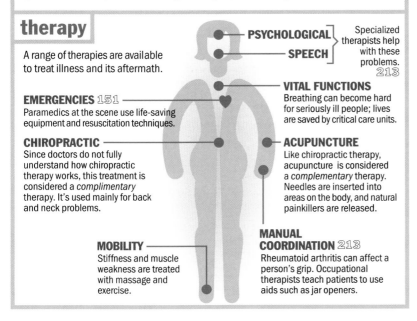

PSYCHOLOGICAL
SPEECH
Specialized therapists help with these problems. 213

VITAL FUNCTIONS
Breathing can become hard for seriously ill people; lives are saved by critical care units.

EMERGENCIES 151
Paramedics at the scene use life-saving equipment and resuscitation techniques.

CHIROPRACTIC
Since doctors do not fully understand how chiropractic therapy works, this treatment is considered a *complimentary* therapy. It's used mainly for back and neck problems.

ACUPUNCTURE
Like chiropractic therapy, acupuncture is considered a *complementary* therapy. Needles are inserted into areas on the body, and natural painkillers are released.

MOBILITY
Stiffness and muscle weakness are treated with massage and exercise.

MANUAL COORDINATION 213
Rheumatoid arthritis can affect a person's grip. Occupational therapists teach patients to use aids such as jar openers.

Here is an overview.

Treatment milestones

1900	Psychoanalysis developed
1901	Radium discovered: led to cancer treatment
1904	Discovery of 4 major blood groups: safe transfusions
1921	Insulin discovered: life-saving diabetes treatment
1928	First antibiotic, penicillin, discovered
1940	Penicillin used to treat infections
1943	Kidney dialysis machine
1950	Chemotherapy used for leukemia
1954	First kidney transplant
1959	Flexible fiberoptic endo-scope allows treatment without open surgery
1967	First heart transplant
1976	Angioplasty for widening narrowed arteries—less invasive than bypass
1986	First heart-lung-liver transplant
1987	Fluoxetine, one of a new class of antidepressants
1990	First attempts at gene replacement therapy
1994	Superglue used to close wounds
1997	Robot arm holds instru-ments during minimally invasive surgery

9 How will this treatment affect my lifestyle? Are there any complementary treatments that might help?

10 If a treatment involves surgery:
- Is there an alternative to surgery?
- How many of these procedures have you done in the last month? Last year?
- Do you keep track of outcomes?
- What's your complication rate?
- Who else is on the surgical team? (i.e., anesthesiologist, surgical nurse, etc.)

11 If a close family member of yours was in my situation, which treatment option would you recommend and why?

12 How much will this treatment cost compared to alternative treatments? How much will I have to pay toward the cost?

Scientists have researched the way in which people change their lifestyle. A study by the University of Rhode Island found that there are **5 stages** in changing health behaviors:

precontemplation: when there is no desire to change

contemplation: when there is a desire to change, but nothing is done about it

preparation: when initial steps are taken, such as buying a book or joining a program

action: when steps are taken to change lifestyle

maintenance: when the changes become a permanent part of daily life

? Which conditions respond well to lifestyle changes?

They include:

GERD (gastroesophageal reflux disease)

heart disease

high blood pressure

high cholesterol

Heart and blood vessel diseases account for more premature deaths each year than nearly all other illnesses combined. Yet heart disease is preventable (even reversible) for most people.
Source: WebMD.

What to do

GERD 123 may happen less often or disappear completely if you make simple changes in your daily routine. The goal is to eliminate factors that cause **reflux.**

Some common foods and drinks relax the lower esophageal sphincter (LES), increasing the risk of reflux.

So avoid these triggers: alcohol, chocolate, carbonated drinks, coffee, tea, soft drinks with caffeine, spicy foods, fatty foods, citrus fruits and juices, tomatoes and tomato sauces. **Don't eat within 2–3 hours of bedtime. Sleep with your head raised a few inches.**

Stop smoking: cigarettes contain chemicals that relax the LES as they pass from the lungs to the blood.

Lose weight 127 : obesity increases pressure in the abdomen. This forces the contents of the stomach past the LES.

Avoid tight-fitting belts or garments around the waist. They may squeeze the stomach and cause stomach contents to pass the LES.

Source: Yahoo! Health.

What to do

Pace yourself: don't do everything all at once. Gradual change will have a more permanent effect than drastic changes. Don't think of your new diet or exercise regimen as being temporary; **it's a new, healthier way of life.**

Reduce saturated fat and cholesterol in your diet.

Eat more foods rich in **carbohydrates and fiber** (fruits, vegetables, whole grains).

Maintain a **healthy weight.** (And keep a diary, so you *know* what you are eating.)

Exercise more.
47

Regular exercise helps lower cholesterol and lose weight, which further lowers cholesterol.

These changes are good for everyone in your family. As well as lowering your cholesterol level, they'll lower family members' risk of developing chronic heart disease, cancer, high blood pressure and obesity.

ACTION ITEMS Supporting your loved ones

Many diseases and conditions require one or more lifestyle changes for proper control or recovery and a healthy life. And, lifestyle changes are often the most difficult adjustments for any of us to make. Habits are formed over a lifetime and generally are not easily changed, even if we've been diagnosed with an illness and told by our doctor that they should be changed. As a family member or friend, you can help make these changes easier on your loved ones.. Here are just a few of the many ways you can help:

1 Talk about it.
Caring for yourself when you have a health issue can add stress to your life and cause feelings of anger, fear, sadness or depression. Encourage your family member or friend to share feelings about their illness with you, their healthcare team or a support group.

2 Learn more. 328
Show your loved one that you care by learning more about their condition and how it is treated.

3 Participate.
Attend medical appointments and educational sessions with your loved one. Learn how to monitor their condition, administer treatments and handle possible crises.

What to do

First, do everything listed on the opposite page, under high cholesterol.

Eat less salt.

Drink less alcohol. 49
(No more than one or two drinks a day)

Get your blood pressure into line with the new national blood pressure guidelines. Manage the stress in your life.

It's easier to prevent heart disease than to reverse it. If you do have to take medication to reduce blood pressure, these lifestyle changes will make your medications more effective.

Blood pressure: the new guidelines

The higher of the two numbers ("systolic") is the pressure when the heart is beating. **120** / **80** normal
The lower number ("diastolic") is the pressure between heartbeats when the heart is at rest.

$\frac{120\text{-}139}{80\text{-}89}$ pre-hypertension

Recommended lifestyle changes: lose excess weight; exercise more; quit smoking; eat more fruit and vegetables; cut salt

$\frac{140\text{-}159}{90\text{-}99}$ stage 1 hypertension

Recommended: the lifestyle changes; one or more drugs (probably a diuretic) to reach 140/90

$\frac{160+}{100+}$ stage 2 hypertension

Recommended: the lifestyle changes; drug treatment (probably two) to bring numbers down to 140/90

Source: *New York Times*; JAMA.

DIET 43 isn't just about avoiding certain foods. **What you eat as a replacement is vital.** If you change from a high-fat, high-cholesterol diet that's rich in animal protein, to a low-fat, plant-based diet, you eat less disease-promoting food, but you benefit from 1,000 substances that help protect you from heart disease (as well as cancer). Eating fruit, vegetables, grains, beans and soy decreases cardiac risk.

3 grams a day of **flax seed** may reduce the risk of sudden heart attack by more than **50%**

Remember: diet is only a part of your lifestyle change. Studies show that people who are lonely and depressed are more likely to get sick. They are more likely to smoke, overeat (and drink) and work too hard as a way of coping with depression. They may die earlier than people who feel loved and connected to their community.

Source: WebMD Health.

In certain cases, changing the way you live and eat may help keep you off medication.

---

4 **Give encouragement.**
Encourage your loved one to stick with their new practices without nagging or becoming a policeman. Motivational calendars or diaries can be helpful for tracking progress.

5 **Change your diet.** 43
Making changes in how one eats is probably one of the most difficult behavioral changes. You can help by learning about your loved one's recommended meal plan and by eating and avoiding the same foods. Most meal plans for people with health conditions are healthy and can be prepared for the entire family.

6 **Exercise together.**
Physical activity is often also recommended. The health benefits of exercise include the control of blood sugar levels, blood pressure and body weight. Support your loved one by offering to exercise with them when possible. Before beginning, confirm that the exercise your loved one is undertaking has been recommended by his or her physician.

7 **Help get the tools they need.**
Make sure your loved one has the items needed for the regimen: appropriate shoes for exercising, healthy food choices and proper health-monitoring supplies.

All in the family

Below are some common families of drugs (and the problems for which they are often used).

INFECTION
Antibiotics (bacteria)
Antivirals (viruses)

CARDIOVASCULAR
ACE Inhibitors (congestive heart failure, hypertension 111)
Alpha Blockers (hypertension, benign prostatic hyperplasia)
Beta Blockers (hypertension, arrhythmias, migraine)
Diuretics (hypertension, edema)
Digitalis (heart failure, atrial fibrillation)
Nitrates (angina)
Statins (high cholesterol)

BLOOD
Anticoagulants (embolism, myocardial infarction, atrial fibrillation)
Thrombolytics (acute myocardial infarction, stroke 115, pulmonary embolism)

RESPIRATORY
Decongestants (congestion)
Expectorants (cough from upper respiratory infection)
Bronchodilators (asthma 97)

DIGESTIVE
Antiemetics (nausea, vomiting)
Antacids (hyperacidity)
Antispasmodics (colitis, cramps)
H2 Antagonists (ulcers, acid reflux 123)
Proton Pump Inhibitors (ulcers, acid reflux)

MUSCULOSKELETAL
NSAIDs (rheumatoid arthritis, osteoarthritis 107, pain)
Muscle Relaxants (skeletal muscle spasms)

NERVOUS SYSTEM
Analgesics (pain)
Antianxiety drugs (anxiety)
Antidepressants (depression)

ENDOCRINE
Insulin (diabetes 121)

❓ What are the different ways that drugs can be introduced into the body?

There are many ways, but before any new drug is put on the market, it must be tested and approved by the Food and Drug Administration.

A license is issued once a drug is shown to be safe and effective, and can be withdrawn if unacceptable side effects become evident later.

The drugs are absorbed through the thin mucous membrane directly into the bloodstream.

NASAL
A spray into the nose

BUCCAL
A tablet in the cheek

SUBLINGU
A tablet unde the tongue

SUBCUTANEOUS
Drugs are implanted or injected into fatty tissue just below the skin. They disperse slowly into the bloodstream.

INTRAMUSCULAR
Drugs are injected into a muscle in the upper arm, thigh, or buttock, then dispersed into the bloodstream.

TRANSDERMAL
Drugs are released continuously from an adhesive patch or gel on the surface of the skin.

DERMAL
Topical drug preparations may be applied directly to the skin.

INTRAVENOUS
Drugs are injected directly into a blood vessel, allowing them to take effect very quickly.

ACTION ITEMS

Ask questions

Here's what you should ask before starting a new medication:

1. **Why has this medication been prescribed?**

2. **What can I expect this medication to do for me and how does it work?**

3. **Are there any behavioral or dietary changes I could make to treat this problem?**

4. **What might happen if I don't take this medicine?**
   This is the question that helps with the risk-benefit analysis.

5. **What are the short and long-term side effects?**

6. **Which side effects signal dangerous reactions, and what should I do if they occur?**

7. **How will this interact with other drugs I am taking?**

8. **Can you give me any written information so I can learn more about this drug?**
   Ask for the drug class and for the generic name. Knowing the drug class can be helpful in case information arises about another drug in the same class that may have parallels to your own.

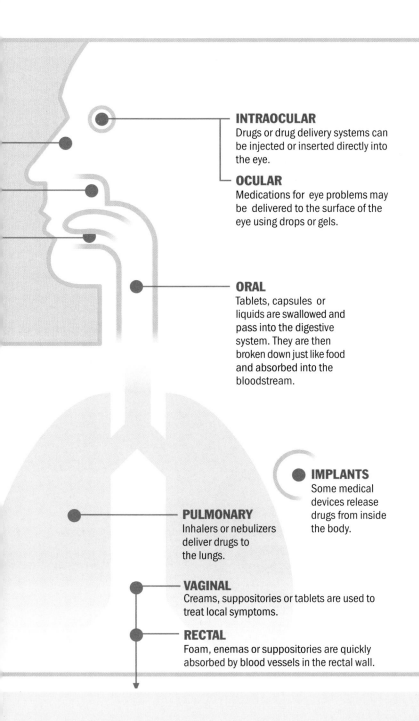

INTRAOCULAR
Drugs or drug delivery systems can be injected or inserted directly into the eye.

OCULAR
Medications for eye problems may be delivered to the surface of the eye using drops or gels.

ORAL
Tablets, capsules or liquids are swallowed and pass into the digestive system. They are then broken down just like food and absorbed into the bloodstream.

IMPLANTS
Some medical devices release drugs from inside the body.

PULMONARY
Inhalers or nebulizers deliver drugs to the lungs.

VAGINAL
Creams, suppositories or tablets are used to treat local symptoms.

RECTAL
Foam, enemas or suppositories are quickly absorbed by blood vessels in the rectal wall.

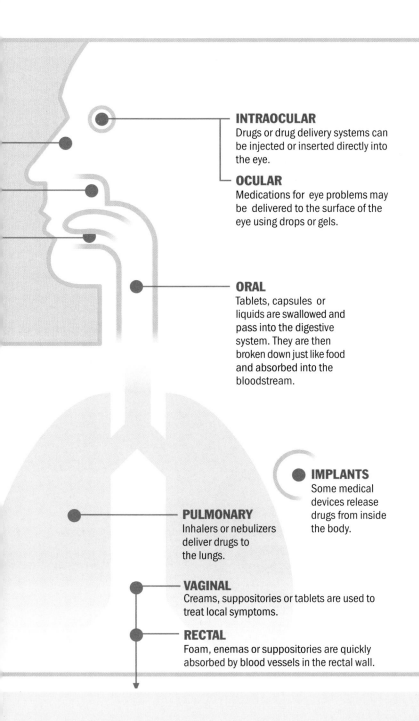

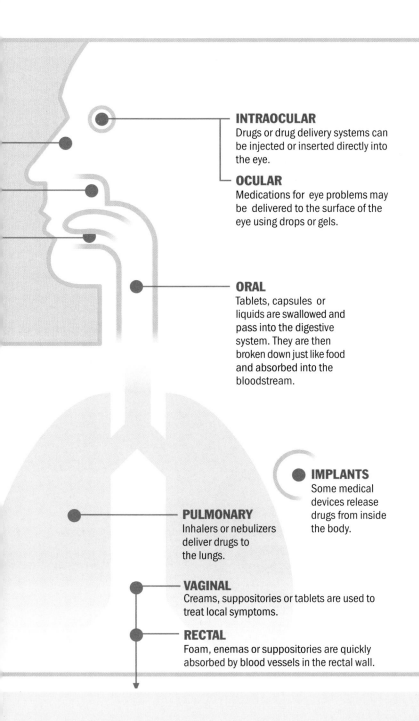

How are drugs used as treatment?

Drugs can be delivered to the body in a variety of ways.

Ranging from eye drops to suppositories, the drug delivery method used for treatment is often chosen based on how the drug is metabolized 198 and area of the body that the drug is targeting.

Sources: Drugs: Prescription, Non-prescription & Herbal.

---

9 **What is the dose and how many times a day should I take it?**

10 **At what times should I take it?**
Pull out your pill planner and ask the doctor to pencil in the best times.

11 **Should I take this medication with food or without?**
Also ask if there any foods or beverages, like grapefruit juice or alcohol, that may interact with your new medication.

12 **When can I expect to see results? Can I measure the effects myself?**

13 **When should I stop taking the medication or when should I have my progress reviewed?**

14 **What should I do if I forget a dose?**
It's important to ask because the answer will change depending on the drugs you take. A dose should be skipped in some cases and taken as soon as you remember in others.

15 **Can I get a refill and how often?**

TIP
If your weight changes by more than 10% (up or down), you may need your medication dosing re-evaluated by your doctor.

12 of the most commonly performed surgical procedures

Be sure to discuss specific procedures and risks with your doctor prior to any surgical procedure.

HEART BYPASS 75
The Procedures
Mammary artery bypass graft (used for one blockage)
- An incision is made along the breast bone, in the center of the chest.
- One of the mammary arteries within the chest, usually the left, is used to create the bypass.
- The chosen artery is then cut below the site of the block.
- The upper end of the artery is left attached to the subclavian artery and the lower end is tied off.
- The freed end of the mammary artery is connected to the coronary artery at a point beyond the blockage to supply blood to the heart muscle.

Saphenous vein bypass graft (the saphenous vein runs the length of the leg) is used for more than one blockage.
- A long incision is made down the leg.
- The saphenous vein is removed in its entirety.
- The vein is divided into sections so that several coronary arteries can be bypassed.
- Another incision is made along the breast bone, in the center of the chest.
- One end of each section is attached to the aorta (main artery in body).
- The other end is attached to the coronary artery beyond the blockage.

Possible risks*
- Excessive bleeding
- Arrhythmia (heart irregularity)
- Peripheral vascular disease
- Cognitive decline (ability to process mentally day-to-day tasks)
- Death (very rare; usually in the case of an emergency procedure)
- Risks are higher in older patients, especially those that have other complications

GALL BLADDER REMOVAL
The Procedure
Laproscopic cholecystectomy
- Four small incisions are made in the abdomen.
- One hole is made near your navel so that the laparoscope can be inserted (carbon dioxide is administered first so that the surgeon may see inside the cavity).
- Instruments are then inserted into three different insertions to grasp and retract the gallbladder, freeing it from your body; two holes are made on the right side below the ribcage, and one hole is made in the upper abdomen.

Possible risks
- Adverse reactions to anesthesia
- Excessive bleeding
- Damage to the bile duct
- Bile leakage into the abdomen
- Pain in your right shoulder as a result of the operation

APPENDECTOMY
The Procedure
Traditional, open surgery
- Requires a single, four-inch abdominal incision.
- Surrounding blood vessels are tied off.
- The appendix is removed.
Laparoscopic surgery
- Requires a few, small incisions.
- Laparoscope is inserted into the primary incision to create a magnified view of the abdomen.
- Instruments are then inserted into the remaining incisions.
- Surrounding blood vessels are tied off.
- The appendix is removed.
Possible risks
- Excessive bleeding
- Adverse reactions to the anesthesia such as problems breathing

TONSILLECTOMY
The Procedure
- A tube is passed through the nose and down the trachea (allows breathing and for the back of the throat to be packed with absorbent material so th blood does not escape down the throat).
- The mouth is held open by a gag (stainless steel instrument).
- One tonsil is grasped with a forceps and pulled toward the front of the mouth stretching it.
- An incision is made through the mucous membra lining the mouth close to the body of the tonsil.
- The tonsil is then removed.
- Bleeding is stopped by securing the vessel in force and tying it off (if it is large) or cauterizing it (if it small).
- This is repeated on the other tonsil.
Possible risk
- Hemorrhaging

ANGIOPLASTY 75
The Procedures
Percutaneous transluminal coronary angioplasty
- A guided wire is inserted through the femoral arte in the groin and moved until it reaches the afflicte coronary artery.
- A deflated balloon catheter is passed up the wire until it reaches the desired location.
- It is then inflated to widen the narrowed area.
- This step is repeated several times to compress th deposits.
Stent assisted coronary angioplasty 259
- All of the above methods are followed.
- A stent (circular piece of wire mesh) is inserted after to keep the artery open.
- When the stent is released from the catheter it expands to become as wide as the artery.
Possible risks
- Damage to the wall of the coronary artery
- Weakening of the wall of the coronary artery
- Heart attack

HERNIA
The Procedures
Herniorrhaphy (most common)
Traditional repair
- A cut is made in the skin over the hernia, the intes is pushed back, and the weakened or torn muscl repaired with stitches.
Laparoscopic repair
- After a small incision, a laparoscope is inserted.
- Instruments are then inserted into several other, sr incisions to repair the hernia.
Hernioplast
- An incision is made at the site of the hernia, and small piece of mesh is inserted into the abdomin cavity covering the area of defect.
- It is then held in place with staples and accepted the body's tissue.
Possible risks
- Breathing problems
- Trouble urinating due to injury of the intestine or bladder (very rare)
- Excessive bleeding
- Formation of scar tissue

PROSTATECTOMY 95
The Procedures
Partial prostatectomy (part of the prostate gland is removed).
- A retroscope is administered through the urethra until it reaches the prostate gla
- A diathermy wire is then pushed along the retroscope and used to cut away excess prostate tissue, which widens the urethra.
- A catheter is administered to facilitate urination and bladder irrigation.
- An irrigation system is attached to the catheter to wash out prostate tissue and keep blood clots from forming.
Suprapubic (radical) prostatectomy
- An incision is made just above the pubic bone, in the lower abdomen.
- The entire prostate gland (the tumor), the seminal vesicles and the neck of the bladder are removed.
- The bladder neck is reconstructed and rejoined to the urethra.
- A catheter is administered to facilitate urination and bladder irrigation.
Perineal (radical) prostatectomy
- A curved incision is made between the back of the scrotum and the anus (then the operation is same as a retropubic prostatectomy).
Possible risks
- Excessive bleeding (less common in partial prostatectomies)
- Impotence (more common in older men)

ELECTIVE (COSMETIC) SURGERY
The Procedures
- **Rhinoplasty** reshapes the nose by reducing or increasing the size, removing a hump, changing the shape of the tip or ridge, narrowing the span between the nostrils or by changing the angle between the nose and the upper lip.
- **Liposuction** removes fat deposits that have not successfully been depleted by exercise and diet.
- **Blepharoplasty** correct drooping, upper eyelids and puffy bags below the eyes by removing fat, skin and muscle.
- **Augmentation mammaplasty** enhances the size of the breast using saline implants (the implant can be inserted directly under the breast tissue or under the chest wall).
- **Rhytidectomy** improves sagging, facial skin and jowls, as well as the loose area of the neck by removing fat, tightening muscles and redraping skin.

Possible risks
- Swelling
- Bruising
- Bleeding
- Tenderness/sensitivity in area of procedure
- Tightness
- Asymmetry
- Scarring

BACK SURGERY 135
The Procedure
- An incision will be made in the midline until the vertebrae and laminae are exposed.
- The muscle that is attached to the vertebrae will be temporarily separated.
- Using bone-cutting forceps, part, or all, of the protruding part of two adjacent vertebrae will be removed, as well as the arch on the side of the disk protrusion exposing the membrane that surrounds the spinal chord.
- Gently, the membrane is pushed to the opposite side of the enclosing vertebrae so that the nucleus pulposus is exposed.
- All of the protruding material is removed. (The vertical ligament that runs through the vertebral column may need to be severed; in rare cases the laminae may need to be removed from the adjacent vertebrae – this may make the spine unstable in supporting the body's weight and a fusion may need to be performed.)
- **If a fusion is necessary**, the disk(s) will need to be removed and the now adjacent bone surfaces will need to be roughened so that they heal together (at times reinforcing strips of bone taken from the fibula or elsewhere may be inlaid, or metal rods may be inserted to promote fusion).
- The muscles are now returned to their normal locations and the wound is closed.
- A catheter may be administered to help with urination.

Possible risks
- Excessive bleeding
- Blood clots
- Recurrent disk herniations
- Nerve damage (low risk)

> According to *Business Week*, "overdone" surgeries include: C-section, gallbladder removal, hysterectomy and surgery for back pain.

A **laparoscope** is a thin tube with an attached light source and video camera. The magnified images are shown on a monitor allowing for guided exploration during the procedure.

A **retroscope** is a straight tubular instrument that offers fiberoptic vision.

*The risk of infection is always possible.

LASIK EYE SURGERY
The Procedure
- You will lie back in a reclining chair located in an exam room.
- A numbing drop will be administered to each eye (anesthetic) and the area around the eye will be cleaned.
- A mild sedative may be administered.
- A lid speculum will be used to keep your eyelids open.
- A device will then cut a hinged flap of corneal tissue off the outer layer.
- The laser will reshape the underlying corneal tissue and the flap will be replaced (it will quickly adhere to the cornea; there are no stitches).
- A clear plastic or perforated metal shield will be placed over the eye to protect the flap (must be worn to protect from daily activities).

Possible risks
- Inability to drive at night
- Need for glasses to aid in vision
- Inability to wear contacts
- Ocular infection
- Loss of visual acuity to the point of functional blindness (very low risk)

CESARIAN SECTION 207
The Procedure
- A small external horizontal (or sometimes vertical) incision will be made in your lower abdomen.
- A second incision is made in your uterus, along the same line as the external incision. Your baby is delivered through this opening.

Possible risks
- Adverse reactions to anesthesia may result in breathing problems
- Infection of the bladder or uterus
- Injury to the urinary tract
- Injury to the baby

HYSTERECTOMY
The Procedures
Abdominal extraction
- Incision will be made vertically on the midline (slightly off-center incision from the navel to the pubis), or on the transverse (bikini incision made above the pubic hair).
- The vertical incision is easier for the surgeon, but the horizontal incision leaves a less conspicuous scar (neither results in less pain or healing time).
- Muscle fibers are then split and pulled apart with retractors to reveal the uterus. The uterus is held under tension so that the weight is taken off the body.
- Blood and urinary vessels are cut away from the uterus and tied off.
- The uterus is severed from the cervix and extracted (the ovaries, cervix and fallopian tubes are then removed if necessary).

Laparoscopic-assisted vaginal hysterectomy (LAVH)
- A laparoscope is inserted through one incision located on the curve of the navel.
- Instruments are inserted through the two remaining incisions (one above the pubic hair and one to the lower side of the navel) to cut away the uterus from blood and urinary vessels.
- The vessels are then tied off.
- The uterus is severed from the vaginal wall and extracted through the vagina.

Possible risks
- Excessive bleeding
- Deep vein thrombosis, DVT (blood clots in the legs that can break off and move toward the lungs causing a pulmonary embolism)
- Damage to the rectum or bladder
- Vaginal dryness
- Emotional distress

Almost **75%** of surgeries are outpatient.

58% of surgical procedures performed are on women.

Surgical procedures are performed **34%** more often on women than men.

Sources: hospitalmanagement.net; University of Maryland Medicine

> The combination of oxygen-rich air, flammable materials and heat from certain surgical equipment causes about 100 fires a year in operating rooms nationwide according to the Joint Commission on Accreditation of Healthcare Organizations (JCAHO). These fires, more often occurring for head and neck surgeries where draping can trap gases, cause as many as 20 injuries and one or two deaths annually.

A new baby! Mary just knew she was pregnant again and now a home test kit confirmed it. "Our first baby, Molly, was born four years ago and we've tried ever since to have another one. My husband and I are thrilled!" she said.

Mary's excitement quickly turned to worry. She was reminiscing about Molly's birth by cesarean. 205 "I had all kinds of complications," she said, her forehead creasing into worry lines. "I had a cesarean because Molly was coming out bottom first. I ended up with an infection and had to stay in the hospital for two weeks! On top of it, the cesarean cost more than we expected."

Given her concerns, Mary picked up the phone and scheduled an appointment with Dr. Savannah, her gynecologist. "I was depressed after Molly's birth because I didn't want a cesarean. I know it was necessary for Molly's health, but with this preg-

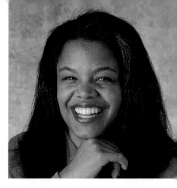

Mary used a birthing plan to give herself comfort about trying to avoid a cesarean.

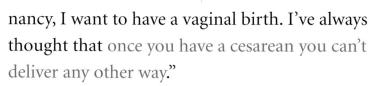

nancy, I want to have a vaginal birth. I've always thought that once you have a cesarean you can't deliver any other way."

At their appointment, Dr. Savannah told Mary that she had an excellent chance of successfully giving birth vaginally. They talked about the pros and cons of cesareans. Dr. Savannah explained that in situations that compromised the baby or mother's health, like with a prolapsed umbilical cord or abnormally attached placenta, a cesarean was necessary. Together they created a birthing plan 209—a document that outlined Mary's preferences for her labor, delivery and postpartum care.

"Now that I know more, I feel better about whatever happens," Mary said. "My doctor knows what I want, but if there's a good reason to have a c-section, we'll deal with it. The bottom line is I want to do what's best for me and my child."

Why you might need a cesarean:

35% **Prior cesarean delivery**

30% **Dystocia (slowed labor process) or cephalopelvic disproportion (your pelvis is too small for your baby's head to pass through)**

12% **Breech presentation (baby is coming out bottom first)**

9% **Problems with baby's heart rate**

Sources: The Risks of Lowering the Cesarean-Delivery Rate, The New England Journal of Medicine, January 1999; C-section: A safe birthing option, MayoClinic.com.

Talk to your doctor before your delivery and discuss at what point you both think this type of operation is necessary for your and baby's health.
Source: Why is a Cesarean Delivery Done?, WebMD.

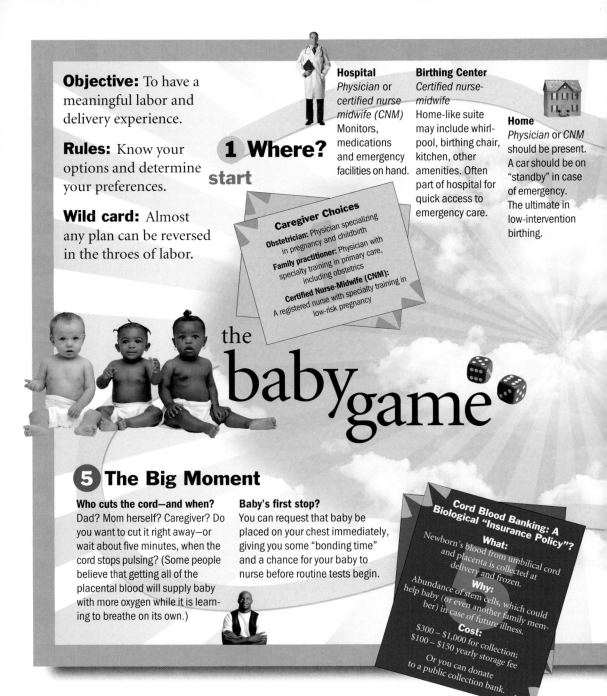

Objective: To have a meaningful labor and delivery experience.

Rules: Know your options and determine your preferences.

Wild card: Almost any plan can be reversed in the throes of labor.

1 Where?
start

Hospital
Physician or certified nurse midwife (CNM) Monitors, medications and emergency facilities on hand.

Birthing Center
Certified nurse-midwife Home-like suite may include whirl-pool, birthing chair, kitchen, other amenities. Often part of hospital for quick access to emergency care.

Home
Physician or CNM should be present. A car should be on "standby" in case of emergency. The ultimate in low-intervention birthing.

Caregiver Choices
Obstetrician: Physician specializing in pregnancy and childbirth
Family practitioner: Physician with specialty training in primary care, including obstetrics
Certified Nurse-Midwife (CNM): A registered nurse with specialty training in low-risk pregnancy

the
babygame

5 The Big Moment

Who cuts the cord—and when?
Dad? Mom herself? Caregiver? Do you want to cut it right away—or wait about five minutes, when the cord stops pulsing? (Some people believe that getting all of the placental blood will supply baby with more oxygen while it is learn-ing to breathe on its own.)

Baby's first stop?
You can request that baby be placed on your chest immediately, giving you some "bonding time" and a chance for your baby to nurse before routine tests begin.

Cord Blood Banking: A Biological "Insurance Policy"?
What:
Newborn's blood from umbilical cord and placenta is collected at delivery and frozen.
Why:
Abundance of stem cells, which could help baby (or even another family mem-ber) in case of future illness.
Cost:
$300 – $1,000 for collection; $100 – $150 yearly storage fee Or you can donate to a public collection bank.

ACTION ITEMS
Creating a "birth plan"

Several months before birth, some expectant mothers begin drawing up a "birthing plan"—a document that outlines their preferences for the man-agement of labor, delivery and postpartum care. Birthing plans are not written in stone, of course. The health of mother and baby during labor override any previously stated preferences.

Sample birthing plans

www.babycenter.com
www.birthplan.com
www.childbirth.org

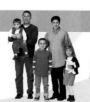

Emergency Consideration

If you need an emergency C-section, will the hospital allow your husband/support person to come into the O.R. with you? Ask your caregiver.

Lights, Cameras, Action?

Decide ahead of time how much you'll want to see (or not see) a year from now. Check with facility about camera and lighting policies.

What birthing options does a woman have?

2 Who Will Be There?

- Spouse/baby's father
- Mom
- Sister
- Other kids
- In-laws
- Best friend
- **Doula***
- Two or more people**

* **Doula** (pronounced "DOO-lah"): a non-medical person trained to comfort and support women during labor and childbirth, especially helpful if the mother doesn't have good support. Studies show that doula care can shorten labor and decrease need for C-section.

** If you wish to have several people present, consider a birthing center or home birth.

3 Childbirth Classes

Lamaze:
Special breathing techniques; mental focus on external object. Open to pain medications during labor.

Bradley:
Normal breathing; inward focus on self. Pain medications discouraged. 12 two-hour classes usually required.

Hospital or birthing center:
Methods taken from a range of birthing approaches.

4 Pain Relief

I want to go "natural"
- Massage
- Acupressure
- Water: Jacuzzi, shower, bath

Bring on the meds!
- Epidural (blocks regional nerve paths)
- "Walking" epidural (permits mobility)
- I.V. pain killers (e.g., Demerol)

Women have an array of choices in planning for childbirth—from the practitioner and type of pain relief right down to the lighting and background music.

Source: Understanding Children, understandingchildren.com, TOP and Civitas.

Go to the Head of the Class

Childbirth classes help fathers feel more involved in the pregnancy—especially if they have been unable to attend doctor visits. Ask if your classes offer a special "dad's only" session.

C-sections and Pain Relief: What You Should Know

- Cesarean deliveries account for about 23% of births in U.S.
- Epidurals are used for many C-sections. (Mom stays awake.)
- General anesthesia, which is faster-acting, is used in emergency C-sections. (Mom is asleep.)
- Medications for incision pain will not enter the first breast fluid baby drinks (**colostrum**). But once regular breast milk comes in fully a couple days later, you should not take any pain meds without consulting your doctor.

TIP

With a birthing plan on record, the mother shouldn't have to communicate her wishes while in labor, or if caregivers change at the last minute.

Birthing plans address issues great and small

- Your own clothes vs. hospital gowns
- Music and dimmed lights
- Clear fluids vs. ice chips for hydration
- Continuous vs. intermittent monitoring of baby
- Medical vs. non-medical pain relief
- Position for pushing
- Episiotomy* vs. natural tearing
- Emergency contingencies
- Shared vs. private hospital room (Note: Insurance may not fully cover a private room.)

*Episiotomy: An incision made during delivery to widen the vaginal opening

Other resources

- Support during labor
  Doulas of North America
  www.dona.com
- Breast-feeding support
  La Leche League
  www.lalecheleague.org
- Childbirth education
  The Bradley Method
  www.bradleybirth.com

  ICEA (International Childbirth Education Association)
  www.icea.org

  Lamaze International
  www.lamaze-childbirth.com

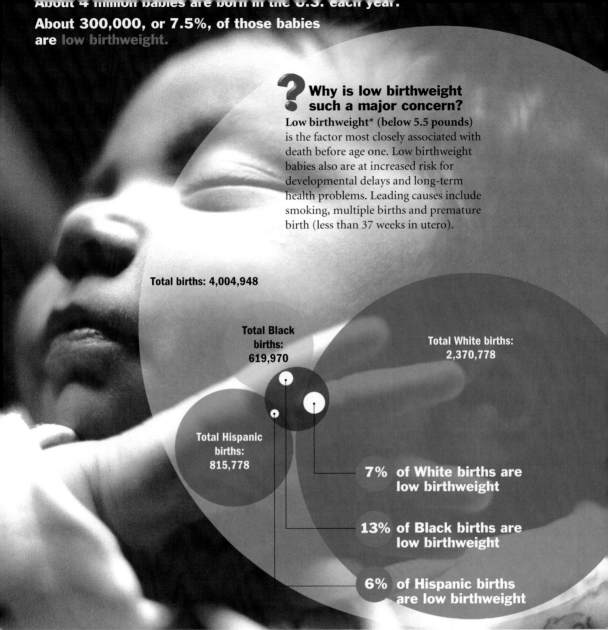

? Why is low birthweight such a major concern?

Low birthweight* (below 5.5 pounds) is the factor most closely associated with death before age one. Low birthweight babies also are at increased risk for developmental delays and long-term health problems. Leading causes include smoking, multiple births and premature birth (less than 37 weeks in utero).

Total births: 4,004,948

Total Black births: 619,970

Total White births: 2,370,778

Total Hispanic births: 815,778

7% of White births are low birthweight

13% of Black births are low birthweight

6% of Hispanic births are low birthweight

*The average weight of a child born at full term is 7.5 pounds. (US)

ACTION ITEMS

What about alcohol consumption?

? I drank alcohol on a few occasions before I learned that I was pregnant. Could this have harmed my baby?

Many women go into their first prenatal exam with this question weighing heavily on their mind—most leave the visit feeling reassured. A few drinks in the early weeks of pregnancy are unlikely to have harmed the baby. However, a woman should stop drinking as soon as she discovers that she is pregnant.

? Having a glass of wine with dinner is okay, isn't it?

Experts now believe that even moderate alcohol consumption—defined as one or two drinks a day or occasional binging on five or more drinks—can increase the risks for miscarriage and other complications. Moreover, there is growing evidence linking moderate drinking with a phenomenon known as **fetal alcohol effect,** a less severe problem than **fetal alcohol syndrome** but still characterized by developmental and behavioral problems as the child grows.

A Day of Births, U.S.: Every **8 seconds** a baby is born. ■ Every **60 seconds** a baby is born to a teen mother. ■ Every **2 minutes** a low birthweight baby is born. ■ Every **3½ minutes** a baby is born with a birth defect. ■ Every **hour** three babies die. ■ Every **24 hours** 406 babies are born to mothers who received late or no prenatal care. Calculations by the March of Dimes Perinatal Data Center

Miscarriage: Loss of pregnancy in first five months. ■ 80% occur in first 12 weeks. ■ Occurs in 15 to 20% of *known* pregnancies. ■ Most are caused by chromosomal abnormalities that prevent normal development of baby. ■ Vast majority of women who miscarry have healthy pregnancies later.

Causes of infant death
Infant deaths in 1999: About 28,000

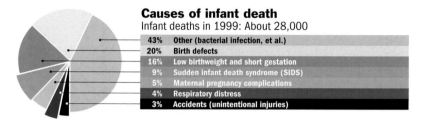

%	Cause
43%	Other (bacterial infection, et al.)
20%	Birth defects
16%	Low birthweight and short gestation
9%	Sudden infant death syndrome (SIDS)
5%	Maternal pregnancy complications
4%	Respiratory distress
3%	Accidents (unintentional injuries)

The vast majority of babies are born perfectly healthy.

Of the problems that do occur, many stem from genetics or random chromosomal abnormalities, and are well beyond the control of the pregnant woman. Other problems, however, are direct consequences of the mother's risky behavior during pregnancy.

Source: Understanding Children, understandingchildren.com, TOP and Civitas.

U.S. Ranks 27th in Infant Mortality
Deaths per 1,000 live births

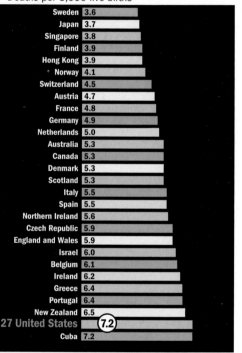

Sweden	3.6
Japan	3.7
Singapore	3.8
Finland	3.9
Hong Kong	3.9
Norway	4.1
Switzerland	4.5
Austria	4.7
France	4.8
Germany	4.9
Netherlands	5.0
Australia	5.3
Canada	5.3
Denmark	5.3
Scotland	5.3
Italy	5.5
Spain	5.5
Northern Ireland	5.6
Czech Republic	5.9
England and Wales	5.9
Israel	6.0
Belgium	6.1
Ireland	6.2
Greece	6.4
Portugal	6.4
New Zealand	6.5
27 United States	7.2
Cuba	7.2

Mom's risky behavior, baby's increased risks

Alcohol
Even one drink per day can increase risks of miscarriage, stillbirth, childhood leukemia, multiple deformations, permanent facial alterations, learning delays and behavioral problems.

Cigarettes
Increased risk of SIDS (sudden infant death syndrome) and low birthweight.

Marijuana
More difficult pregnancy and labor for mom; respiratory distress for baby at birth.

Cocaine
Risk of infant stroke at birth, excessive crying; later behavioral problems.

Resources and support

Many of the national resources listed here offer referrals to local chapters and meetings. Some hold online meetings as well.

Alcohol

● Alcoholics Anonymous
www.alcoholics-anonymous.org

● The National Clearinghouse for Alcohol and Drug Information
800.729.6686

Smoking

● Smoking
www.nicotine-anonymous.org

Cocaine, marijuana and other drugs

● Narcotics Anonymous
www.na.org

● Cocaine Anonymous
www.ca.org

Partner abuse

● National Domestic Violence Hotline
800.799.SAFE, ext. 7233
www.ndvh.org

Miscarriage/pregnancy loss

● **Surviving Pregnancy Loss: A Complete Sourcebook for Women and Their Families**
Rochelle Friedman and Bonnie Gradstein

What are the major types of rehabilitation therapy?

There are three : **physical therapy, occupational therapy** and **speech and language therapy.**

Physical therapy

WHEN IT'S USED	WHAT'S INVOLVED
To restore muscle strength and flexiblity.	**EXERCISE** The goal here is to strengthen weak muscles and increase flexibility. This form of therapy is needed after a prolonged period in bed or after a leg has been immobilized following an operation.
To improve mobility after an injury, illness or surgery.	**HEAT AND COOLING TREATMENTS** **Hot** packs transmit heat to muscle injuries and joint stiffness caused by arthritis or excessive exercise. Blood flow is stimulated, tense muscles are relaxed and pain is relieved. Ice or **cold** packs may be used to reduce pain and swelling.
To relieve pain after after an injury, illness or surgery.	**MASSAGE** Muscles are kneaded or stroked using circular or long sweeping motions. This stimulates the blood flow, thus reducing inflammation and fluid retention.
To prevent complications after an injury, illness or surgery.	**HYDROTHERAPY** Hydrotherapy takes places in a heated pool, using water to support the body. This makes movements easier, and provides gentle resistance.
To prevent chronic conditions from worsening.	**ELECTRICAL STIMULATION** A mild electric current is passed through pads applied to the surface of the skin. This generates heat that relieves stiffness and improves mobility in joints.

HOW LONG?	
If you have suffered a minor injury, you may only need a short course of physical therapy to get your mobility back. After a major illness or surgery, however, you may need long-term treatment.	**ULTRASOUND** Gel is applied to the skin, and high-energy sound waves are used to create heat. This eases pain and reduces inflammation. The treatment is used on ligament, tendon or muscle tissues, usually over several sessions. Some people experience a tingling in the affected area after an ultrasound session.

GAIT TRAINING
This helps a patient to walk again after an illness such as a stroke. Part of the training is learning to use walking aids that support the upper body while building strength in the legs.

CHEST PHYSICAL THERAPY
This is used to prevent chest infections in older people after major surgery or children with cystic fibrosis where mucus collects in the lungs and leads to infection. The therapy involves breathing and coughing exercises to fill the lungs with air. If your child needs regular chest physical therapy, you can learn the technique and do it at home.

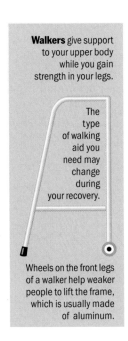

Walkers give support to your upper body while you gain strength in your legs.

The type of walking aid you need may change during your recovery.

Wheels on the front legs of a walker help weaker people to lift the frame, which is usually made of aluminum.

ACTION ITEMS Check your physical therapy coverag

Ask your human resources director or insurance company the following questions to determine if your current benefits package gives you access to appropriate physical therapy services:

1 **Is your physical therapy benefit "bundled" with those of other providers of care?**
Physical therapy services should be listed separately in the benefit language so that access to necessary services is not compromised.

2 **Does the benefit language permit access to physical therapists for each condition during the year?**

Benefit language should permit treatment of more than one condition in a calendar year (eg, ankle fracture in January and low back injury in July).

3 **Does the benefit language permit access to physical therapists for each episode of care?**
A person may require more than one episode of care for the same condition. For example, someone with arthritis may receive physical therapy intervention for knee weakness in an attempt to avoid surgery. While this is often successful, some patients may still require surgery for the knee condition (e.g., total knee replacement), which may require

Occupational therapy

WHEN IT'S USED	WHAT'S INVOLVED
To encourage and restore independence to those with physical or mental health problems. 61	An occupational therapist will probably visit you at your home to see how you manage with everyday routine tasks, such as bathing or dressing. Then a program of therapy will be advised.

WHEN IT'S USED

To encourage and restore independence to those with physical or mental health problems. 61

To help with simple tasks that are difficult due to a disorder such as MS or arthritis 107 or following a stroke. 115

To help children with learning difficulties.

HOW LONG?

A therapist will monitor your progress to ensure the treatment is working well. Occupational therapy may help restore your independence fairly rapidly.

WHAT'S INVOLVED

An occupational therapist will probably visit you at your home to see how you manage with everyday routine tasks, such as bathing or dressing. Then a program of therapy will be advised.

PRACTICAL WORK
To build muscle strength, stamina and concentration, an occupational therapist will suggest a practical activity such as cooking or a handicraft. If you find it hard to write after a stroke, the therapist might recommend woodworking to help strengthen muscle and improve fine muscle control.

HELP WITH EQUIPMENT
Occupational therapists have extensive knowledge of a wide range of equipment to help you regain your independence. Slings can support parts of the upper body. If you need to use a walking aid, there are a variety of models to suit your strength and match the stage of your recovery. You may need to adapt parts of your home by installing handrails or even a stairlift, and you may need to use adapted utensils for everyday tasks such as opening jars or special devices to help you dress or eat.

What are rehabilitation therapies?

Rehabilitation therapies help us regain abilities or functions that have been lost due to accidents, illness or surgery.

Speech and language therapy

WHEN IT'S USED

To help those who have problems with verbal communication, stuttering or comprehension problems from a stroke 115 or other problem. Early treatment for children is important so that social problems do not arise.

HOW LONG?

In some cases, just a few weekly sessions may be all that is necessary. More serious problems will require regular sessions over months or years.

WHAT'S INVOLVED

PLAY
Children are often treated for speech problems by using games that encourage them to use both verbal and nonverbal communication. Parents are taught how to encourage speech development at home by playing naming games.

EXERCISES
Larynx (voice box) problems can be overcome by specific exercises to improve articulation. Fluency problems are addressed by exercises that control your speech and make you feel less tense. After a stroke, a patient may need to do exercises such as describing a picture to help retrieve words.

ARTIFICIAL DEVICES
If the larynx has been removed due to cancer, you may be taught to speak by using a device that generates sounds when held against the neck, or you may be fitted with an implant inserted between the windpipe and the esophagus that uses inhaled air to produce sounds.

post-operative physical therapy treatment. The benefit language should support each "episode of care."

 Does the benefit language ensure coverage that facilitates restoration of function?
Benefit language that restricts physical therapy care to a 60- or 90-day period imposes an arbitrary limit on recovery. In determining an appropriate physical therapy benefit that will allow an individual to return to his or her previous level of function, benefit language should reflect the normal amount of time that it takes to recover from an injury or from surgery.

 Does the benefit language ensure coverage that promotes functional independence for those with chronic conditions?
Someone who has a chronic condition may need to be seen periodically by a physical therapist. The physical therapist will determine if the individual's home program, equipment or adaptive devices should be modified. (For instance, children requiring orthotic devices will need modifications to those devices as they grow.) Benefit language should ensure that someone with a chronic condition may receive the kind of care that promotes personal safety and the greatest degree of function possible.

Source: American Physical Therapy Association, apta.org.

Acknowledging that you are depressed is one of the most difficult steps in the healing process.

But with the rise in use of Prozac and other anti-depressants, **fewer people** are getting an important part of the treatment for depression: face to face therapy—what used to be called the "talking cure."

Between 1987 and 1997, the percentage of patients in therapy dropped from 71.1% to 69.2%.

Pills are a lot less expensive than therapists.

But critics say that throwing pills at problems ignores the underlying causes.

Source: TIME.

First, make an appointment with your primary care doctor. A complete physical exam will help rule out any physical problems that may be contributing to your depressive symptoms.

Describe your symptoms to your doctor or another health care provider you trust. He or she may be able to provide inform-ation or prescribe an appropriate antidepressant. He may also have information about mental health professionals with whom he works closely

Talk to friends or family. Seek their help in finding a therapist. Sometimes the best help in finding a therapist is from someone who's already gone to one.

If you don't have a primary health care provider or someone who can recommend a therapist, **contact your local community mental health agency.** You can usually find these community organizations in your local phone book.

Source: Women's Health Interactive.

ACTION ITEMS Finding the right counselor

Here are some resources that should help you connect with a counselor:

National Mental Health Association
This is often the best place to start. Check your yellow pages for a listing or call the National Mental Health Association at 800.969.NMHA.

Your local health department's Mental Health Division.
These services are state-funded and are obligated to first serve individuals who meet "priority population criteria" as defined by the state Mental Health Department.

Other mental health organizations

A family services agency
Some examples are Catholic Charities, Family Services and Jewish Social Services.

Your family physician

Psychiatric hospitals
Look for accreditation by the Joint Commission on Accreditation of Health Care Organizations.

Hotlines and crisis centers
Check your local yellow pages or call directory assistance for listings.

Clergy

Your hospital's emergency room

? What are some different types of mental health professionals?

All of these should have a state license to practice.

A **psychiatrist** is a medical doctor with speacial training in the diagnosis and treatment of mental and emotional disorders. Like other physicians, psychiatrists are qualified to prescribe medication. **Child/ adolescent psychiatrists** have special training in the diagnosis and treatment of emotional and behavioral problems in children and adolescents.

Source: National Mental Health Association.

A **psychologist** is a mental healthcare provider with an advance degree from an accredited graduate program in psychology. He or she is trained to make diagnoses and provide individual and group therapy.

A **clinical social worker** is a counselor with a masters degree in social work from an accredited graduate program, who can make diagnoses and provide individual and group counselling.

Some warning signs of mental illness

- Marked personality change
- Inability to cope with problems and daily activities
- Strange ideas or delusions
- Excessive anxiety
- Prolonged feelings of sadness
- Marked changes in eating or sleeping patterns
- Thinking or talking about suicide
- Extreme highs and lows
- Abuse of alcohol or drugs
- Excessive anger or hostility
- Violent behavior
- Irrational fears

If you notice any of these symptoms, you should seek psychiatric evaluation. If you need help right away, go to a hospital emergency room. Also, many psychiatrists make themselves available to handle emergency cases.

Source: American Psychiatric Association.

? When should you seek counseling?

Professional counselors offer help in addressing many situations that cause emotional distress, including, but not limited to:

- **Anxiety, depression 129 and other mental and emotional problems and disorders**
- **Family and relationship issues**
- **Substance abuse 53 and domestic violence**
- **Eating disorders**
- **Career change and job stress** 67
- **Social and emotional difficulties related to disability and illness**
- **Adapting to life transitions**
- **The death of a loved one**

You may feel some anxiety about going to a therapist for the first time.

It's quite normal. Remind yourself that you are taking care of yourself and your mental health. However, you don't have to stay with a therapist if you begin to feel uncomfortable over time. **Your needs and feelings should always come first during therapy.**

Source: Women's Health Interactive.

How is counseling used as treatment?

There are times when you may need help addressing problems and issues that cause you emotional distress or make you feel overwhelmed.

You should consider counseling when you're having difficulties at work, your ability to concentrate is diminished or your level of pain becomes too uncomfortable.

Source: American Counseling Association, counseling.org.

Once you've been given a referral by one of the resources above:

❶ Make the call.

❷ Spend a few minutes asking about their approach to working with patients and their philosophy of treatment.

❸ Ask if they have a specialty or concentration.

❹ If you feel comfortable talking to them, the next step is to make an appointment.

❺ On your first visit, the counselor or the doctor will want to get to know all about you in order to assess your situation and develop a treatment plan.

❻ If you don't feel comfortable, talk about your feelings. Don't be afraid to contact another counselor. Feeling comfortable with the professional you choose is very important to the success of your treatment.

For more information contact:
National Mental Health Association
1.800.969.NMHA
TTY 1.800.433.5959
www.nmha.org

Source: National Mental Health Association.

A've got yellow ones, purple ones, fat ones and skinny ones. You name 'em, I've got 'em," says Maria displaying a palm full of pills. "I take so many medications that I can't keep them straight. And that almost got me into trouble."

Maria, 64, is a widow who lives alone in a tidy Brooklyn apartment and sometimes struggles to manage three chronic illnesses. The strain shows on her pale face as she talks about her situation. She's had asthma ⑨⑦ since childhood, then in her late 50s was diagnosed with a heart condition and depression. "I was doing OK with the asthma, but after adding two more conditions, things started getting out of control," she said.

She recalled a recent health crisis. "I didn't realize how important it was to follow my doctor's instructions or get my prescriptions filled at the same pharmacy. I took over-the-counter weight loss

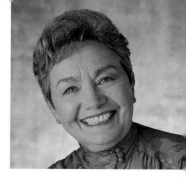

Maria found out the hard way that managing multiple medications is serious business.

tablets to lose weight quickly, not knowing that it could cause any problems."

After taking the supplements, Maria's heart rate dramatically increased. Fearing a heart attack, she called her doctor and learned she was suffering a reaction from combining medications.

"That's when I realized I needed some help," Marie said. "First, I went to my pharmacist and consolidated all my records. She signed me up for refill reminders by email and explained the importance of giving my doctors full disclosure."

Marie bought a pillbox timer that sounds alarms for each medication. And, one of her doctors explained Health Hero, a monitoring system that makes it easy for Maria to inform her doctor about any changes in her health.

"I feel much better being organized," Maria said. "And, it really helps to know I'm not alone."

What are some common chronic illnesses?

Mental Disorders
Affect about **44.3 million Americans** each year. Depression affects nearly **18.8 million** American adults. Bipolar disorder and schizophrenia affect some **4.5 million.**

Alzheimer's Disease 109
Affects more than **4 million Americans.**

Chronic Obstructive Pulmonary Disease (COPD)
This includes illnesses such as emphysema, chronic bronchitis and asthma, and is responsible for more than **100,000 deaths** each year.

Diabetes 121
An estimated **16 million Americans** have diabetes, and **one-third of them don't know it.** It's the seventh leading cause of death among Americans and is the leading cause of blindness, kidney failure and amputations below the waist.

Osteoporosis
Occurs when calcium loss causes bones to become brittle. This condition results in **1.5 million fractures each year.** Half of people who fracture a hip because of osteoporosis are unable to walk without assistance, and a quarter of them require long-term care.

Sources: National Center for Chronic Disease Prevention and Health Promotion; Mayo Clinic Family Health Book, Second Edition, National Institute of Mental Health.

Epilepsy
A neurological condition that affects about **2.3 million Americans.** About 181,000 people are diagnosed with epilepsy and seizures each year.

Cardiovascular Disease 75

Kills almost a million Americans every year and is the leading cause of death among both men and women across all racial and ethnic groups. Includes high blood pressure, heart disease and stroke. About **58 million Americans** live with some form of the disease.

Arthritis 107

One of every six people —nearly **43 million Americans** have this disease.

Cancer 87
Second leading cause of death among Americans, will cause an estimated **550,000 US deaths** this year. Approximately 8.4 million Americans alive today have a history of cancer.

How can chronic illnesses affect a person's everyday life?

Living with chronic illness affects you in many ways. It can hinder your ability to work, limit your physical activities and add enormous stress to your life.

Common stress signals can include: **pain or body aches, anxiety, headaches, irritability and difficulty sleeping.** Don't wait until you feel you can't cope any longer. Long-term stress can lead to depression and feelings of hopelessness.

> Seek help early and take one step at a time.
>
> Managing your stress will help you feel more in control of your situation.
>
> Seek a support group.
>
> Talk to your doctor or ask her to recommend a mental health care provider.
>
> Don't try to cope alone.

Sources: clevelandclinic.org; *Coping with the Stress of Chronic Illness*, Gretchen Malik, Suite101.com, HealingWell.com.

Where can I find support for my chronic condition?

Living with a chronic illness is challenging physically and emotionally, but you can find local support groups that meet in person and over the Internet. Associations for specific illnesses, such as the American Heart Association and the American Diabetes Association, provide support groups, educational information and even recipes for special diets.

Find strength and support in knowledge. Learning as much as possible about your illness puts you in charge of your health. Find information at the library, on the

---

ACTION ITEMS   Resources

National Guidelines Clearinghouse (NGC)
A database of practice guidelines. These guidelines, developed by national experts, are the essential aspects of good care for specific illnesses and conditions. Diabetes, hypertension and arthritis are all conditions that have guidelines. You can find these guidelines through NGC or sometimes through the main support organizations for specific conditions, such as the American Heart Association. Talk to your doctor about the guidelines he or she uses in your care.

www.guideline.gov

Friends Health Connection
Linking people who share or have overcome the same chronic illness, injury or disability. 800.48.FRIEND (800.483.7436)
www.48friend.org

National Center for Chronic Disease Prevention and Health Promotion
A great source for statistics, educational information and resources.
www.cdc.gov/nccdphp

? What is the impact of chronic health conditions in America?

Chronic diseases such as heart disease, cancer and diabetes are leading causes of disability and death in the United States.

Every year, chronic diseases claim the lives of more than 1.7 million people in the US That means 7 of every 10 Americans who die each year die from a chronic illness. Chronic diseases cause major limitations in daily living for more than 1 of every 10 Americans—

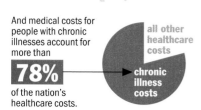

that's
25 million chronically ill people.

And medical costs for people with chronic illnesses account for more than

78% of the nation's healthcare costs.

all other healthcare costs

chronic illness costs

Sources: National Center for Chronic Disease Prevention and Health Promotion, *Chronic Conditions: Making the Case for Ongoing Care, 2002;* Partnership for Solutions, Johns Hopkins University, for The Robert Wood Johnson Foundation.

! CONSUMER ALERT

Are you getting the right treatment and care for your chronic illness? About one-third of chronically ill people in America aren't.

Our healthcare system currently isn't designed to provide coordinated, ongoing care and services to the growing number of people with chronic illnesses. Healthcare financing and delivery systems have been slow to respond to the changing environment. The healthcare system does not place a high priority on prevention efforts, providers are not adequately trained to address chronic conditions and health care payers are paying for duplicate and inappropriate services.

Sources: *Chronic Conditions: Making the Case for Ongoing Care, 2002;* Partnership for Solutions, Johns Hopkins University, for The Robert Wood Johnson Foundation; *A Portrait of the Chronically Ill in America, 2001;* FACCT—Foundation for Accountability and The Robert Wood Johnson Foundation.

What should I know about chronic illness?

Broadly defined, chronic illness is a condition that is prolonged, does not resolve on its own and is rarely completely cured.

Internet 325 and at your doctor's office.

Pick a doctor 229 who has experience in treating your condition and who has a good rapport with you. Make sure he listens to you and clearly explains your situation and options.

It is crucial that you monitor and manage your chronic condition. Active involvement in managing your condition and good self care can improve your health, reduce mortality and disability, increase productivity and lower health care costs.

Research your condition and learn how to track changes in key indicators of your health, such as changes in your blood sugar or cholesterol. Report any changes to your health care provider. Follow your provider's

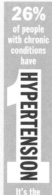

26% of people with chronic conditions have

HYPERTENSION 1

It's the #1 chronic condition.

advice about diet and nutrition. Ask questions if you are concerned or want additional guidance .

Ask your doctor about new technology or pocket diaries that can help you better manage your condition. Visit the websites of associations for specific illnesses, such as the National Arthritis Foundation, for specific tips and programs. Ask your local pharmacist about devices 265 to monitor cholesterol, blood pressure monitors, blood sugar or other indicators and symptoms of your condition. Find a support group of people who share your condition and ask them about how they monitor their care.

Sources: AARP; *Patients as Effective Collaborators in Managing Chronic Conditions,* Center for the Advancement of Health, July 1999.

Healthfinder
A Web site for consumer health information, including information on many chronic illnesses, such as arthritis, diabetes and heart disease.
www.healthfinder.gov

American Chronic Pain Association
A support system for people with chronic pain.
The ACPA
PO Box 850
Rocklin, CA 95677
800.533.3231
www.theacpa.org

National Chronic Care Consortium
An alliance of individuals and organizations across the health care industry that seeks to improve care for people with chronic illnesses.
www.nccconline.org

Pain is an unpleasant sensory and emotional experience associated with actual or potential tissue damage. Pain is the body's mechanism for self-preservation. It acts as a warning to indicate harm or potential danger to tissues in our bodies. However, when pain persists or reoccurs over a long period of time (more than six months) it is considered chronic pain.

More than 75 million Americans suffer chronic pain.

Source: The American Association of Neurological Surgeons.

? What is the difference between acute and chronic pain?

Acute pain is of short limited duration, and is usually the result of an injury, surgery or medical illness. As the healing process takes place, the pain generally disappears.

Chronic pain is of longer duration than acute pain, sometimes lingering long after the original injury has healed. It can be made much worse by environmental and psychological factors, and often causes great problems for patients.

Treatments for the two kinds of pain are quite different.

? How is chronic pain pain managed?

The main goal is to improve function, enabling infdividuals to work, attend school and participate in day-to-day activities. Sometimes relaxation and the use of imagery can provide relief. Sufferers should remember that most pain is at least partiallytreatable in some way.

Source: National Institute of Health.

? What are some common illnesses that cause long-term pain?

Arthritis 107 Conditions such as osteoarthritis, rheumatoid arthritis, and gout cause joint pain in the extremities. Millions of Americans suffer from some form of arthritic condition.

Back pain 135 A very common type of back pain called **sciatica,** can send shooting pain down the leg. Other pack pains can be attributed to discs which have degenerated over time.

Cancer 87 The effects of cancer on the body, the growth of a tumor and the treatment of cancer can all cause pain.

Shingles A neurological disorder that affects the skin with agonizing pain, shingles appears to be almost resistant to treatment. Prompt treatment with antiviral agents is important to stop the infection. Other painful disorders of the skin include **vasculitis** (inflammation of the blood vessels), **herpes simplex, skin tumors, cysts** and **neurofibromatosis** (tumors caused by a neurogenetic disorder).

Spinal stenosis This is a narrowing of the canal surrounding the spinal cord, and occurs naturally with aging. It causes weakness in the legs and leg pain usually felt while the person is standing up.

Central and thalamic pain syndromes These are conditions where abnormal signals are relayed to and from the brain; for instance, touch can be perceived as intense burning. These conditions affect 100,000 Americans with MS, Parkinson's, amputated limbs, spinal cord injuries and stroke.

Source: National Institute of Neurological Disorders and Stroke.

ACTION ITEMS

Resources

NIH Neurological Institute
The National Institute of Neurological Disorders and Stroke is the leading federal supporter of research on brain and nervous system disorders. The Institute also sponsors an active public information program about diagnosis, treatment and research on painful neurological disorders.
800.352.9424; TTY 301.468.5981
www.ninds.nih.gov

Additional information about pain research supported by the NIH may be obtained from:
National Institute of Dental and Craniofacial Research
301.496.4261
www.nidcr.nih.gov

Private organizations providing services and information on pain include:

American Chronic Pain Association (ACPA)
Provides self-help coping skills and peer support to people with chronic pain. Sponsors local support groups throughout the US and provides assistance in starting and maintaining support groups.
800.533.3231
www.theacpa.org

American Pain Foundation
This non-profit information, education and advocacy organization works to raise public awareness, promote research and advocate increased access to effective pain management.
888.615.PAIN (7246)
www.painfoundation.org

❓ What drugs can treat chronic pain?

Many medicines can treat pain, but they may have serious side effects, so listen to your family doctor when he talks to you about dosage and useage.

Drugs are not the only way to reduce pain. Getting your mind off the pain with relaxation techniques can help to control it. So even if you are taking pain medication, you should try to find methods of stress reduction.

Acetaminophen (Tylenol). This helps many kinds of chronic pain. But many prescription medicines have acetaminophen in them, so if you already take Tylenol, you could end up having a larger dosage than you thought.

Anti-inflammatory drugs Examples include **aspirin, ibuprofen** (Motrin) and **naproxen** (Aleve). These medicines can be taken daily; they build up in the blood to levels that fight the pain of inflammation (swelling).

Narcotics These can be addictive, so a doctor will be very careful when prescribing them. There is a difference between physical dependence and psychological addiction. Physical dependence means your body gets used to the drug and needs the drug for it to work. Psychological addiction is the desire to use a drug even if there is no need for pain relief.

Many drugs that are used to treat other illnesses can also treat pain. For example **carbamazepine** is a seizure medication that can treat pain in some people, and **amitripyline** is an antidepressant that can help relieve chronic pain for some sufferers.

Source: American Academy of Family Physicians.

❓ What non-traditional methods are used to treat long-term pain?

No therapy for pain has caused as much controversy recently as **Accupuncture,** the 2,000 year-old Chinese technique of inserting fine needles under the skin. The needles are manipulated by a practitioner to produce pain relief that can last for hours or even days. Opinion is divided as to whether accupuncture really works. Some specialists say that patients report relief when the needles are placed near the site of the injury, rather than at the points shown on Chinese charts.

In **transcutaneous electrical nerve stimulation (TENS)**, brief pulses of electricity are applied to nerve endings under the skin. This yields excellent pain relief in some chronic pain patients.

Brain stimulation is another method for controlling pain, especially the severe pain of advanced cancer. It is done through electrodes surgically implanted in the brain. The patient determines how much and when the stimulation is needed.

Placebo effects For years doctors have known that a simple sugar pill can make people feel better—even after major surgery. It has now been shown that the effect may be neurochemical, and that those who respond to placebos are actually tapping into their brain's endorphin systems, though how they do it is yet to be discovered.

Source: National Institute of Neurological Disorders and Stroke.

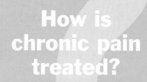

❓ How is chronic pain treated?

Chronic pain can often be managed with a combination of drugs and non-traditional therapies.

Arthritis Foundation
This volunteer-driven organization works to improve lives through leadership in the prevention, control and cure of arthritis and related diseases. Offers free brochures on types of arthritis, treatment options and management of daily activities.
800.283.7800
www.arthritis.org

National Chronic Pain Outreach Association (NCPOA)
This national information clearinghouse on chronic pain services patients and medical professionals.
540.862.9437
www.chronicpain.org

National Foundation for the Treatment of Pain
This not-for-profit organization provides support for patients suffering from intractable pain, and for their families, friends and physicians. They offer a patient forum, advocacy programs, support resources and direct medical intervention.
831.655.8812
www.paincare.org

Mayday Fund [For Pain Research]
This private foundation dedicated to the alleviation of human physical pain works to increase awareness and provide objective treatment information.
212.366.6970
www.painandhealth.org

Source: National Institute of Neurological Disorders and Stroke (NINDS).

? What is long-term care?

Long-term care includes a wide range of medical and support services for people with degenerative conditions such as Parkinson's or stroke, people with a prolonged illness such as cancer or people with a cognitive disorder such as Alzheimer's. Because of the nature of these illnesses long-term care might more correctly be termed custodial care. It involves giving a patient assistance with everyday activities that normal, healthy people take for granted: **getting out of bed, walking to the bathroom, using the toilet, having a shower, getting dressed, eating breaakfast.**

Because this type of care is full-time it can be very expensive. It is provided in nursing homes, your own home, assisted living facilities and adult day care centers.

The cost of staying in a nursing home is rising at nearly

4

times the rate of inflation.

Source: The Wall Street Journal.

? Why is there a growing need for long term care?

Because people are living longer.

By the year 2050, the number of people over 65 will double.

The 80+ segment of the population is the fastest-growing portion of the US population.

As people take care of themselves with a healthy diet and exercise, theyt live longer. However the longer they live the more likely they are to suffer from diseases such as Alzheimer's.

Americans over 65 face a 40% risk of entering a nursing home for long-term care.

In addition, families don't look after their aged parents in the same way they used to. Many women are in the work force, and divorce rates are approaching 50%, which means that many families are no longer equipped to look after older relatives.

? What's the best care choice for me?

A nursing home cares for people who cannot be cared for at home or in the community. If you cannot take care of yourself due to physical, emotional or mental problems, nursing homes provide a wide range of personal care and health services. Much of this care is custodial, or non-skilled.

Nursing homes usually provide 24-hour medical care as well as meals, activities and some personal care. You may have to pay extra for other services or special medical needs. Make sure you know what is included and what is not in your monthly fee.

A nursing home is not the only choice you have. Depending on your needs and resources, there are other kinds of long-term living and care choices available. You can get long term care at:

home
accessory dwelling units (ADUs)
subsidized senior housing
community centers
assisted living facilities
retirement communities

You may need to get help from family and friends, community services and professional care agencies.

To find out what long-term care is available in your state, call your local Area Agency on Aging. You can find the telephone number at www.aoa.gov

Source: Centers for Medicare and Medicaid Services.

ACTION ITEMS Nursing Home Checklist

Basic Information on the Nursing Home
❑ Medicare 297 and Medicaid 303 -certified
❑ Has the level of care needed
❑ Has an available bed
❑ Has special services if needed
❑ Located close enough to visit

Residents' Appearance
❑ Residents clean, well-groomed

Nursing Home Living Spaces
❑ Clean and well-kept, a comfortable temperature. acceptable noise levels, good lighting
❑ Smoking not allowed or restricted to certain areas
❑ Furnishings sturdy, attractive and comfortable

Staff
❑ Good relationship between staff and residents
❑ Training and continuing education for staff
❑ Background checks on all staff
❑ Full-time Registered Nurse 231 present at all times
❑ Same team of nurses and Certified Nursing Assistants (CNAs) work with the same resident 4 to 5 days per week
❑ CNAs work with a reasonable number of residents
❑ CNAs involved in care planning meetings
❑ A full-time social worker on staff
❑ A licensed doctor on staff daily and reachable at all times

If you own a single-family unit, you may want to convert part of it to a separate living space with its own cooking area and bathroom. Check with your local zoning office to see if ADUs are allowed in your area

There are federal and state programs to help older people with low to moderate incomes. Some programs also help with meals, housekeeping, shopping, and laundry. Rents are usually a percentage of your income.

A variety of community services can help you with your day-to-day activities. Some, such as volunteer groups that help with shopping or transport, may be free. Most commuties offer: adult day care, a meals program, senior centers and help with legal questions and bill paying.

These facilities help with activities of everyday living, such as bathing, dressing and using the bathroom. They may also help with taking medicine and additional services such as making appointments or cooking. Re sidents often live in their own room or apartment within a building or group of buildings, and they have some or all of ther meals together. Some assisted living facilities have health services on site. The term "assited living" may mean different things in different facilities, so check what services are provided in any facility you see.

Continuing care retirement communities (CCRCs) are retirement communities with more than one kind of housing and different levels of care. Where you live depends on the level of care you need. In the same community, there may be individual homes or apartments for those who still live at home, and assisted living facility for people who need some level of daily care and a nursing home for those who need a higher level of care. You move from one level to another based on your needs, but you stay in the same CCRC.

Source: Centers for Medicare and Medicaid Services.

What do long-term care services cost? 305

In 1999, The Wall Street Journal reported that a year in a **nursing home** cost more than **$40,000 and could exceed $100,000** in some parts of the country. Home care is also very expensive: a home health aide coming to **your home** every other day for a **4-hour visit can easily cost $1,800 a month.** If the visit rises to an 8-hour day, the costs rise to $7,200 a month.

Costs for **assisted living facilities** vary greatly and depend on the size of the unit, the services provided and the location. An average monthly fee for rent and other services is about **$1,900**.

Sources: mrltc.com,
The National Center for Assisted Living.

High quality long-term care is available if you plan for it in advance and choose a facility that will meet your needs.

There are about **33,000 assisted living facilities** in the US, with about **800,000** people in them.

Residents' Rooms
❏ Personal belongings and/or furniture permitted in residents' rooms
❏ Storage space available in residents' rooms
❏ Window in the bedroom
❏ Access to a personal telephone and television
❏ A choice of roommates
❏ Water pitchers reachable by residents
❏ Policies/procedures in force to protect residents' possessions

Hallways, Stairs, Lounges and Bathrooms
❏ Exits clearly marked
❏ Quiet areas for visits with friends and family
❏ Smoke detectors and sprinklers installed
❏ All areas designed for wheelchair use
❏ Handrails and grab bars where needed

Menus and Food
❏ Choice of foods at each meal, snacks available
❏ Staff help for residents at mealtimes if needed

Activities
❏ A variety of activities for residents
❏ Outdoor areas and staff to help residents go out
❏ An active volunteer program

Safety 65 and Care
❏ Emergency evacuation plan; regular fire drills
❏ Preventive care available (e.g., yearly flu shots)
❏ Access to resident's personal doctors
❏ Association with nearby hospital for emergencies
❏ Care plan meetings held at convenient times
❏ All Federal and State requirements met

Source: Centers for Medicare & Medicaid Services (CMS).

? How much training does it take to become a doctor?

4 years of **regular college** (most medical schools require a minimum of 3 to 4 years)

4 years of **medical school**

Then **residency training**, which might also include training in a particular specialty, and can take up to **10** years.

There are two types of medical school in the US: **allopathic** and **osteopathic.** Allopathic students receive a medical doctorate (MD); osteopathic students receive a doctorate in osteopathic medicine (DO). The main difference is that osteopathic schools tend to concentrate on training physicians to be primary care practitioners.

The first two years of medical school are **basic science courses**, including:
anatomy
neuroanatomy
histology
embryology
behavioral sciences
genetics
physiology
biochemistry
microbiology
pharmacology
pathology

Source: Emedicine.

The third and fourth years at medical school consist of **clinical sciences.**

During the third year, students treat patients under close supervision of fully trained physicians, rotating through specialties such as:
pediatrics
internal medicine
general surgery
gynecology
psychiatry
family practice
emergency medicine

The fourth year at medical school is one of about 50 **elective choices**, such as:
orthopedic surgery
plastic surgery
ophthalmology
neurosurgery
oncology
radiation oncology
cardiology
neonatology
endocrinology

After graduating from medical school with a medical degree, students advance to **residency training,** where they are supervised by fully trained physicians for 3 to 5 years.

There are 24 specialities recognized by the American Board of Medical Specialties. These specialties cover all aspects of medical treatment from allergies to urology.

Most of this residency training is in teaching hospitals and clinics. The hours are long (regularly 100+ a week), and pay is modest. They are often required to work through the night and the following day so that they can experience first-hand the critical 36 hours of patient care after admittance to a hospital.

When the 3-5 years of residency training is completed, physicians are considered specialists and are "board eligible." They can take difficult written and oral board exams, and if successful, can state they are **"board-certified."**

About 30% of fully trained doctors go on to do an **additional 1-6 years** of training to become sub-specialists within their chosen field.

And, of course, after all this is completed, doctors have to constantly keep up with new advances in their field.

ACTION ITEMS
Questions you should ask

Today, patients take an active role in their healthcare. You and your doctor should work in partnership to achieve your best possible level of health. An important part of this relationship is good communication. Here are some questions you can ask your doctor to get the discussion started:

About diagnostic tests...
- What kinds of tests will I have?
- What do you expect to find out from these tests?
- When will I know the results?
- Do I have to do anything special to prepare for any of the tests?
- Do these tests have any side effects or risks?
- Will I need more tests later?

About a disease or condition...
- What is my diagnosis?
- What caused my condition?
- Can my condition be treated?
- How will this condition affect me now and in the future?
- Should I watch for any particular symptoms and notify you if they occur?
- Should I make any lifestyle changes?

About treatment...
- What is the treatment for my condition?
- When will the treatment start, and how long will it last?
- What are the benefits of this treatment, and how successful is it?

? What about bedside manners?

The National Board of Medical Examiners is conducting a trial to make sure that student doctors know how to deal with patients effectively. Specially trained actors play the parts of patients with different illnesses, and the students must interview them and report their findings to a supervisor. The actors likewise report their impression of the student doctors' "bedside manner." If this pilot program is successful, the test will become a requirement for all medical students as early as 2004.

Source: *New York Times*.

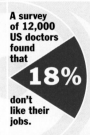

A survey of 12,000 US doctors found that **18%** don't like their jobs.

This disatisfaction may reflect problems with managed care and insurance companies' attempts to limit a doctor's autonomy. As a result, the study notes that many health plans have now eased restrictions on doctors.

Source: Journal of the American Medical Association.

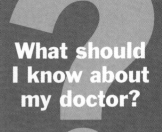

What should I know about my doctor?

Doctors are highly trained healthcare professionals. Getting them to communicate with you about your care may require asking a few questions. 147

? How much does the average doctor earn?

Earnings and expenses for a family practice doctor

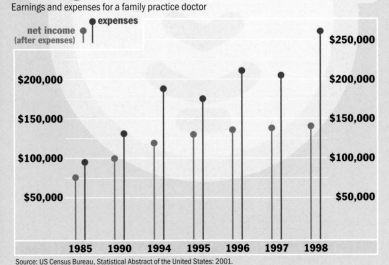

net income (after expenses) | expenses

| | 1985 | 1990 | 1994 | 1995 | 1996 | 1997 | 1998 |

$250,000
$200,000
$150,000
$100,000
$50,000

Source: US Census Bureau, Statistical Abstract of the United States: 2001.

- What are the risks and side effects associated with this treatment?
- Are there foods, drugs or activities I should avoid while I'm on this treatment?
- If my treatment includes taking a medication, what should I do if I miss a dose?
- Are other treatments available?

Understanding your doctor's responses is essential to good communication.

Here are a few more tips:

- If you don't understand your doctor's responses, ask questions until you do understand.

- Take notes, or get a friend or family member to take notes for you. Or, bring a tape-recorder to assist in your recollection of the discussion.
- Ask your doctor to write down her instructions to you.
- Ask your doctor for printed material about your condition.
- If you still have trouble understanding your doctor's answers, ask where you can go for more information.
- Other members of your healthcare team, such as nurses and pharmacists, can be good sources of information. Talk to them, too.

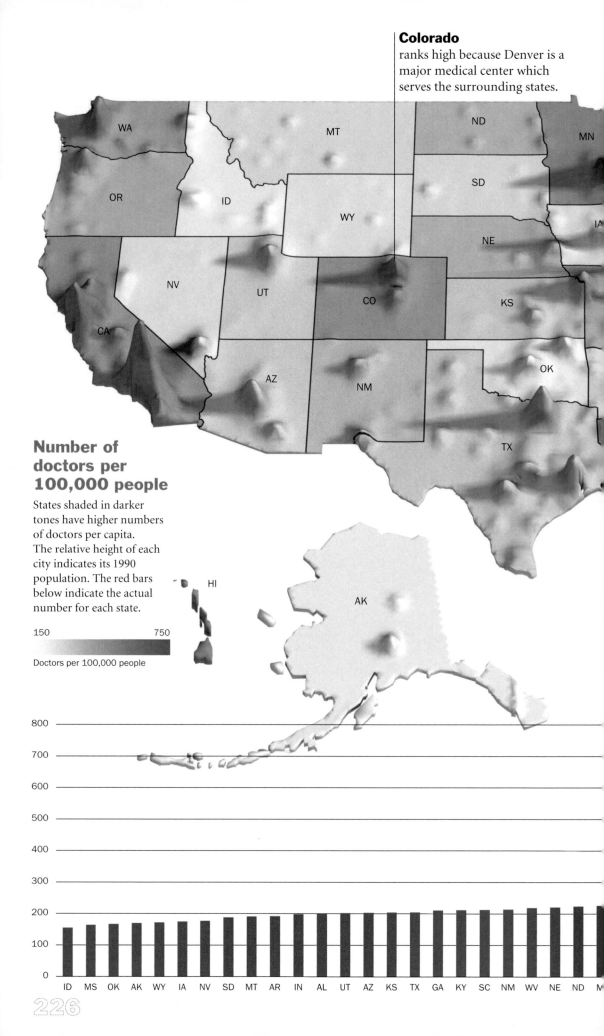

Colorado

ranks high because Denver is a major medical center which serves the surrounding states.

Number of doctors per 100,000 people

States shaded in darker tones have higher numbers of doctors per capita. The relative height of each city indicates its 1990 population. The red bars below indicate the actual number for each state.

150   750

Doctors per 100,000 people

On average, the US has about
1 doctor for every
384 people.

VT NH
ME
MI
NY
MA
RI
CT
IN OH PA
NJ
IL
DC
WV
DE
KY VA
MD
TN
NC
SC
MS AL GA
FL

Generally, the states on the west coast including Hawaii, and those on the east coast, from Massachusetts to Maryland.

Physician supply is not the sole criterion for judging adequacy of health care; there are other demographic and socioeconomic variables that affect both availability and quality. The ratio of physicians to population, however, is certainly one of the most commonly used indicators.

Large numbers of doctors are concentrated in certain medical meccas, most of them metropolitan areas, while many rural areas remain underserved.

Maryland and Washington, DC
benefit from a number of major civilian and military medical facilities, as well as being home to the National Institutes of Health.

Mississippi
has a large rural population of African Americans with low income.

Florida
has a large population of affluent retirees needing medical facilities.

Approximately **1 in 4 doctors** in the US are women (205,903 total.)
Source: ama-assn.org.

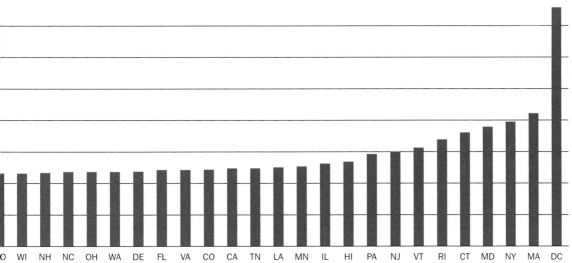

O WI NH NC OH WA DE FL VA CO CA TN LA MN IL HI PA NJ VT RI CT MD NY MA DC

> **Superior general medical knowledge and training are the core elements of a good doctor.**

❓ What should I look for in a doctor?

Don't choose a doctor solely based on location, one referral or board certification. Look for a doctor who provides high-quality healthcare—one who keeps up to date with current medicine, who practices evidence-based medicine, who wants to communicate well with you and who will work in partnership with you. It's important to carefully choose your doctor because the quality of care provided by doctors varies.

Trust is a key part of your relationship with your doctor. You depend on your doctor for treatment and to give you guidance and tools you need to take care of yourself. Research has shown that patients who say they trust their doctor and feel their doctor knows them well are different from those who do not— they are more satisfied with their care, they are more likely to follow their doctor's instructions and they are more likely to report improvements in their health.

Sources: FACCT, *CompareYourCare*; Safran DG, et al., *Linking Primary Care Performance to Outcomes of Care*.

❓ How do I find the best doctors?

Research! Ask questions! Do some homework. Look for a doctor who:

- **Has significant training** and background in the areas you need.
- **Treats you as a partner** sharing information with you and working with you to make decisions.
- **Listens** to you and has your trust.
- **Encourages you** to ask questions.
- Treats you with **respect.**
- **Explains** information clearly.
- Practices **evidence-based** medicine (their advice is based on the best medical research).
- **Suggests** medical decisions based your needs.
- **Keeps current** with new research and recommended practices.
- Is using **technology** (the Internet, email, etc.) to improve patient care and get you the best and most current information.
- Has **privileges** at the hospital of your choice.

Sources: Agency for Healthcare Research and Quality; FACCT, *What Do Patients Want in the Doctor/Patient Relationship?*

❓ What type of doctor do you need?

A general or primary care doctor (your regular doctor) is the one you see most often and is usually a general practitioner, family practitioner, pediatrician or internist. These doctors see you for regular physicals, for minor illness like colds or the flu and for minor injuries, such as a cut that needs stitching.

Your doctor may need to send you to a doctor that is specially trained in a certain aspect of medicine. There are

24 specialty areas

that require training beyond medical school and internships.

THE 24 AREAS OF MEDICAL PRACTICE

Neurological surgery	BRAIN
Psychiatry & neurology	MENTAL STATE
Opthalmology	EYES
Otolaryngology	HEAD & NECK
Anesthesiology	
Allergy & immunology	
Plastic surgery	
Thoracic surgery	CHEST & HEART
Internal medicine	ALL ADULT DISEASES
Dermatology	SKIN
Urology	KIDNEYS & BLADDER
Pathology	BLOOD & BIOPSIES
Colon & rectal surgery	
Obstetrics & gynecology	PREGNANCY & CHILDBIRTH
Orthopedic surgery	BONES
Surgery	
Physical medicine & rehabilitation	FOR PEOPLE WITH DISABILITIES
Preventive medicine	DISEASE PREVENTION
Emergency medicine	
Family practice	TOTAL HEALTH CARE
Medical genetics	MONITORING THIS NEW FIELD
Pediatrics	FOR CHILDREN
Radiology	X-RAYS & THERAPY
Nuclear medicine	X-RAYS & THERAPY

ACTION ITEMS

Rate your doctor

Research shows that when people trust their doctor and feel that their doctor knows them well they are more satisfied with their care. If you're not sure how well you trust your doctor, ask yourself these questions and rate your doctor based on the following scale:

Poor   Fair   Good   Excellent

1 How would you rate your doctor's knowledge of what worries you the most about your health?

2 How thorough is your doctor's knowledge of you as a person (your values and beliefs)?

3 Thinking about the personal aspects of the care you receive from your doctor, how would you rate your doctor's caring and concern for you?

4 How would you describe your trust level on your doctor's judgment about your medical care?

Your answers will give you an idea of how well this relationship is working. If you don't feel comfortable with your doctor or question the treatment recommended for you, you may want to find another doctor.

Source: CompareYourCare; FACCT-Foundation for Accountability.

How do I know if a doctor provides quality care?

It can be hard to learn who provides the best care. Most professional societies don't disclose information about doctors' performance. Similarly, while you can call a doctor referral service at a hospital, these services usually refer you to a doctor on staff at the hospital. Find out if a local consumer group has rated doctors in the area where you live. Call the local medical society to learn if they'll release any information about the doctor you're considering.

- Call the American Board of Medical Specialties at **800.733.2276** to find out if the doctor is board-certified.

- Find your state's Department of Medical Examiners, usually located in your state capital. They grant licenses to doctors and monitor their performance. Find out where they went to school, what their specialty is

and if they've had any disciplinary action.

- A board-certified doctor has completed specialty training and passed an exam that assesses his knowledge, skills and experience to provide quality patient care in that specialty.

Sources: *Finding the Best Doctor for You*, Mark S. Vass; Agency for Healthcare Research and Quality.

If you need a specialist, check out this new doctor as thoroughly as you did your general doctor. **Find out:**

- **How experienced** is this doctor in the specific treatment that you need or ailment you have?

- **How long** has this doctor been in practice?

- Has this doctor ever had **any disciplinary or malpractice actions?**

- If you're considering surgery or some other procedure, find out **how many of the specific procedures the doctor has performed** and if he does them on a regular basis.

- Is this doctor **board-certified** (has advanced training and passed a written examination to demonstrate competence)? Find out by searching on **www.abms.org** .

- How many **patients with your particular condition** has the specialist treated?

- Does this doctor **participate in quality improvement projects** in his clinic or hospital?

- Does the doctor **keep a database** of patients to learn how they progress over time and remind them of follow-up steps?

- Does he **use computerized medical records** to reduce errors and keep all your information organized? 261

Source: Metro Medicine.

Gather basic information

Make a list and call doctors' offices. Ask the office staff if the doctor is accepting new patients and then:

- Which insurance plans do you accept?

- What are your office hours?

- How long does it take to get an appointment?

- Who do I see if my doctor isn't available?

- With which hospitals are you affiliated?

- Can I schedule a "get acquainted" meeting?

Source: healthatoz.com; American Heart Association.

Trust on your part, and expert knowledge of your health on your doctor's part add up to a good doctor/patient relationship.

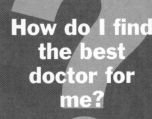

How do I find the best doctor for me?

By doing your homework.

It takes work to find a doctor who is right for you, but it is well worth the effort.

CONSUMER ALERT

People with chronic conditions are not advised by their doctors to make healthy behavior changes about two-thirds of the time; they don't get enough information to manage their own health about one-third of the time; they don't get tests and treatments recommended for their conditions about one-half of the time. To get quality care, choose a good doctor and know what to expect from him or her.

Source: A Portrait of the Chronically Ill in America, 2001, The Robert Wood Johnson Foundation and FACCT — Foundation for Accountability

---

American Medical Association Physician Finder
American Medical Association
515 N. State Street
Chicago, IL 60610
312.464.5000
www.ama-assn.org/aps/amahg.htm

Agency for Healthcare Research and Quality
2101 E. Jefferson St., Suite 501
Rockville, MD 20852
301.594.1364
www.ahrq.gov

Administrators in Medicine (AIM)
DocFinder
www.docboard.org

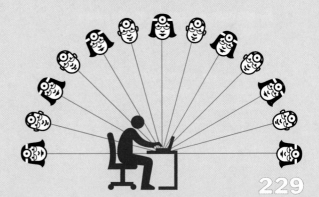

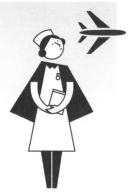

What are the different types of nurse?

Registered nurses (RNs) have graduated from a 2- or 4-year nursing program, have passed state board exams, and are licensed by the state.

Licensed practical nurses (LPNs) are state-licensed caregivers who have been trained to care for the sick. Advanced practice nurses have education and clinical experience beyond the basic training and licensing required of all RNs.

Nurse practitioners (NPs) are RNs with master-level educations. The profession includes these specialties: family (FNP), pediatric (PNP), adult (ANP) and geriatric (GNP). Nurse practitioners can prescribe medications independently in some states, with a co-signer in others.

Clinical nurse specialists (CNSs) are RNs with graduate training in a specialized clinical field such as cardiac, psychiatric or community health.

Certified nurse midwives (CNMs) are RNs with graduate training in women's healthcare needs, including primary prenatal, labor and delivery and post partum care.

Certified registered nurse anesthetists (CRNAs) are RNs with graduate training in the field of anesthesia.

"Airline stewardess" first appeared as a job title in the 1940 US Census, but only as a subsection of **nurses,** since stewardesses were required to be medically trained at that time.
Source: *The Wall Street Journal.*

Nursing is the largest US healthcare occupation: there were 2.2 million registered nurses in 2000.

About a quarter of RNs work part-time.

How much training does it take to become a nurse?

In all states, students must graduate from one of the 1,700 approved nursing programs and pass a national licensing exam to get a nursing license. Nurses may be licensed in more than one state, either by examination or by endorsement of a license from another state. All states require periodic license renewal and that may involve further education.

There are **two major educational paths** to registered nursing:

Bachelor of science degree in nursing
These programs are offered by colleges and universities and take **4-5 years.**

Associate degree in nursing
More than half of all RN programs are at this level. They are offered by community and junior colleges and take **2-3 years.**

Nursing education includes classroom instruction and supervised clinical experience in hospitals and other health facilities.
Students take courses in: anatomy, physiology, microbiology, chemistry, nutrition, psychology, sociology and nursing.

Supervised clinical experience in hospitals includes: pediatrics, psychiatry, maternity and surgery. Most programs also include experience in nursing homes, public health departments and ambulatory clinics.

Source: US Department of Labor.

ACTION ITEMS

Using a nurse practitioner

Many people find it beneficial to use a nurse practitioner (NP) as their primary healthcare provider. Get the answers to these questions if you're considering making the switch.

1 Do you have any serious health issues?
Family practice advanced nurses can treat acute illnesses such as upper respiratory diseases, ear infections, rashes, urinary tract infections and a multitude of other acute illnesses. They can also assist with management of chronic illnesses such as asthma or allergies. If you or someone in your family has severe problems that require highly specialized medical care, you may need to seek the care of a doctor. If you are

unsure about your specific illness and want to know if a nurse practitioner can help, ask your doctor.

2 What are the nurse practitioner's credentials?
If you want to verify an NP's credentials, check with the American College of Nurse Practitioners (ACNP). Also ask NPs about specific qualifications, education and training.

3 What are your states regulations concerning nurse practitioners?
NPs are licensed in all 50 states and follow the rules and regulations of the Nurse Practice Act of the state where they work. Although they can prescribe most medications, some states

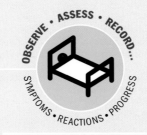

what jobs do nurses do?

Registered nurses (RNs) work to promote health, prevent disease and help patients cope with illness. They are advocates and health educators for patients, families and communities. When providing direct patient care, nurses observe, assess and record symptoms, reactions and progress, and provide nursing treatment and patient education. They assist physicians during treatments and and examinations. They administer medicines and assist in convalescence and rehabilitation.

Office nurses care for outpatients in doctors' offices, clinics and emergency medical centers. They prepare patients for examinations, give injections, dress wounds and maintain records.

Other jobs include: **nursing home care, home health nursing** (for example, caring for recovering patients), **public health nursing** (working to improve the overall health of a community), **occupational health** or **industrial nursing** (nursing at work sites for employees, customers and others with minor illnesses and injuries).

OBSERVE · ASSESS · RECORD...
SYMPTOMS · REACTIONS · PROGRESS

Most nurses work in hospitals, where they are staff nurses providing bedside nursing care and carrying out medical regimens.

How much do nurses earn?

Median earnings in the sectors employing the largest numbers of nurses in 2002

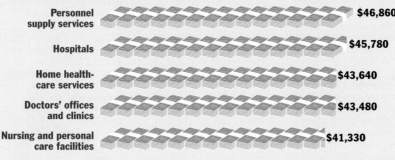

Personnel supply services	$46,860
Hospitals	$45,780
Home health-care services	$43,640
Doctors' offices and clinics	$43,480
Nursing and personal care facilities	$41,330

Source: US Department of Labor.

What should I know about nurses?

Nursing care in a hospital is a critical element in your care and recovery.

For a list of graduate nursing programs write to:
American Association of Colleges of Nursing, 1 Dupont Circle NW, Suite 530, Washington DC 20036

Information on registered nurses is available from:
American Nurses Association, 600 Maryland Avenue SW, Suite 530, Washington DC 20024

---

require a doctor to co-sign prescriptions.

 What is your healthcare attitude?
Nurse practitioners are trained with an emphasis on disease prevention, reduction of health risks and thorough patient education. If your attitude is on the side of prevention, a NP may make a good healthcare partner.

Do you wish it were easier to get an appointment with your doctor?
Many people get their first exposure to an NP when their doctor is booked and they are referred to an NP in the same office. Some practice independently, and you can make appointments with them directly.

 Do you wish that your doctor would spend more time with you?
Often, nurse practitioners are able to take more time with their patients covering issues that are often considered routine.

 Will I save money by using an NP?
Research shows that using NPs can provide satisfying, high-quality and cost-effective care.

 Will your health insurance provider cover care from a nurse practitioner?
Most health plans cover NPs, but check with your insurance company to be sure.

Source: www.kidshealth.org.

What is a physician assistant?

Physician assistants (**PAs**) provide healthcare services under the supervision of physicians. They must graduate from an accredited PA program and pass a national certification examination. PAs work as members of a healthcare team, taking medical histories, examining and treating patients, ordering and interpreting lab tests and x-rays and making diagnoses.

PAs treat minor injuries by suturing, splinting and casting. They record progress notes, instruct and counsel patients and order or carry out therapy. In 47 states and Washington, DC, PAs may prescribe medications.

In rural or inner city clinics, where a doctor is present for one or two days each week, PAs may be the principal care provider. In these situations, PAs may make house calls or go to hospitals and nursing homes to check on patients and report back to the doctor.

There were about 40,500 certified PAs in clinical practice in 2000.

% of PAs in the offices of doctors dentists, etc. — **56**

% of PAs in hospitals — **32**

12

% of PAs in schools, prisons, public health clinics, etc.

What is a pharmacist?

Pharmacists dispense drugs prescribed by physicians and provide information to patients about medications. Pharmacists understand the use, effects, side effects and composition of drugs— their chemical, biological and physical properties—and they advise patients, doctors and other health practioners about these factors.

Pharmacists who work in home healthcare monitor drug therapy and prepare infusions—solutions that are injected into patients—and other medications for use in the home.

There were about 217,000 pharmacists in 2000, more than half worked in drug store chains or similar outlets.

Most **pharmacists keep confidential computerized records of patients' drug therapies** to ensure that harmful drug interactions do not occur.

Pharmacists are responsible for the accuracy of every prescription that is filled, but they often rely on pharmacy technicians and pharmacy aides to fill them.

What is an emergency medical technician? 151

Depending on the nature of the emergency, **EMTs and paramedics** (who are EMTs with additional advanced training) are dispatched to the scene by a 911 operator. They often work wth police and fire departments. On the scene, they determine the patient's condition and try to see if there are pre-existing medical problems. EMTs give emergency care at the scene and transport the patient to a medical facility, if necessary.

Emergency treatments for more complicated problems are carried out under the direction of doctors by radio during transport.

The National Registry of Emergency Medical Technicians lists EMTs by four levels of qualification. The lowest level is First Responder (EMT-1). Many policemen and firefighters have this level of training. The highest level is EMT-Paramedic (EMT-4). These may administer drugs orally and intravenously, interpret EKGs and perform other important medical procedures.

There were about 172,000 EMTs and paramedics working in 2000. Most career EMTs work in big cities, while in smaller towns and the country, many are volunteers. These part-timers work for their local fire departments or hospitals.

What is a physical therapist? 213

Physical therapists (**PTs**) provide services that help restore function, improve mobility, relieve pain and prevent or limit permanent physical disabilities of patients suffering from injuries or disease. Patients include accident victims and people with low back pain, arthritis, heart disease, fractures, head injuries and cerebral palsy.

Treatment often includes exercise. The PT will encourage patients to use their own muscles to increase flexibility and range of motion. The ultimate goal is to improve the way a patient functions at work and at home.

PTs also use electrical stimulation, hot packs or cold compresses and ultrasound to relieve pain. They also teach patients to use assistive devices such as crutches, prostheses and wheelchairs, and to exercise at home to expedite their recovery.

Some PTs treat a wide range of ailments, others specialize in areas such as **cardio fitness, pediatrics, geriatrics, orthopedics, neurology** and **sports medicine.**

ACTION ITEMS
Learn more

- **American Academy of Physician Assistants**
  950 North Washington Street
  Alexandria, VA 22314
  703.836.2272
  www.aapa.org

- **National Commission on Certification of Physician Assistants**
  157 Technology Parkway, Suite 800
  Norcross, GA 30092
  www.nccpa.net

- **American Optometric Association**
  243 North Lindbergh Boulevard
  St. Louis, MO 63141
  www.aoanet.org

- **Association of Schools and Colleges of Optometry**
  6110 Executive Boulevard, Suite 510
  Rockville, MD 20852
  www.opted.org

- **American Dental Association**
  211 E. Chicago Avenue
  Chicago, IL 60611
  312.440.2500
  www.ada.org

- **American Dental Education Association**
  1625 Massachusetts Avenue NW
  Washington, DC 20036
  www.adea.org

❓ What is a radiologic technologist?

Radiologic technologists and technicians take x-rays and administer nonradioactive materials into patients' blood streams for diagnostic purposes.

Experienced radiographers may perform more complex imaging procedures. **CT technologists** operate computerized tomography scanners to produce cross-sectional images of patients.

Magnetic resonance imaging (MRI) technologists operate machines using strong magnets and radio waves rather than radiation to create an image.

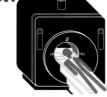

Radiologic technologists must follow physicians' orders precisely and conform to regulations concerning use of radiation to protect themselves, their patients and coworkers from unnecessary exposure.

There were about 167,000 radiographers in 2000, more than half in hospitals. Most of the rest are in doctor's offices and clinics.

❓ What is an optometrist? 161

Optometrists conduct more than 70% of primary eye examinations in thiscountry. Doctors of optometry are independent, primary health care providers who examine, diagnose, treat and manage diseases and disorders of the visual system, the eye and associated structures as well as diagnose related systemic conditions. Optometrists prescribe eyeglasses, contact lenses, low-vision aids, vision therapy and medications used to treat many eye diseases. Optical services including eyeglass and

contact lens sales are a part of many optometric practices.

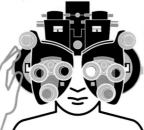

Optometric specialties include elder vision, occupational vision, vision-related learning disabilities, sports vision and low-vision services.

Source: American Optometric Association.

❓ What is a dentist?

Dentists diagnose, prevent, and treat problems of the teeth and the tissue surrounding them. They remove decay, fill cavities, examine x-rays, place protective plastic sealant on children's teeth, straighten teeth and repair fractured teeth. They perform corrective surgery on gums and supporting bones to treat gum disease. They extract teeth and make models for dentures to replace missing teeth.

Dentists provide instruction on diet, brushing, flossing and use of fluorides. They administer anesthetics and write prescriptions for antibiotics and other medications.

Most dentists are general practitioners. Others practice in one of nine specialty areas:
Orthodontists straighten teeth by applying pressure to the teeth with braces or retainers.
Oral and maxillofacial surgeons operate on the mouth and jaws.
Pediatric dentists focus on dentistry for children.
Periodontists treat gums and bones supporting the teeth.
Prosthodontists replace missing teeth with permanent fixtures, such as crowns and bridges or removable fixtures, such as dentures.
Endodontists perform root canal therapy.
Oral pathologists study oral diseases.
Oral and maxillofacial radiologists diagnose disease through imaging technologies.
Public health dentists promote dental health within the community.

Who else helps us with our healthcare?

There is a wide variety of healthcare professionals, other than doctors and nurses, who contribute to your medical well-being. The more you know about what they do, the better prepared you are to be proactive in your healthcare.

● **American Society of Radiologic Technologists**
15000 Central Avenue SE
Albuquerque, NM 87123
www.asrt.org

● **American Registry of Radiologic Technologists**
1255 Northland Drive
St. Paul, MN 55120
www.arrt.org

● **American Association of Colleges of Pharmacy**
1426 Prince Street
Alexandria, VA 22314
www.aacp.org

● **National Associations of Boards of Pharmacy**
700 Busse Highway
Park Ridge, IL 60068
www.nabp.net

● **National Association of Emergency Medical Technicians**
408 Monroe Street
Clinton, MS 39056
www.naemt.org

● **National Registry of Emergency Medical Technicians**
PO Box 29233
Columbus, OH 43229
www.nremt.org

● **American Physical Therapy Association**
1111 North Fairfax Street
Alexandria, VA 22314
www.apta.org

Even after 30 years together, Paul would often boast, "Nora's the most beautiful woman I've ever seen." The couple met on a blind date and married three months later. They bought a home in Phoenix and raised two sons. They loved their life together. That life changed when Nora developed Alzheimer's.

It began with memory loss. Nora forgot lunch plans with friends. Paul became more concerned when she couldn't remember simple words like toothbrush. The petite blonde would jab at her mouth in frustration and say, "You know, that thing." Her symptoms grew steadily worse.

"I always thought we'd grow old together," Paul said. "We'd be one of those couples who travel around in an RV, stopping whenever and wherever we wanted."

As Nora's care became more difficult, Paul with-

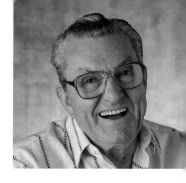

Paul needed help when caring for his wife became too stressful.

drew, not wanting to burden anyone else. He no longer saw friends or played golf, his favorite pastime. The stress of caregiving was taking its toll. He became depressed and developed frequent headaches.

Relief came from the couple's oldest son Ben. He found a respite service in their area that would give his father some much-needed time for himself.

"I didn't know that these kind of services existed," Paul said. Once he started looking, he was amazed at the many resources in his community. He and his son discussed a plan for making Paul's life more manageable. Paul saw a doctor about his depression and organized regular respite and visiting nurse services. And, his two sons offered to stay with their mother more often.

"I know I won't always be able to care for Nora at home," Paul said sadly. "But it's important to me that I do it as long as possible."

Respite care provides a temporary break for caregivers. Sometimes covered by health insurance, respite services means someone comes into your home to care for your loved one or you take him or her to a facility while you spend time on your own. Emergency respite is offered in some nursing homes and residential care facilities when a caregiver becomes ill. There are also programs for adult day services that include meals and recreation.
Source: National Respite Network and Resource Center.

Visiting nurses provide full service home healthcare for patients. A team of nurses and therapists provides a variety of services. Your team could include a home care nurse, a physical therapist and a speech pathologist or a psychiatric nurse and a medical social worker. Care depends on individual patient needs and is coordinated with the patient's physician. They are often available 24 hours a day.
Source: Visiting Nurses Association.

❓ What is the impact of being a caregiver?

Caregiving isn't easy emotionally or physically. Most people provide care out of love and commitment. But constant stress, few resources and long hours can cause depression and feelings of isolation.

1 Feelings reported by people caring for their parent

- **96%** LOVING
- **90%** APPRECIATED
- **84%** PROUD
- **53%** WORRIED
- **37%** FRUSTRATED
- **28%** SAD or DEPRESSED
- **22%** OVERWHELMED

Sources: Family Circle and Kaiser Family Foundation; The Robert Wood Johnson Foundation; FACCT—Foundation for Accountability.

2

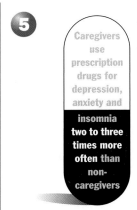

Research says that about

50%

of caregivers are clinically depressed

129

Source: *The Gerontologist.*

---

3 Stress...

...in family caregivers is inversely correlated to income: the less income a caregiver has, the more stress he or she is likely to experience.

Source: *In the Middle: A Report on Multicultural Boomers Coping with Family and Aging Issues,* AARP.

4 Older people experience the **death of a spouse** 61 differently depending on if they provided care or not. Those who had provided care and felt stressed from their caregiving actually showed improved health behaviors and no increase in distress after their spouse's death. People who had not provided care for their spouse reported an increase in depression and weight loss.

Source: Schulz, R. et al. *Involvement in Caregiving and Adjustment to Death of a Spouse.* JAMA.

5

Caregivers use prescription drugs for depression, anxiety and **insomnia two to three times more often than non-caregivers**

Source: *Caregiver Well-Being: A Multidimensional Examination of Family Caregivers of Demented Adults,* The Gerontologist.

---

6 Only **43%** of caregivers feel involved in healthcare decisions for the person they are caring for. Less than half of caregivers feel that the care recipient's healthcare provider is helpful in clarifying treatment goals and helps the caregiver understand the care recipient's treatment.

Source: The Robert Wood Johnson Foundation and FACCT, *A Portrait of Informal Caregivers in America, 2001.*

ACTION ITEMS
Find out more about caregiving

AoA National Family Caregiver Support Program
www.aoa.dhhs.gov/carenetwork/default.htm

AARP
Education and information about caregiving, long-term care and aging
601 E Street, NW
Washington, DC 20049
800.424.3410
www.aarp.org

National Family Caregivers Association(NFCA)
Educates, supports, empowers and advocates on behalf of caregivers
www.nfcacares.org

National Alliance for Caregiving
Provides support to family and professional caregivers
www.caregiving.org

Family Caregiver Alliance (FCA)
FCA is the lead agency in California's system of Caregiver Resource Centers
690 Market Street Suite 600
San Francisco, CA 94104
415.434.3388 or 800.445.8106 (CA only)
email: info@caregiver.org
www.caregiver.org

Take charge of your life and don't let your loved one's illness always take center stage.

•

Set aside time for your own needs. Be good to yourself.

•

Watch out for signs of depression, and get professional help when you need it.

•

Accept offers of assistance.

•

Educate yourself about your loved one's condition. Information is powerful. Be an advocate. Demand involvement in and information about treatment decisions.

•

Grieve for your losses, but also allow yourself to have new dreams.

•

Seek support from other caregivers.

•

Have a back-up when you need a break.

•

Stand up for your rights as a caregiver and citizen.

•

Source: National Family Caregivers Association, Caregiving Resources, sfcacares.org.

Who are the people most likely to need a caregiver?

1 out of every 2 people in America has a chronic condition. 219

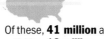

Of these, **41 million** are limited in their daily activities. **12 million** are unable to go to school, to work or to live independently.

Source: *Chronic Care in America* Institute for Health & Aging, Univ. of CA/SF for the Robert Wood Johnson Foundation.

Nearly half of people age 75 and older say their daily activities are adversely impacted from an ongoing physical, mental or emotional problem. 61

Source: *Chartbook on Trends in the Health of Americans*, National Center for Health Statistics.

Where can I get information and support?

There is sporadic help for caregivers, depending upon where you live and the age of the care recipient. Most federal or private health insurance does not pay for in-home help unless a doctor orders it. Even then, services are often limited to short periods of time. However, many states have programs that cover an array of services from respite to help with bathing. You probably will have to do some digging to find services, but learning about resources in your community is worth the effort. The more support you and your loved one have, the better the caregiving situation.

● **Contact** your county or state department of senior services or aging, area social service agencies, your local hospital's social work department, adult day centers and the local chapter of the health association that focuses on your loved one's condition. Ask if they offer support programs and how to apply for them.
● **If you are caring for a child**, check with the local school or county children's agency.
● Check the **local university and hospital** to see if they have a caregiver program. The federal government funds large research centers in many diseases, which may include support and some services for caregivers.
● Check your local paper for listings of **classes and workshops for family caregivers.**
● Ask your **doctor's office** about resources in the community.
● Find **local support groups** of caregivers. These are people who are sharing the same experiences and generally know community resources. Ask your doctor about where to find one or call a national disease organization.

Source: National Family Caregivers Association.

What should I know about caregiving?

Informal caregivers are unpaid individuals, such as family, neighbors or friends, who provide help to people unable to care for themselves.

They number over 50 million, and the value of their free services is estimated to be $257 billion a year.

Source: National Family Caregivers Association.

Friends Health Connection
Links persons with illness or disability and family caregivers with others in similar situations
800.384.7436
www.48friend.org

A Guide to Improving Doctor/Caregiver Communication
Designed to help improve communication between family caregivers and health care professionals
www.nfcacares.org

Caregiver Resource Directory
A practical guide offering resources, facts and advice about caregiving
www.stoppain.org/caregivers/resource_form.html

Well Spouse Foundation
Offers support to husbands, wives and partners of people with chronic illnesses and disabilities
30 East 40th Street PH
New York, NY 10016
800.838.0879
www.wellspouse.org

Northwest Covenant Medical Center
25 Pocono Road
Denville, NJ 07834
973.625.9565
www.selfhelpgroups.org

❓ Are hospitals accountable to any governing body?

There is no one entity that oversees hospitals, though both state and federal agencies play some role. All hospitals must receive a license to do business from the state in which they operate. Various states require hospitals to have certain policies in place. Your state health agency can tell you about the requirements in your area.

The federal government oversees the Medicare program, and in order to receive Medicare payments, hospitals are required to undergo a review and approval process (called accreditation) by a national, private organization called the **Joint Commission on Accreditation of Healthcare Organizations (JCAHO)**. Since Medicare payments account for almost half of most hospitals' income, the majority of hospitals seek accreditation. In some states, the JCAHO review is the only criteria necessary for operation.

Seventy percent of JCAHO's income depends on payments from the hospitals that ask for its approval. Representatives of major health care organizations govern JCAHO, and the organization has no accountability to the government or the public. Of America's nearly 6,000 hospitals, only about one percent fail the JCAHO's accreditation test; so look for other evidence of a hospital's quality besides its accreditation status!

❓ Is your hospital approved by JCAHO? Check it out.

A list of JCAHO accredited hospitals and their survey results, including past performance reports, are posted in the "Quality Check™" section of the JCAHO's Web site at

www.jcaho.org
Or call **630.792.5800.**

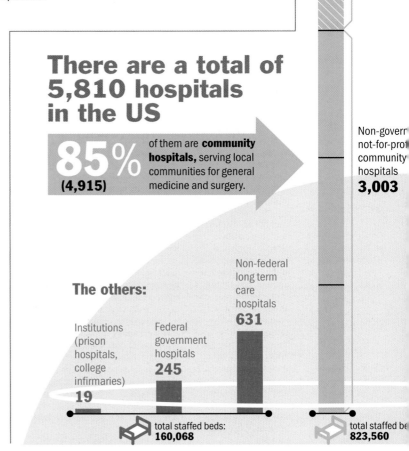

There are a total of 5,810 hospitals in the US

85%
(4,915)
of them are **community hospitals,** serving local communities for general medicine and surgery.

For-profit community hospitals
749

State and local government hospitals
1,163

Non-government not-for-profit community hospitals
3,003

The others:

Institutions (prison hospitals, college infirmaries)
19

Federal government hospitals
245

Non-federal long term care hospitals
631

total staffed beds:
160,068

total staffed beds:
823,560

ACTION ITEMS
Questions to ask about your hospital

General Information

● Is the hospital approved by an accrediting body, such as the Joint Commission on Accreditation of Healthcare Organizations?
  ☐ Yes ☐ No

● Is the hospital clean?
  ☐ Yes ☐ No

● What kind of hospital is it? Do they specialize in certain areas of care?
  ☐ Yes ☐ No

● Is your doctor affiliated with your hospital?
  ☐ Yes ☐ No

Specific Needs

● Do you have a medical condition that needs specialized care? If so, does this hospital provide the services you need?
  ☐ Yes ☐ No

● If you need surgery, does the hospital have a good success record with this procedure?
  ☐ Yes ☐ No

? What is a teaching hospital?

Doctors, nurses and dentists train in teaching hospitals. Under the guidance of experienced professionals, these students work directly with patients. Over 75,000 medical and dental residents train in teaching hospitals every year. These hospitals also are home to medical researchers looking for answers to our most challenging medical questions, like how we can cure diseases or prevent people from getting them.

These facilities are often state-of-the-art and offer highly specialized services (burn care units, transplant services, pediatric intensive care units, open-heart surgery and trauma centers). **One in five hospitals is a teaching hospital.** You're most likely to find teaching hospitals in urban areas, where 90% are located.
Source: Advancing Health In America, Trend Watch.

? What's the difference between general and specialized hospitals?

Most hospitals are "general" hospitals that care for a full range of medical conditions. "Specialized" hospitals limit their treatment to particular conditions, diseases or populations. For example, you can find hospitals that specialize in treating cancer, rehabilitation, and psychiatric illnesses; and others that care just for children or the elderly.

When faced with a decision about which hospital to use, keep in mind that a general hospital may not offer the offer the most up-to-date treatment for all conditions. Talk to your doctor about which hospital is best for your situation.
Source: Health Pages.

Total admissions to all US hospitals
(2001)

34,890,750
👤👤👤👤👤👤👤👤👤👤👤👤👤👤👤👤👤👤👤👤👤👤👤

Total annual expenses for all US hospitals (2001)

$395,391,209,000

Source: American Hospital Association.

? What's different about rural healthcare?

🌳 **Rural areas have about half as many physicians as urban areas to serve a given population base.** Nearly 90% of all specialists practice in urban areas, leaving rural America largely unserved.

🌳 **Rural residents are less likely to have employer-provided healthcare coverage.**

🌳 **Rural residents are twice as likely as urban residents to die in motor-vehicle accidents.**

🌳 **Rural residents tend to be poorer.** On average, percapita income is $7,417 lower than in urban areas. The disparity in incomes is greater for minorities. Nearly 24% of rural children live in poverty.

🌳 **Medicare payments to rural hospitals and physicians are less than those given to urban hospitals for the same services.** This might help explain why more than 470 rural hospitals have closed in the past 25 years.

Source: National Rural Health Association.

What should I know about my hospital?

You should know specifics about the quality of your hospital.

There are factors beyond accreditation that can be even more important.

70% of specialty or "boutique" hospitals are owned partly or entirely by doctors.
Source: The Wall Street Journal.

● Does the hospital have written information on patients' rights and responsibilities?
☐ Yes ☐ No

● Does the hospital have social workers on staff?
☐ Yes ☐ No

Patient Safety

● Is the ICU staffed with doctors trained to treat critically ill patients?
☐ Yes ☐ No

● Does the hospital use a computerized prescription entry system to reduce medication errors?
☐ Yes ☐ No

Discharge Planning

● Does the hospital provide discharge plans?
☐ Yes ☐ No

● Does the hospital give you information or training to continue your care after you leave the hospital?
☐ Yes ☐ No

Sources: JCAHO; Leapfrog Group.

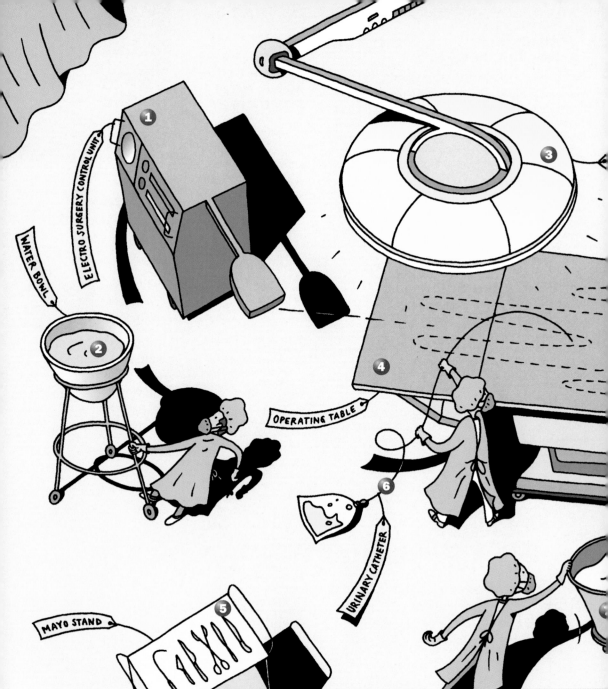

WATER BOWL

ELECTRO SURGERY CONTROL UNIT

OPERATING TABLE

URINARY CATHETER

MAYO STAND

ACTION ITEMS   What is all that stuff?

1 Electrosurgical Machine
This machine uses high-frequency electrical signals to cauterize, or seal off, blood vessels or to cut through tissue with minimal bleeding.

2 Water Bowl
Sterile water used to moisten swabs and instruments during surgery is held in this bowl.

3 Operating Room Light
This light, positioned over the operating table, provides bright light with no shadows to give surgeons excellent viewing capabilities.

4 Operating Table
The table can be raised, lowered and tilted in any direction to position the patient for surgery.

5 Urinary Catheter
Also called a foley catheter, this flexible plastic tube used to drain the patient's bladder helps monitor a patient's fluid status and kidney function.

6 Mayo Stand
Sterile instruments are arranged for access during surgery on this stainless steel table.

7 Kick Bucket
This bucket, positioned on the floor to be away from the surgical field, is used to collect used sponges.

8 IV (Intravenous) Line
This flexible plastic tube inserted into a vein delivers blood, fluids, nutrients and/or medications.

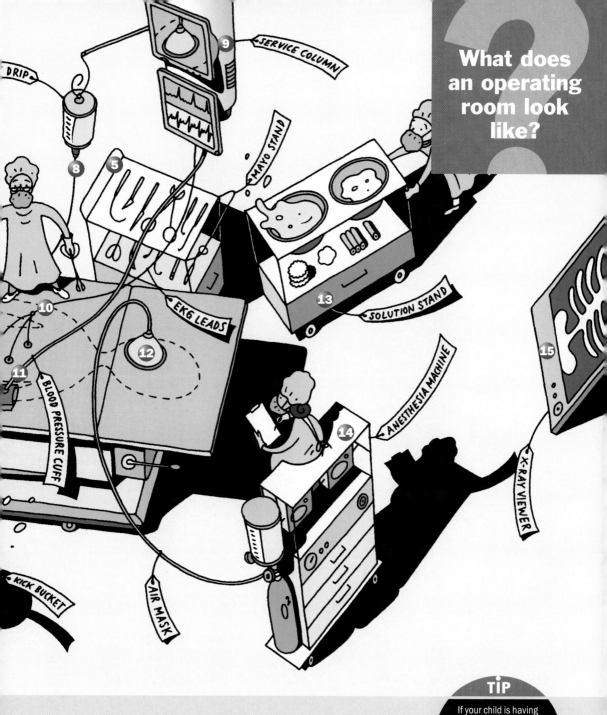

TIP

If your child is having an operation, ask if he can visit the hospital to play with surgical gloves, mask and cap so they are not so scary later.

9 Service Column
A service column provides gas and electrical power to an OR in one convenient, central location.

10 EKG Leads
These wires connect small, round electrode pads adhered to the patient's chest to a monitor which displays heart rate and rhythm.

11 Blood Pressure Cuff
During surgery, an automated blood pressure cuff automatically inflates to measure blood pressure at regular intervals.

12 Air Mask
This mask, attached to the anesthesia machine, delivers the appropriate mix of gases for anesthetizing the patient.

13 Solution Stand
Fluid used to sterilize the patient's skin is kept handy to the OR staff in the stainless bowls on a solution stand.

14 Anesthesia Machine
Located at the head of the operating table, this machine, connected to the air mask, assists breathing and has built in monitors that help control the mixture of gases.

15 X-Ray Viewer
This screen displays x-rays and other scans so the surgeons can reference them during an operation.

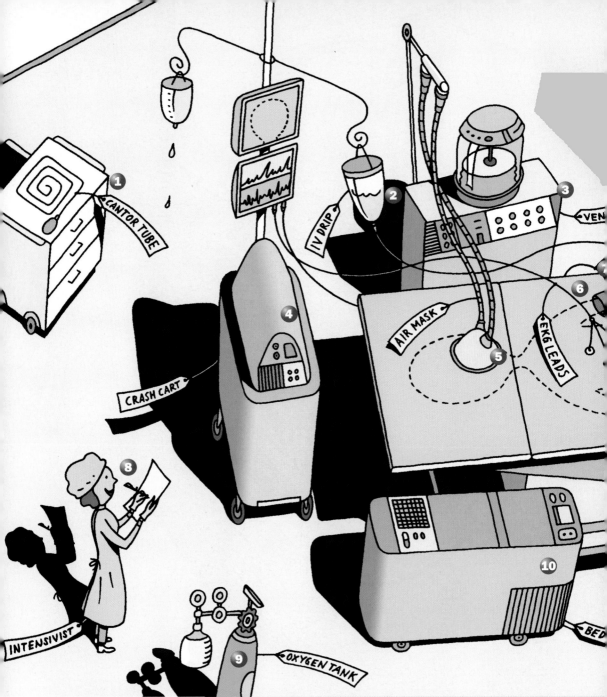

CANTOR TUBE

IV DRIP

VEN-

AIR MASK

EKG LEADS

CRASH CART

INTENSIVIST

OXYGEN TANK

BED

ACTION ITEMS   Know your way around

1 Cantor Tube
Also called a nasal-gastric or NG tube, this tube inserted through the nose can aspirate, or suck out, gastric fluid.

2 IV (Intravenous) Line
This flexible plastic tube inserted into a vein delivers blood, fluids, nutrients and/or medications.

3 Ventilator
Also called respirator, this machine, connected by a mask, an endotracheal tube (breathing tube) through the mouth or a tracheostomy tube through the neck, "breathes" for a patient who can't breathe on his own.

4 Crash cart
Used if a patient's heart or lungs stop working, this cart, also called a resuscitation cart, has all the drugs and equipment necessary for advanced life support and CPR.

Air Mask
5 This mask delivers humidified, oxygenated air.

EKG Leads 165
6 These wires connect electrodes on the patient's chest to a monitor showing heart rate and rhythm.

7 Blood Pressure Cuff
Positioned around the patient's arm, this cuff periodically measures the patient's blood pressure.

8 Intensivist
Intensivists are highly trained doctors familiar with the complications that can occur in the ICU.

242

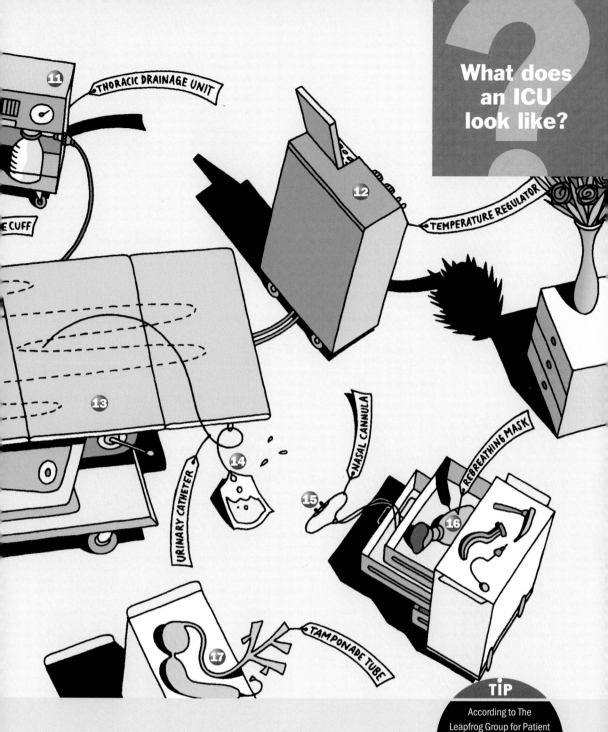

THORACIC DRAINAGE UNIT

CUFF

TEMPERATURE REGULATOR

URINARY CATHETER

NASAL CANNULA

REBREATHING MASK

TAMPONADE TUBE

TIP

According to The Leapfrog Group for Patient Safety, hospitals with intensivists have lower rates of surgical mortality.

⑨ Oxygen Tank
This tank stores oxygen which is added to the patient's air supply.

⑩ Bed Controls
These controls reposition the ICU bed to facilitate care and comfort the patient.

⑪ Thoracic Drainage Unit
This drainage unit connected by a tube from the chest, removes air and fluid from the thorax, the area between the patient's head and waist.

⑫ Temperature Regulator
This machine regulates the patient's body temperature by circulating heated or cooled saline.

⑬ ICU Bed
The ICU bed can be adjusted to prevent bed sores or stiffened for CPR compressions.

⑭ Urinary Catheter
This plastic tube is used to drain the patient's bladder and monitor kidney function.

⑮ Nasal Cannula
These prongs on tubing connected to an oxygen tank add oxygen to air breathed through the nose.

⑯ Breathing Bag
Used for short-term, manual resuscitation, this bag, which can be used with a mask or breathing tube, is squeezed to push oxygen into the lungs.

⑰ Tamponade Tube
This apparatus helps prevents cardiac shock by draining fluid from the pericardium, the sack around heart.

don't like hospitals," said Henry, a 55-year-old mechanic. "It just reminds me that I have a heart condition and I might end up there one day. But when my friend Joe had a heart attack 77 I just had to go visit him. I'm glad because I learned a lot from his experience."

At the hospital, Joe was pale but feisty. He told Henry he was transferring to another hospital the next day. Henry was puzzled. "Aren't all hospitals the same?" he asked Joe. "Why move to a hospital 30 miles farther away?"

"They don't listen to me here," Joe explained. "I keep asking about these pills the nurses give me and I can't get an answer. I want to know what I'm taking. Plus, my wife did some research and we compared nearby hospitals. I found out that this other hospital specializes in taking care of people with heart problems."

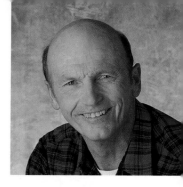

Henry learned from his friend that choosing a hospital shouldn't be done by location alone.

A month after Joe returned home, he went into the hospital again, this time for a planned procedure, coronary bypass surgery. He'd studied the rates of death shortly after surgery at various hospitals and chose one that performed a high volume of the surgery he needed.

"Practice makes perfect," he told his wife. "I want a surgeon and a hospital that specializes in this type of surgery and makes far fewer preventable mistakes."

A few months later, Henry experienced chest pains and was being sent to the hospital by his doctor for testing. Based on his friend's experience and research, he, too, requested the hospital in the next town. As he registered, he tried make his wife feel better about the distance, "This place can take better care of me. I feel much better knowing I'm in expert hands."

You'll find hospital ratings on these Web sites:
healthscope.org (California only)
healthgrades.com
myhealthfinder.com (New York only)
healthcarechoices.org

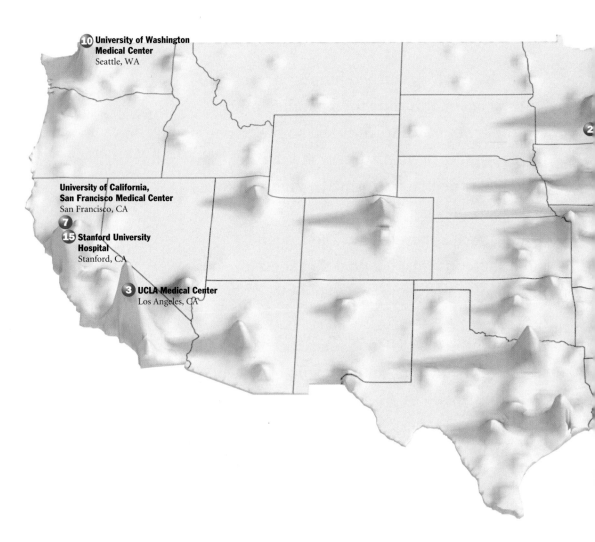

University of Washington
Medical Center
Seattle, WA

University of California,
San Francisco Medical Center
San Francisco, CA

Stanford University
Hospital
Stanford, CA

UCLA Medical Center
Los Angeles, CA

2003 US News Honor Roll Hospitals Overall

1

Johns Hopkins Hospital

32 points in
16 specialties

www.jhu.edu

2

Mayo Clinic

28 points in
14 specialties

www.mayo.edu

3

UCLA Medical Center

24 points in
14 specialties

www.clevelandclinic.org

4

Massachusetts General Hospital

24 points in
12 specialties

www.mgh.harvard.edu

5

Cleveland Clinic

23 points in
12 specialties.

www.healthcare.ucla.edu

6

Duke University Medical Center

22 points in
13 specialties

www.mc.duke.edu

7

University of California, San Francisco Medical Center

21 points in
12 specialties

www.ucsf.edu/

8

Barnes-Jewish Hospital

18 points in
12 specialties

www.med.umich.edu

9

University of Michigan Medical Center

16 points in
11 specialties

www.barnesjewish.org

10

University of Washington Medical Center

15 points in
10 specialties

www.brighamandwomens.org

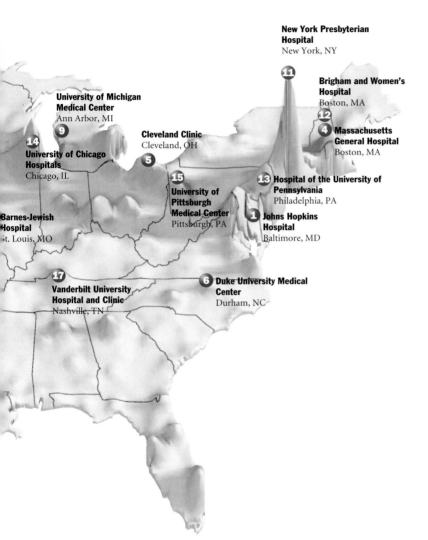

Where the expertise is broadest.

US News & World Report's 2003 rankings identified 17 hospitals that stood out dramatically because of the unusual breath of their expertise—the Honor Roll. They ranked at or near the top in as many as 16 specialties tracked by the survey. Each hospital was then awarded points that created the final ranking shown here. 249

Source: US News & World Report, 14th Annual Honor Roll, 2003.

Map labels:

New York Presbyterian Hospital
New York, NY

University of Michigan Medical Center
Ann Arbor, MI

Brigham and Women's Hospital
Boston, MA

Cleveland Clinic
Cleveland, OH

Massachusetts General Hospital
Boston, MA

University of Chicago Hospitals
Chicago, IL

Hospital of the University of Pennsylvania
Philadelphia, PA

Barnes-Jewish Hospital
St. Louis, MO

University of Pittsburgh Medical Center
Pittsburgh, PA

Johns Hopkins Hospital
Baltimore, MD

Vanderbilt University Hospital and Clinic
Nashville, TN

Duke University Medical Center
Durham, NC

---

11 New York-Presbyterian Hospital

15 points in 9 specialties

www.washington.edu

12 Brigham and Women's Hospital

14 points in 8 specialties

www.nyp.org

13 Hospital of the University of Pennsylvania

13 points in 9 specialties

www.med.upenn.edu

14 University of Chicago Hospitals

10 points in 7 specialties

www.uchospitals.edu

15 (TIE) University of Pittsburgh Medical Center

9 points in 7 specialties

www.stanfordhospital.com

15 (TIE) Stanford University Hospital

9 points in 7 specialties

www.upmc.edu

17 Vanderbilt University Hospital and Clinic

8 points in 6 specialties

www.mc.vanderbilt.edu

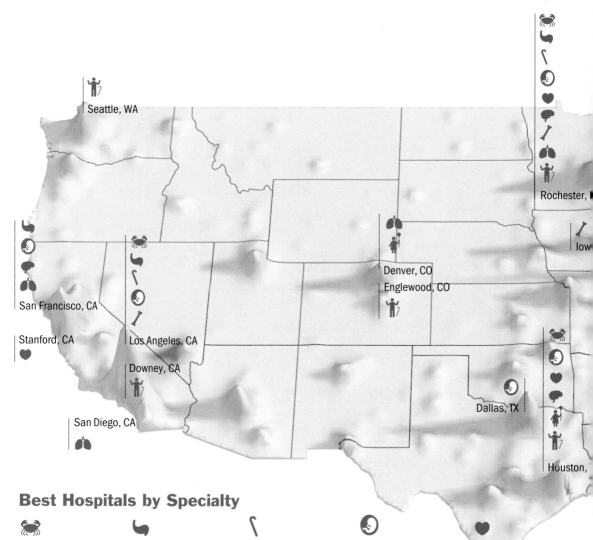

Seattle, WA

Rochester,

Iow

Denver, CO
Englewood, CO

San Francisco, CA

Stanford, CA

Los Angeles, CA

Downey, CA

San Diego, CA

Dallas, TX

Houston,

Best Hospitals by Specialty

Cancer

1. **University of Texas, M.D. Anderson Cancer Center**
   Houston, TX
2. **Memorial Sloan-Ketterling Cancer Center**
   New York, NY
3. **Johns Hopkins Hospital**
   Baltimore, MD
4. **Dana-Farber Cancer Institute**
   Boston, MA
5. **Mayo Clinic**
   Rochester, MN
6. **University of Chicago Hospitals**
   Chicago, IL
7. **Duke University Medical Center**
   Durham, NC
8. **UCLA Medical Center**
   Los Angeles, CA
9. **University of Michigan Medical Center**
   Ann Arbor, MI
10. **H. Lee Moffet Cancer Center**
    Tampa, FL

Digestive Disorders

1. **Mayo Clinic**
   Rochester, MN
2. **Johns Hopkins Hospital**
   Baltimore, MD
3. **Cleveland Clinic**
   Cleveland, OH
4. **Massachusetts General Hospital**
   Boston, MA
5. **Mt. Sinai Medical Center**
   New York, NY
6. **University of Chicago Hospitals**
   Chicago, IL
7. **UCLA Medical Center**
   Los Angeles, CA
8. **Duke University Medical Center**
   Durham, NC
9. **University of California, San Francisco Medical Center**
   San Francisco, CA
10. **University of Pittsburgh Medical Center**
    Pittsburgh, PA

Geriatrics

1. **UCLA Medical Center**
   Los Angeles, CA
2. **Johns Hopkins Hospital**
   Baltimore, MD
3. **Mt. Sinai Medical Center**
   New York, NY
4. **Massachusetts General Hospital**
   Boston, MA
5. **Duke University Medical Center**
   Durham, NC
6. **Mayo Clinic**
   Rochester, MN
7. **Cleveland Clinic**
   Cleveland, OH
8. **Yale-New Haven Hospital**
   New Haven, CT
9. **St. Louis University Hospital**
   St. Louis, MO
10. **University of Michigan Medical Center**
    Ann Arbor, MI

Gynecology

1. **Johns Hopkins Hospital**
   Baltimore, MD
2. **Mayo Clinic**
   Rochester, MN
3. **Brigham and Women's Hospital**
   Boston, MA
4. **University of Texas, M.D. Anderson Cancer Center**
   Houston, TX
5. **UCLA Medical Center**
   Los Angeles, CA
6. **Duke University Medical Center**
   Durham, NC
7. **Massachusetts General Hospital**
   Boston, MA
8. **Parkland Memorial Hospital**
   Dallas, TX
9. **Cleveland Clinic**
   Cleveland, OH
10. **University of California, San Francisco Medical Center**
    San Francisco, CA

Heart & Heart Surgery

1. **Cleveland Clinic**
   Cleveland, OH
2. **Mayo Clinic**
   Rochester, MN
3. **Massachusetts General Hospital**
   Boston, MA
4. **Brigham and Women's Hospital**
   Boston, MA
5. **Duke University Medical Center**
   Durham, NC
6. **Johns Hopkins Hospital**
   Baltimore, MD
7. **Texas Heart Institute**
   Houston, TX
8. **Emory University Hospital**
   Atlanta, GA
9. **Stanford University Hospital**
   Stanford, CA
10. **Barnes-Jewish Hospital**
    St. Louis, MO

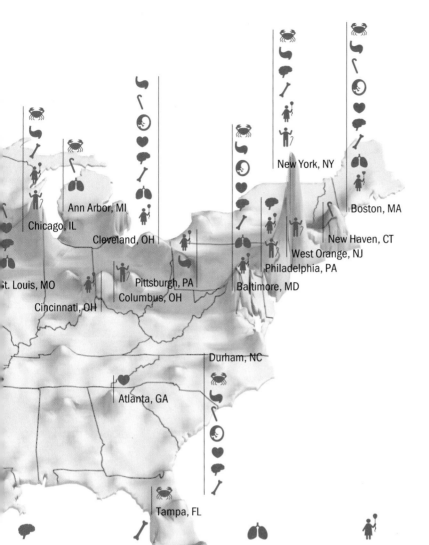

Not always where you'd expect.

US News & World Report ranks "America's Best Hospitals" each year to identify the top hospitals by specialties from cancer to urology. More than 6,000 medical centers were rated against a wide range of criteria and their performance in one or more specialties was evaluated. Rankings for 10 of 17 specialties are shown here. 251

Source: US News & World Report, 14th Annual Honor Roll, 2003

New York, NY

Ann Arbor, MI

Chicago, IL

Boston, MA

Cleveland, OH

New Haven, CT

West Orange, NJ

Philadelphia, PA

St. Louis, MO

Pittsburgh, PA

Columbus, OH

Baltimore, MD

Cincinnati, OH

Durham, NC

Atlanta, GA

Tampa, FL

Neurology and Neurosurgery

1 **Mayo Clinic**
Rochester, MN

2 **Massachusetts General Hospital**
Boston, MA

3 **Johns Hopkins Hospital**
Baltimore, MD

4 **New York Presbyterian Hospital**
New York, NY

5 **Cleveland Clinic**
Cleveland, OH

6 **University of California, San Francisco Medical Center**
San Francisco, CA

7 **Barnes-Jewish Hospital**
St. Louis, MO

8 **UCLA Medical Center**
Los Angeles, CA

9 **Hospital of the University of Pennsylvania**
Philadelphia, PA

10 **Methodist Hospital**
Houston, TX

Orthopedics

1 **Mayo Clinic**
Rochester, MN

2 **Hospital for Special Surgery**
New York, NY

3 **Massachusetts General Hospital**
Boston, MA

4 **Johns Hopkins Hospital**
Baltimore, MD

5 **Cleveland Clinic**
Cleveland, OH

6 **Duke University Medical Center**
Durham, NC

7 **UCLA Medical Center**
Los Angeles, CA

8 **University of Iowa Hospitals and Clinics**
Iowa City, IA

9 **Brigham and Women's Hospital**
Boston, MA

10 **University of Chicago Hospitals**
Chicago, IL

Respiratory Disorders

1 **National Jewish Center**
Denver, CO

2 **Mayo Clinic**
Rochester, MN

3 **Johns Hopkins Hospital**
Baltimore, MD

4 **Barnes-Jewish Hospital**
St. Louis, MO

5 **Massachusetts General Hospital**
Boston, MA

6 **University of California, San Francisco Medical Center**
San Francisco, CA

7 **University Hospital**
Denver, CO

8 **Cleveland Clinic**
Cleveland, OH

9 **UCSD Medical Center**
San Diego, CA

10 **University of Michigan Medical Center**
Ann Arbor, MI

Pediatrics

1 **Children's Hospital**
Boston, MA

2 **Children's Hospital of Philadelphia**
Philadelphia, PA

3 **Johns Hopkins Hospital**
Baltimore, MD

4 **Children's Hospital**
Denver, CO

5 **Children's Hospital of New York Presbyterian**
New York, NY

6 **University Hospitals of Cleveland (Rainbow Babies and Children's Hospital)**
Cleveland, OH

7 **Children's Hospital**
Pittsburgh, PA

8 **Texas Children's Hospital**
Houston, TX

9 **Children's Hospital Medical Center**
Cincinnati, OH

10 **Children's Memorial Hospital**
Chicago, IL

Rehabilitation

1 **Rehabilitation Institute of Chicago**
Chicago, IL

2 **The Institute for Rehabilitation and Research**
Houston, TX

3 **University of Washington Medical Center**
Seattle, WA

4 **Mayo Clinic**
Rochester, MN

5 **Kessler Institute for Rehabilitation**
West Orange, NJ

6 **Craig Hospital**
Englewood, CO

7 **New York University Medical Center (Rusk Institute)**
New York, NY

8 **Ohio State University Medical Center**
Columbus, OH

9 **Rancho Los Amigos National Rehabilitation Center**
Downey, CA

10 **Thomas Jefferson University Hospital**
Philadelphia, PA

Though you may not realize it, you do have a choice of hospitals.

When you select a health plan or primary care doctor or specialist, often you're choosing a hospital—the hospital that your health plan, doctor or medical group uses. It's your health at stake, so be sure to choose wisely.

Answering these questions can help you find the best one for your needs.

? Does the hospital meet national quality standards?

A "seal of approval" by the Joint Commission on Accreditation of Healthcare Organizations (JCAHO) means the hospital meets certain quality standards. Some hospitals get better marks than others. Would you prefer a hospital that meets all accreditation standards or one that meets only some of the standards?

? Is my doctor permitted to admit patients to the hospital?

If not, you would be under the care of another doctor while at the hospital. Ask your doctor about his or her affiliations with hospitals in your area.

? What programs does the hospital have to improve patient safety and reduce medical errors?

Some hospitals are working to better protect patients from medical errors. Is yours? Here are some examples of hospital practices that can improve patient safety. **Ask your hospital what they do to protect their patients.**

Computer Physician Order Entry (CPOE)
Can't read your doctor's handwriting? Maybe your hospital pharmacist can't either and that's a recipe for disaster. With computerized prescription systems, a doctor enters the medication you need into a computer and the prescription is automatically checked for potential mistakes or problems.

Studies show that a computerized prescription system can reduce serious medication mistakes by up to

86%

Practice Makes Perfect
Some hospitals have more experience with certain procedures. "General" hospitals handle a wide range of routine conditions, such as hernias and pneumonia. "Specialty" hospitals have a lot of experience with certain conditions (such as cancer) or certain populations (such as children). You also may want to find out if the hospital has a team of health professionals that specializes in working with your condition or the treatment you need.

Source: Agency for Healthcare Research and Quality, ahrq.gov.

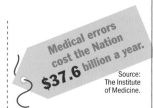 Medical errors cost the Nation **$37.6** billion a year.
Source: The Institute of Medicine.

ICU Physician Staffing (IPS)
"Intensivists" are physicians specially trained to care for critically ill patients in Intensive Care Units (ICUs). Studies reveal that at least one in ten patients who die every year in ICUs would have had an increased chance to live if intensivists had been present in the ICU. **Ask if these types of physicians are available in the ICU at the hospital you're checking out.**

Source: The Leapfrog Group for Patient Safety.

? Does my health plan cover care at the hospital?

If not, you'll have to pay all of the costs for your care. If going to a certain hospital is important to you, keep that in mind when choosing your doctor and/or health plan. In general, you will go to the hospital where your doctor has "privileges" (is permitted to admit patients). Ask your health plan about their affiliations with hospitals.

Source: Agency for Healthcare Research and Quality, ahrq.gov.

ACTION ITEMS

Resources

healthfinder®
Healthfinder is a gateway to reliable consumer health information from the federal government and other organizations.
www.healthfinder.gov

The Leapfrog Group for Patient Safety
See how your hospital scores on patient safety.
www.leapfroggroup.org

Health Grades®
View hospital ratings in detailed consumer reports.
www.healthgrades.com

Health Care Choices
Find report cards for hospitals in many states.
www.healthcarechoices.org

Health Scope
Health Scope provides detailed ratings of California hospitals in many aspects of care and treatment.
www.healthscope.org

What criteria can I use to compare hospitals?

 Look at hospital report cards developed by state health organizations and consumer groups to learn about hospital quality.

 Some states have laws that require hospitals to report data on the quality of their care. This information is provided to the public so consumers can compare hospitals. Pennsylvania, California and Ohio have these laws.

 Consumer groups publish guides to hospitals and other healthcare institutions in various cities. You can find out what's available where you live by calling your state department of health, healthcare council or hospital association.

Ask your doctor, relatives, friends and neighbors about their experiences with the hospital you are considering.

Source: Agency for Healthcare Research and Quality, ahrq.gov.

When should I consider leaving my area when I need hospital services?

When you need the specialized care that some hospitals provide.

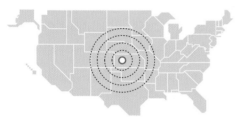

For example, if you need cancer care and you don't feel satisfied that your community hospital is the best choice for you, talk to your doctor or insurance provider about options outside your local area. You or your doctor may be able to make a case to the health plan about why another hospital is better for you.

What's tiering?

Some health insurance plans are reducing costs for employers by introducing **tiering** programs that give consumers their choice of hospitals based on cost and quality.

Members health plans pay less when they choose from the **preferred list** versus the **non-preferred list.** Many larger health plans are experimenting with this concept. Each has its own pricing plan for members and requirements for hospitals to get on the **preferred list.** Generally, hospitals are **tiered** into two or three categories. In a two-tier program you have the choice of hospitals on the **A** list at either no additional cost or a lower co-payment. Or you can choose from the **B** list, with a higher co-payment.

Hospitals get on the **A** list as a reward for improving quality, patient safety and efficiency. The hospital may receive a lower payment, which they make up through increased business from being on the **A** list. This means that the consumer actually pays less for better quality healthcare. However, some programs are based on cost alone. If you choose a hospital on the **A** list because it's less expensive, you need to make sure that the quality of the hospital of your choice is equal to its higher cost alternative.

Sources: *Kiplinger Report; The Atlanta Business Journal.*

How do I find the best hospital for my needs?

The important thing to remember is that you have a choice. You don't have to go to the nearest facility or the one that's considered the "biggest and best."

The hospital you choose could be the difference between life and death.

Source: All Hospitals Are Not Created Equal, thehealthpages.com.

Health-Mart
Find comparison information on how Medicare patients are treated in hospitals.
601.209.9196
www.health-mart.net

Joint Commission on Accreditation of Healthcare Organizations (JCAHO)
Is your hospital accredited?
630.792.5000
www.jcaho.org

> **CONSUMER ALERT**
> **DID YOU KNOW?**
> As many as 98,000 people die each year from preventable mistakes (medical errors) that occur in hospitals. That's more than die from motor vehicle accidents, breast cancer or AIDS.
> **WHAT CAN I DO?**
> Protect yourself by finding the best facility before you need to go into the hospital. Be proactive. Some hospitals perform better than others in areas vital to your well being.
> Sources: Institute of Medicine, To Err Is Human: Building a Safer Health System, 2000.

Animals, vegetables, minerals—and US!

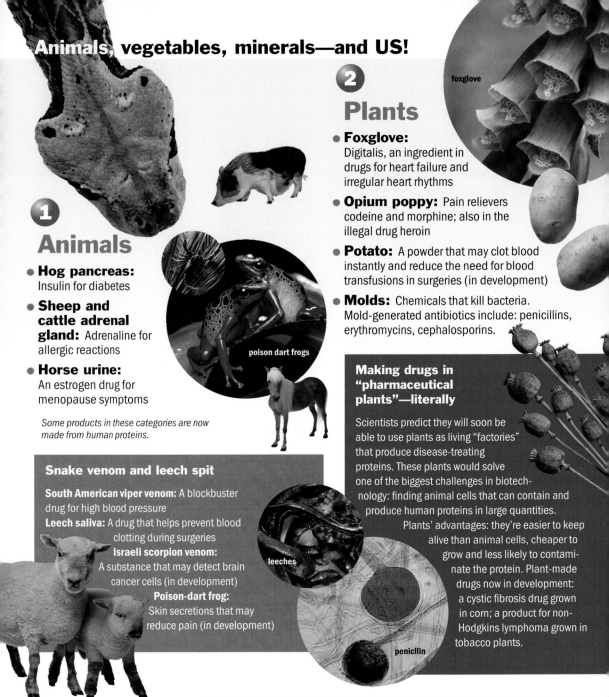

② Plants

- **Foxglove:** Digitalis, an ingredient in drugs for heart failure and irregular heart rhythms
- **Opium poppy:** Pain relievers codeine and morphine; also in the illegal drug heroin
- **Potato:** A powder that may clot blood instantly and reduce the need for blood transfusions in surgeries (in development)
- **Molds:** Chemicals that kill bacteria. Mold-generated antibiotics include: penicillins, erythromycins, cephalosporins.

foxglove

① Animals

- **Hog pancreas:** Insulin for diabetes
- **Sheep and cattle adrenal gland:** Adrenaline for allergic reactions
- **Horse urine:** An estrogen drug for menopause symptoms

Some products in these categories are now made from human proteins.

poison dart frogs

Making drugs in "pharmaceutical plants"—literally

Scientists predict they will soon be able to use plants as living "factories" that produce disease-treating proteins. These plants would solve one of the biggest challenges in biotechnology: finding animal cells that can contain and produce human proteins in large quantities. Plants' advantages: they're easier to keep alive than animal cells, cheaper to grow and less likely to contaminate the protein. Plant-made drugs now in development: a cystic fibrosis drug grown in corn; a product for non-Hodgkins lymphoma grown in tobacco plants.

Snake venom and leech spit

South American viper venom: A blockbuster drug for high blood pressure
Leech saliva: A drug that helps prevent blood clotting during surgeries
Israeli scorpion venom: A substance that may detect brain cancer cells (in development)
Poison-dart frog: Skin secretions that may reduce pain (in development)

leeches

penicllin

ACTION ITEMS

Weighing home remedies & folk cures

As a rule, try a home remedy only if the condition will not worsen by delaying standard medical treatment. The remedies cited below are not intended as medical advice.

Search your pantry for healing "staples"

- **Oatmeal:** Use in baths to relieve sunburn pain. Pour the uncooked flakes into a piece of nylon stocking, tying the hose at both ends. As you fill the bathtub, let the water pour through the nylon.

- **White vinegar:** Use on insect bites and stings, sunburn, itchy rashes. Dissolve a tablespoon of vinegar in a quart of water, refrigerate and soak a cloth to apply to the affected area.

- **Honey:** Apply to minor cuts and burns to relieve pain and speed healing. Cover with gauze. Eat a spoonful to stop hiccups.

- **Tea bags:** To heal cold sores, steep tea bag in boiling water and apply (4-5 days). To stop bleeding of minor cuts, dampen with cold water and apply.

③ Minerals

- **Lithium:** Drugs for manic depression. The lightest metal, lithium is also used in manufacturing of glass, ceramics, aluminum and batteries.

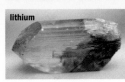

lithium

- **Magnesium:** Constipation and heartburn relief. This element is found in some minerals (dolomite) and sea water. Named after "Magnesia," a region of Greece.

- **Kaolin:** Diarrhea remedies. This white clay is also used in making china.

- **Calcium:** Indigestion relief; osteoporosis prevention. Also used in making bricks, cement, lime, glass, paper and other materials.

Minerals used in drugs are typically in the form of a salt, a chemical combination of a mineral and one or more other elements.

④ Humans

- **Blood:** Factor VIII, used to treat hemophiliacs. Extracted from blood donations of healthy people.

- **Urine:** Follicle stimulating hormone (FSH), used to enhance ovulation. Derived from the urine of postmenopausal women.

The Human Genome Project

The human **genome** is the complete set of coded instructions for making and maintaining a person. Current and potential uses:

Genetic testing 29: Tests available now can predict rare diseases caused by a single gene mutation (e.g., Lou Gehrig's Disease; forms of muscular dystrophy). Many diseases, however, involve the mutation of more than one gene; designing tests for these will require more knowledge.

Drug tolerance: Experts believe our genes determine our response to medications and hope to use this knowledge to prevent toxic drug reactions.

Disease treatment: Gene therapy will involve using normal genes to replace defective, disease-causing genes.

You'll be surprised to learn what goes into some common medications.
Ancient cultures and pre-industrial societies looked to the world surrounding them—animals, plants, the soil—to treat disease. Today, many of those natural sources or synthetic copies of their compounds are still used to manufacture drugs.

Take chicken soup (with a grain of salt)

Researchers have tried—without success—to prove scientifically that chicken soup fights colds and the flu. Despite the experts' skepticism, true believers cite theories behind chicken soup's supposed powers: Salt and minerals in the soup help the body retain fluids (thereby combating the dehydrating effects of colds); the soup's proteins help the body overcome infection and heal; and steam from the broth clears the sinuses.

Be careful about herbal supplements

"Natural" is not always better—or even safe. Many supplements can interact dangerously with prescription and non-prescription drugs. Since herbal supplements are not regulated by the FDA, it's important to buy from a dependable manufacturer; less established brands may be contaminated with toxic metals or chemicals. If you want to take an herbal remedy, talk with your doctor first. Also: do not try to treat children with herbal remedies unless their doctor approves.

14 years, $800 million to get a drug to market

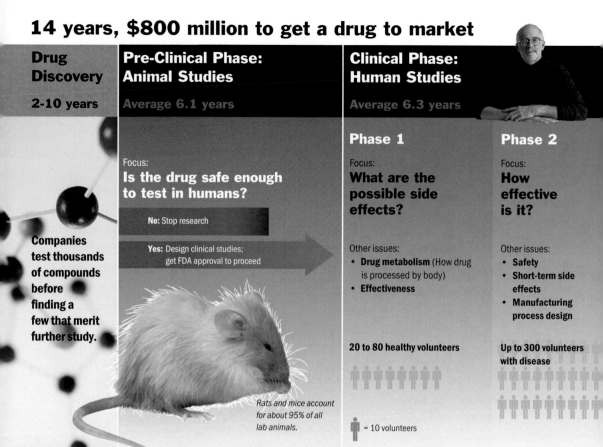

Drug Discovery	Pre-Clinical Phase: Animal Studies	Clinical Phase: Human Studies	
2-10 years	Average 6.1 years	Average 6.3 years	

Drug Discovery

2-10 years

Companies test thousands of compounds before finding a few that merit further study.

Pre-Clinical Phase: Animal Studies

Average 6.1 years

Focus:
Is the drug safe enough to test in humans?

No: Stop research

Yes: Design clinical studies; get FDA approval to proceed

Rats and mice account for about 95% of all lab animals.

Clinical Phase: Human Studies

Average 6.3 years

Phase 1

Focus:
What are the possible side effects?

Other issues:
- **Drug metabolism** (How drug is processed by body)
- **Effectiveness**

20 to 80 healthy volunteers

👤 = 10 volunteers

Phase 2

Focus:
How effective is it?

Other issues:
- **Safety**
- **Short-term side effects**
- **Manufacturing process design**

Up to 300 volunteers with disease

Life of a drug *after* approval

Phase 4 studies

Even after a drug is approved and on the market, companies are sometimes required to continue testing the drug in Phase 4 studies. If problems are detected, the approval can be suspended. After being approved for one disease, companies often test the drug in others; getting FDA approval for additional "indications" can help companies recoup more of their R&D investment.

Generic drugs

Generic drugs have the same active ingredients as their corresponding brand-name drugs. In 1984, generic drugs accounted for 19% of the prescription drug market. In 2000, they accounted for nearly half. Generic drugs cost so much less because they don't undergo the expensive R&D process that brand-name originals do. For FDA approval, generics just need to prove that they are pharmacologically equivalent to the originals. Sales of a brand-name drug can drop by as much as 50 percent if a generic version is developed.

ACTION ITEMS   Joining a clinical trial

Recognize different trial types

Clinical trials are not only about testing new drugs. Some trials focus on other aspects of illness and treatment. And you don't need to be sick to participate; many trials need healthy volunteers.

Trial type
- **Screening:** Methods of checking for disease when there are no symptoms
- **Genetics:** Predisposition to diseases or responses to treatment
- **Prevention:** Methods for preventing disease
- **Diagnostic:** Methods of detecting disease
- **Supportive Care:** Methods for relieving treatment side effects

Ask the right questions

What is required of me?
- How long does the trial last?
- How often do I need to visit the doctor/study center?
- Over the long term, will I have to return for tests and check-ups?

What are the risks?
- What known side effects are there?
- Is there a chance that I'll receive a placebo? If so, will I have the opportunity at a later date to receive the drug?

It takes an average of 14 years and $800 million for a prescription drug to go through the testing and review process. Once a drug is approved, companies often race to recoup their investment before their patent expires and less expensive generic drugs enter the market.

Process of elimination

5,000–10,000 potential drug compounds screened

250 enter preclinical testing (animal studies)

5 enter clinical testing (human studies)

1 gets FDA approval

Phase 3

Focus:

How should the drug be taken?

Other issues:
- **Effects on more populations** (e.g., the elderly; patients with multiple diseases)
- **Effects of different doses**
- **Interactions with other drugs**

Several hundred to 3,000 volunteers

Source: PhRMA 2002 industry profile.

Review and Approval Phase

Average 1.8 years

Focus:

Will the FDA approve the drug?

The company compiles trial data into a **New Drug Application**. Tens of thousands of pages long, an **NDA** could fill two trucks. (Today NDAs are submitted electronically.)

Upon FDA approval, a company may begin to sell the drug.

10 – 15% of NDAs are rejected

Off-label use

Once a drug is available, doctors can prescribe it in any way they deem medically appropriate—even for conditions not specified by the FDA approval. Through off-label use, more patients can benefit from new drugs. However, because off-label treatments haven't undergone the rigorous approval process, there can also be risks. A notorious example: **Fen-Phen**, an unapproved drug combination for obesity, ultimately proved to cause heart and lung problems.

Over-the-counter drugs

Sometimes a company extends a drug's profitability beyond patent expiration by formulating it as an over-the-counter (OTC) drug. Many popular brands are former prescription drugs that underwent the "OTC switch":
- **Heartburn:** Pepcid®, Tagamet®, Zantac®
- **Pain:** Advil®, Aleve®, Motrin®
- **Smoking:** NicoDerm®, Nicorette®, Nicotrol®
- **Allergy:** Claritin®
- **Hair loss:** Rogaine®

Find out who's paying

The trial's sponsor (a drug company or federal agency) usually covers the cost of the drug being tested. But the costs of trial-related routine care—lab tests, x-rays, doctors' visits—are met more variably. Medicare and some state-regulated insurance groups are now required to cover these costs. However, some private insurance companies refuse payment, on grounds that clinical trials are "experimental." Before you enroll, make sure you know who's paying for what. There's also the issue of your personal expenses. Some trial sponsors—but by no means all—will reimburse you for incidentals like travel to the study site or for time missed at work. Some trials pay patients a small fee for participating.

Clinical trial information

- Trials listings

  www.clinicaltrials.gov

  www.nci.nih.gov (cancer trials)

- Food and Drug Administration

  www.fda.gov

TIP

You have many important rights as a trial participant — including the right to leave the trial at any point.

All images courtesy of Philips Medical Systems, a division of Royal Philips Electronics of the Netherlands:

Radiography/X-ray
Digital Chest X-ray

Contrast X-ray
Contrast x-ray image of a colon filled with a barium contrast agent

Angiography
Angiogram showing the aortic birufucation, where arteries branch off to supply blood to the legs

Ultrasound Scanning
3-D ultrasound image of a fetus

Magnetic Resonance Imaging (MRI)
MRI showing soft tissues of the brain and eyes

Computerized Tomography (CT)
Head and neck

Positron Emission Tomography (PET)
PET image showing a tumor in the right lung with multiple secondary tumors

Radionuclide Scanning
SPECT image showing views of the blood distribution in the heart muscle during various phases of the heart beat

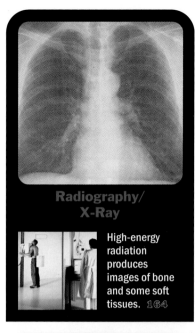

Radiography/X-Ray

High-energy radiation produces images of bone and some soft tissues. 164

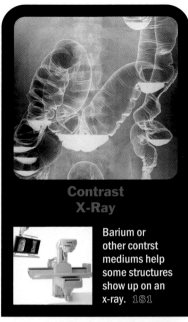

Contrast X-Ray

Barium or other contrst mediums help some structures show up on an x-ray. 181

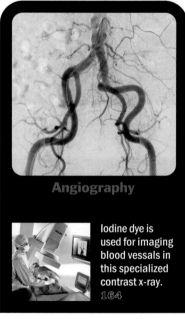

Angiography

Iodine dye is used for imaging blood vessals in this specialized contrast x-ray. 164

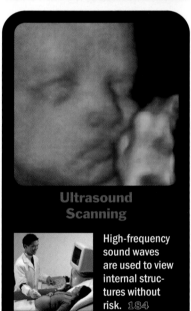

Ultrasound Scanning

High-frequency sound waves are used to view internal structures without risk. 184

ACTION ITEMS

Tips for getting through testing

1 **Know where you're going.**
Ask for the address, phone number and directions for the test location. It's a good idea to call to confirm your appointment a day or two before the scheduled date.

2 **Follow any preparation instructions.**
Some exams require you to limit your intake of food or drink or perform other pre-test procedures. When the appointment is made make sure you ask what preparation, if any, you need, and follow the instructions to the letter. If you don't, you could be turned away, you could suffer side effects or your results could be incorrect or inconclusive.

3 **Be on time.**
It is a good idea to arrive on time or a little early for any testing procedure. This will allow you time to orient yourself, fill out any necessary paperwork and relax before your test.

4 **Learn more about the procedure.**
It is a good idea to educate yourself about any diagnostic imaging test you undergo before your appointment. However, immediately before your examination, the imaging center staff or physicians (called radiologists) may take additional time to explain what will happen during your procedure. Some will even allow you to watch an educational video or give you additional material to read.

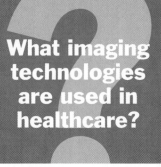
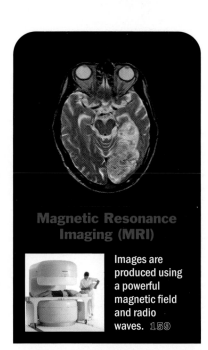

Magnetic Resonance Imaging (MRI)

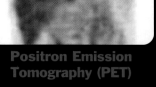

Images are produced using a powerful magnetic field and radio waves. 159

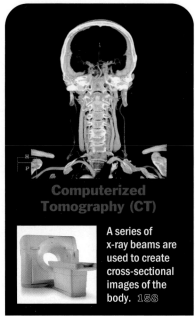

Computerized Tomography (CT)

A series of x-ray beams are used to create cross-sectional images of the body. 158

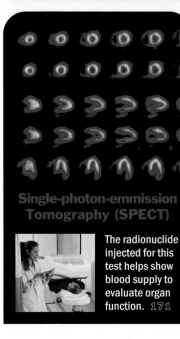

Positron Emission Tomography (PET)

This method of radionuclide scanning reveals cell function levels. 159

Single-photon-emmission Tomography (SPECT)

The radionuclide injected for this test helps show blood supply to evaluate organ function. 171

Imaging technology lets us see inside our bodies without the risk and discomfort of exploratory surgery.

Some tried-and-true and newly developed methods are shown here.

Source: Philips Medical Systems.

5 **Be prepared to answer some questions.**
Some questions you may be asked before having an imaging test may include:
- Are you pregnant?
- Are you allergic to iodine or any medication?
- Have you had any head or heart surgery?
- Do you have any metal objects implanted in your body (such as an artificial hip or pacemaker)?

6 **Follow "patient prep" instructions.**
Exam preparation may require different steps prior to the actual imaging exam. Directions may include taking a special contrast liquid, changing into a medical gown and removing jewelry, hairpins, eyeglasses, hearing aids and removable dental work.

7 **Wait to be released.**

Once the diagnostic imaging test has been performed, you will have a short wait while the technologist and radiologist determine if the images are of the appropriate clarity and orientation. In some cases, the staff may repeat the examination or they may run a different imaging test to gather more information. There is minimal patient recovery for most diagnostic imaging examinations. However, some exams, like x-ray angiography, may require a slightly longer recovery period. If you have been given a sedative as part of the procedure, you may need to have someone else drive you home.

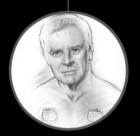

Brain pacemakers create electronic impulses blocking brain signals that cause the symptoms of Parkinson's disease.

Photo courtesy of Medtronic

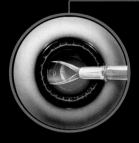

Intraocular lens implants replace the cloudy lenses of cataract patients restoring useful vision.

Photo courtesy of STAAR Surgical

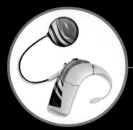

Cochlear implants deliver converted sound to the hearing nerve bypassing auditory damage.

Photo courtesy of Advanced Bionics

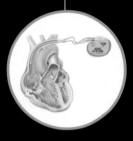

Defibrillators monitor the heart and deliver shocks to correct dangerously fast or irregular rhythms.

Photo courtesy of Guidant

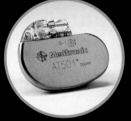

Pacemakers stimulate the heart to correct a pulse that is too slow or irregular.

Photo courtesy of Medtronic

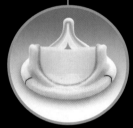

Replacement heart valves are used when the patient's own valve cannot be repaired with surgery.

Photo courtesy of Edwards Lifesciences

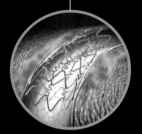

Drug-eluting stents keep clogged arteries open by delivering drugs that prevent scarring.

Photo courtesy of Cordis

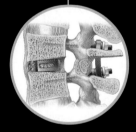

Spinal cages can help stabilize the damage that causes some back pain.

Photo courtesy of DePuy

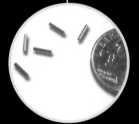

Radioactive seeds are implanted to fight some prostate cancers without radical surgery.

Photo courtesy of Theragenics

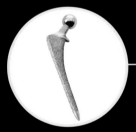

Joint replacements are used to fix damaged hips, knees, ankles, shoulders, elbows, wrists and fingers.

Photo courtesy of DePuy

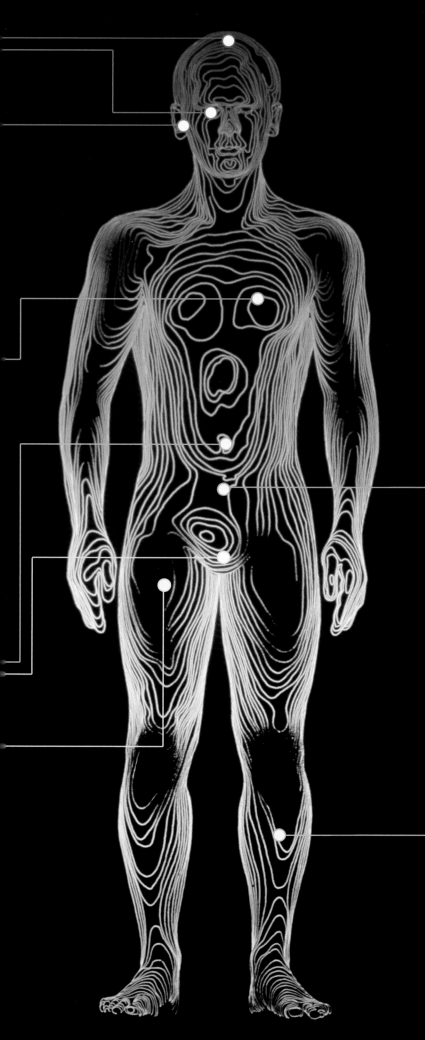

The bionic man has become a reality through a broad spectrum of technologically sophisticated medical devices.

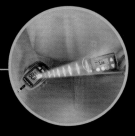

Insulin pumps mimic some actions of the pancreas replacing insulin injections for some people with diabetes.

Photo courtesy of Medtronic

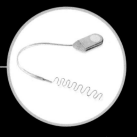

Bone growth stimulators help rebuild broken bones that are not healing properly.

Photo courtesy of EBI

❓ How is Information Technology used to improve the quality of healthcare?

How information is communicated can make a significant difference in the quality of your healthcare. In many ways, the quality of care you receive is dependent on the accuracy of information that your doctor has, the way information passes between your providers and the amount and quality of information you have. Exciting uses of information technology like electronic medical records are helping improve our healthcare, but we still have a long way to go. New technology is expensive and many healthcare facilities and providers have been reluctant to make the investment. Also, the payment structure in the healthcare system doesn't necessarily provide the right incentives for use of such technology. To improve the care you get, ask your providers what kind of technology they are using in their practices.

And take advantage of technology that may be available to treat a condition you have— ask your provider about what is available and do research to learn for yourself.

❓ What are some recent developments in information technology?

Just look at what online pharmacies are doing. For example, Walgreens.com allows you to check online for possible negative interactions between your prescriptions, vitamins, supplements or over-the-counter drugs. You also can email questions to pharmacists and find information on care for hepatitis, cystic fibrosis, multiple sclerosis and other conditions.

Computerized prescription entry systems in hospitals are reducing medical errors significantly—from 55% to 88%, according to recent studies. Instead of writing on paper, a doctor enters a drug order into a computer that is programmed with your personal information. Communication improves in two ways. First, the pharmacist isn't interpreting handwriting and second, the prescribed drug is checked automatically against your health history avoiding any potential severe drug interactions. How serious are these errors? About 20% of these errors are life-threatening and approximately 7,000 people die each year as a result.

Sources: Walgreens, The Leapfrog Group, *Psychiatric Service.*

❓ How is information technology used to improve access to health care?

Sometimes just getting to a doctor or hospital is nearly impossible because of where you live. In fact, nearly 90% of physician specialists practice in cities, leaving rural communities severely underserved. Technology can connect patients with doctors and doctors with specialists, giving people quicker and easier access. Images like x-rays or EKGs can be sent privately over the Internet to specialists for diagnosis. A doctor in rural Washington state can send an image to a colleague in Boston. Then they talk by phone while they are both looking at the same image—and there you have it—real time diagnosis. Another way technology improves access to care is through web sites like California Healthy Families www.healthyfamilies.ca.gov . This site allows people who may be eligible for state-sponsored health insurance (i.e., Medicaid) to register children online, giving eligible children faster coverage. The web site provides program information and help with finding a doctor and other health resources. The program cut eligibility time by 21% and reduced enrollment errors by nearly 40%. The success of the project has encouraged 10 other states to consider Web-based enrollment programs.

Source: iHealth Beat.

❓ How is information technology being used to get patients more involved in health care?

The more information you have, the more likely you are to engage in your health care. Keep your personal health records on your computer and print out copies whenever you need to see the doctor. Order prescriptions online. Technology allows you to monitor your own vital signs at home. People with diabetes can keep an eye on their blood sugar levels. Track your cholesterol level with a hand held monitor that gives you results in three minutes. You can find home screening test kits in your local pharmacy that let you detect a urinary tract infection, monitor fat metabolism or test for colorectal disease.

Source: Wellmed, Walgreens.

ACTION ITEMS

Resources

The Markle Foundation has convened the Connecting for Health Initiative, a public-private collaborative to address the challenges of using information to improve quality, conduct research and empower patients to become full participants in their care and bolster the public health infrastructure.
www.connectingforhealth.org

The California Healthcare Foundation conducts research and commissions surveys and reports on emerging technology trends and related policy and regulatory issues.
www.chcf.org

The eHealth Initiative seeks to improve the quality, safety and cost-effectiveness of health care through information.
www.ehealthinitiative.org

❓ How is technology being used to deliver information?

There is no one central standardized system that collects patient data and provides the information back to whoever needs it. Many countries, such as Canada and Britain, have been building national information systems for healthcare as a way to improve quality and assure that people get the safest and most appropriate treatments. Some countries are mandating the use of electronic medical records. In the US, the federal government has developed a vision and strategic plan for a national health information infrastructure (NHII). As conceived, the NHII would be a comprehensive system that could provide information to improve healthcare. In addition to considering technology, the NHII is looking at values, standards, systems and applications that support individual health, health care and public health. Source: nhii.org.

Information technology has helped in many ways to improve healthcare.

IT has helped to improve communication, reduce errors, aid in diagnosis, reduce distance issues and standardize information.

❓ How is information technology being used to capture and analyze information?

Public health is getting a boost from technology when it comes to early detection of potential widespread health problems. One such system is the Rapid Syndrome Validation Project (RSVP), a web-based program that notifies public health officials when symptoms or illnesses are clustered in the same geographic area. Doctors enter a patient's symptoms into a computer, which then transmits the data to a central database in the local health department. Other bio tech companies have developed and are testing early warning systems as well.

Sources: US News & World Report, cmc.sandia.gov.

Doctors also are using technology to capture information about their practices and patient satisfaction. Patients are given surveys that ask questions about their health problems and how well their physicians are addressing their concerns. The surveys are fed into a computer that in turn gives feedback on individual patient concerns as well as overall patient satisfaction trends. Doctors can then use the information to guide improvement.

Source: American College of Physicians, American Society of Internal Medicine.

❓ Is email being used to help doctor-patient communication?

The jury is still out on physicians communicating with patients through email. First, insurance companies don't pay doctors for time spent writing emails. Then there's the concern by patients and physicians that important information could be lost if meetings aren't face to face. Some simply aren't comfortable with the technology. A 2001 survey found that 23% of doctors email patients. On the other hand, some people find that emailing questions to their doctor saves time and gets them information faster. Nearly 90% of people who use the Internet would like to communicate with their doctors online. A medical group in Portland, Oregon finds email works well for many of the questions, non-urgent requests and messages their practice normally gets by phone or in an appointment. The technology has reduced patient visits by 75%, giving doctors more time to spend with patients in the office.

Sources: KATU News; HarrisInteractive.

About 90% of doctors who go online use the Internet for research purposes. Of these doctors, 78% read journal articles online, 61% use the Internet to communicate with colleagues, and 31% attend online conferences

Source: Harris Interactive.

Telemedicine Information Exchange is a resource for information about telemedicine and telemedicine-related activities.
www.tie.telemed.org

Medical Records Institute provides information about Electronic Health Records.
www.medrecinst.com/index.shtml

Canada Health Infoway Inc. (Infoway) administers Canada's effort to foster and accelerate the development and adoption of sustainable and effective electronic health records with compatible standards and communication technologies.
www.canadahealthinfoway.ca

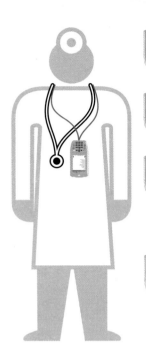

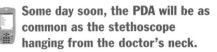
Some day soon, the PDA will be as common as the stethoscope hanging from the doctor's neck.

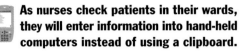
As nurses check patients in their wards, they will enter information into hand-held computers instead of using a clipboard.

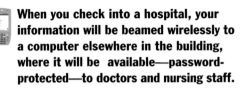
When you check into a hospital, your information will be beamed wirelessly to a computer elsewhere in the building, where it will be available—password-protected—to doctors and nursing staff.

Some hospitals are already using PDAs for writing prescriptions (meaning pharmacists can actually read them!), looking up information in electronic drug reference manuals, keeping records and even previewing operations with patients.

Source: *The New York Times.*

? How are PDAs used for writing prescriptions?

Busy doctors are not easily persuaded to change their old habits. But PDAs allow them to send a prescription directly to their patient's pharmacy; also, to see whether the brand being prescribed is covered by the patient's HMO. Writing prescriptions this way avoids the roughly 50% of all calls to doctors from pharmacists who cannot read the doctors' scribbled handwriting.

Some software allows doctors to enter a patient's name and birth date, to find the appropriate diagnosis from a list of common ones and to enter the prescription and correct dosage from a menu. If there is a dangerous drug reaction with another medication already being taken by the patient, the doctor is alerted.

? How extensive is the use of PDAs in healthcare today?

The medical profession is a latecomer to the world of computing, largely because of reservations about the lack of mobility. But now, small handheld computers (PDAs) can be carried in a doctor's pocket. What's more, a growing number of healthcare information technology applications are coming onto the market. While many doctors are still cautious about how to apply the new technology, about 30% of US doctors own a PDA, and **50% are expected to use one for clinical purposes by 2005.**

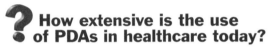

When it comes to using **electronic medical records,** it appears that the US is far behind most European countries. Many people regard keeping good, up-to-date medical records as a useful tool for reducing medical errors.

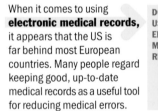

DOCTORS' USE OF ELECTRONIC MEDICAL RECORDS				
SWEDEN	90%	ITALY	37%
NETHERLANDS	88%	LUXEMBOURG	30%
DENMARK	62%	IRELAND	28%
UNITED KINGDOM	58%	UNITED STATES	17%
FINLAND	56%	GREECE	17%
AUSTRIA	55%	SPAIN	9%
GERMANY	48%	FRANCE	6%
BELGIUM	42%	PORTUGAL	5%

Sources: amednews.com, healthdatamanagement.com, rnpalm.com.

ACTION ITEMS   Find out more

Handheldmed, Inc.
www.handheldmed.com

PDA Verticals Corp.
www.healthypalmpilot.com

PalmGear.com
www.palmgear.com

PDA MD
www.pdamd.com

ZDNet
www.zdnet.com

DDH Software, Inc.
www.ddhsoftware.com

Skyscape.com, Inc.
www.skyscape.com

Austin Physician Productivity, LLC
www.statcoder.com

ePhysician, Inc.
www.ephysician.com

ePocrates, Inc.
www.epocrates.com

Cutting Edge Software, Inc.
www.cesinc.com

DC & Co.
www.isilo.com

❓ How can PDA-like devices be used in diagnostic tests?

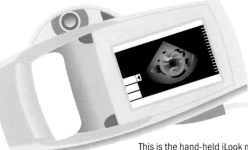

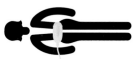

This is the hand-held iLook machine. A quick-look model costs $12,000. One that allows doctors to follow the path of medical devices inserted into the body costs $15,000.
Source: sonosite.com.

The development of miniaturization that has packed the power of a desktop computer into a PDA has produced a new hand-held device for taking ultrasound readings. It weighs three pounds, and measures 11 by 6.5 inches—very small compared to conventional ultrasound machines which weigh 200+ pounds and are mounted on a cart to be moved around.

Battery-powered devices such as this allow specialists to accurately detect abnormalities in the kidneys and arterial system. Cardiologists can now see the heart, not just to listen to it.

Source: *The New York Times.*

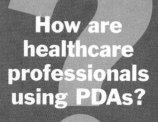

How are healthcare professionals using PDAs?

PDAs are being used more and more in health care.

Their primary uses seem to be as clipboard, prescriptions pad and reference shelf.

PRIVACY ISSUES 41

In the same way that people were initially concerned about privacy when using the Internet, and would be wary of buying anything with a credit card via the web, so patients have expressed nervousness about who might get hold of their medical information once it is recorded and sent to different parts of a hospital system or pharmacy. **The answer to questions about privacy in the medical field are the same as those about privacy in general commerce on the Internet: electronic transactions are generally safer than paper transactions.** Many doctors feel that they are *much* safer, given that one can track who has been looking at medical files on a password-protected and otherwise security controlled computer, while people who have looked at a piece of paper cannot be checked. In addition, paper can more readily be stolen, or easily left by mistake where someone might be tempted to look at it or steal it.

THE BOTTOM LINE

The move to electronic systems will be driven by a number of factors:

- the improvement of patient care
- the reduction of medical errors
- more accurate and faster claims to insurers, saving money

When patients and the medical profession understand these dynamics, handheld computing will become the norm.

Source: *The New York Times.*

LogonHealth Corp.
www.logonhealth.com

AvantGo, Inc.
www.avantgo.com

iScribe, Inc.
www.iscribe.com

DataViz, Inc.
www.dataviz.com

Blue Nomad
www.bluenomad.com

? Can I use technology to monitor my health?

As use of the web and web-enabled cell phones increases, people are finding simple solutions to healthcare needs. The Internet offers patients a wide range of opportunities to research topics such as managing chronic conditions, or looking after the health of distant relatives. The promise of new technology is that it will bring better understanding about healthcare and fewer medical errors.

According to the Institute of Medicine of the National Academy of Sciences, medical errors lead to nearly 100,000 deaths every year. Because of this, people are taking a much more active role in monitoring their health—for instance, keeping better records so that emergency procedures won't lead to the wrong drugs being administered.

Wireless devices are currently used to:

- **retrieve personal health information.** Health insurance, physician contracts, blood type, medications, allergies, immunizations and past medical conditions. You can send emergency information from a cell phone to a fax machine in a hospital or emergency care clinic.

- **check drug interactions** . Consumers can input a drug name and see if it has harmful interactions with medicines you are currently taking.

- **keep track of health conditions.** Blood sugar, heart rate, weight.

- **receive alerts and reminders.** Input medication reminders, doctor's appointments, exercise and diet routines.

? What diseases will a PDA help me manage?

There are **hundreds of software programs** that practically transform your handheld into a medical laboratory. Most work on the Palm operating system, though Pocket PC systems are catching up in the competitive field of personal health management.
Here are two examples:

Diabetes **:** with the help of an attachment, your PDA can measure blood glucose, alert you to when it's time to take insulin and keep a running total of carbohydrate intake. Some software has a food database listing the carbs in common foods.

Heart disease **:** if you travel a lot and want to keep monitoring your heart, you can now take a form of cardiac monitor with you. The FDA has approved a PDA that comes with wires you attach to your chest to record your heart rhythms. If you have a wireless connection on your Palm device, you can send the results directly to your doctor.

Add-ons for your Palm or Pocket PC

ActiveECG www.activecenter.com	Transforms PDAs into a cardiac monitor. Records heart rhythms and can beam them to your doctor.
Diet & Exercise Assistant www.keyoe.com	Tracks your calorie intake and burn rate, based on what you eat and how you exercise.
Freestyle Tracker www.therasense.com	Turns your PDA into a diabetes management system when you slide a test strip with a drop of blood into a module attached to the top.
On-Time-Rx www.ontimerx.com	Sounds an alarm on your PDA when it's time to take your pills or order a refill.
Profile-MD www.e-medtools.com	A record keeper for your prescriptions, allergies, health plan details, doctors' contact numbers, family health history, etc.

Source: *Business Week.*

Pregnancy Assistant for Palm helps track your pregnancy and then becomes a monitor for your contractions during labor.

(Less than half of patients who are prescribed medications are taking them properly, leading to 10% of hospital admissions.)
Source: healthleaders.com.

ACTION ITEMS
Buying a PDA

Consider these points before buying:

1 Color display
Most brands are now available with color displays which give you a clearer display and better readability in low light. However, they may also make your PDA heavier and reduce your battery life. If your software doesn't take advantage of the color display stick with a monochrome model.

2 Memory
You'll want to make sure that the memory in your PDA will be adequate for the software you'll be running. Find out too if you can add more memory later if you need it.

3 Operating system
Although a Pocket PC may be more familiar to you if you're used to Windows, Palm OS is much more efficient and needs less processing power. In general, these devices will be less expensive, use less power and give faster response times.

4 Software
Many basic programs are available to run on both Palm OS and Pocket PCs, but the majority of specialty programs are available for the Palm OS only. Check with the company that makes the software.

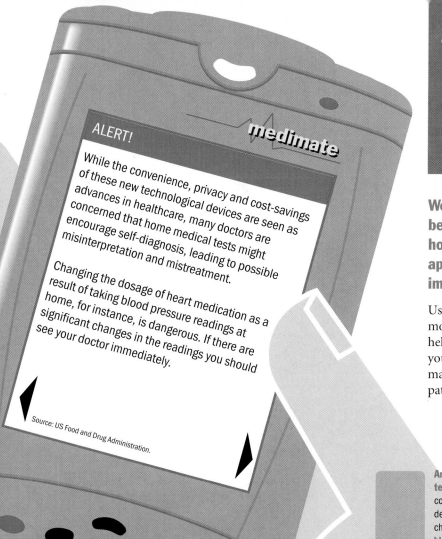

medimate

ALERT!

While the convenience, privacy and cost-savings of these new technological advances in healthcare, many doctors are concerned that home medical tests might encourage self-diagnosis, leading to possible misinterpretation and mistreatment.

Changing the dosage of heart medication as a result of taking blood pressure readings at home, for instance, is dangerous. If there are significant changes in the readings you should see your doctor immediately.

Source: US Food and Drug Administration.

We are only beginning to see how wireless applications will impact healthcare.

Using technology to monitor your health can help put it at the top of your mind and help make you a better patient or caregiver.

Another way to take your temperature. The Japanese company Matsushita has developed a smart toilet that checks your blood pressure, blood sugar and temperature.

5 Size
Before you buy, pick up and hold different types of PDAs. Check them for ease of use, and readability.

6 Data input
For the most part, you must input data into a handheld device with a stylus. Some, however, can be outfitted with a keyboard.

7 Expandability
Being able to add memory and accessories to your PDA will help keep it from becoming obsolete too quickly.

8 Battery life
Monochrome Palm OS PDAs will run the longest on a charged battery. As long as you recharge it regularly there is little chance of being stuck without power. If you want to be able to replace batteries anywhere, buy a device that runs on regular AAA batteries.

9 Market share
Software developers are more likely to write software for the more popular device. And, if you need to share data with others you're more likely to be compatible.

New treatments and therapies can improve the quality of life for people with chronic conditions [219], treat specific symptoms of illness and, sometimes, eradicate certain diseases.

Before the Food and Drug Administration (FDA) approves a new drug and the medical community accepts and uses a new treatment, the therapy undergoes significant testing, usually through clinical trials.

What's a clinical trial?

It is an experiment that tests a drug, medical device or other treatment for safety and effectiveness. During a clinical trial, new information is gained about a drug or treatment—its risks and how well it may or may not work. Participants are assigned randomly to different groups. One group receives the experimental regimen or procedure while the other group does not. The experiment compares the outcomes in the two groups.

Source: Centers for Disease Control.

What are the legal and ethical requirements for clinical trials and experimental medicine?

Using human beings as research subjects has ethical and legal ramifications. Before deciding to participate in any kind of experimental treatment, inform yourself about your rights. The federal government regulates the protection of human research subjects and educates researchers and others about the ethics of experimental research. For example, these regulations require the review and approval of human subject research by an Institutional Review Board (IRB). An IRB is a committee whose primary mandate is to protect the rights and welfare of humans who are the subjects of research. Any health organization that does research (academic hospitals, medical schools, etc) must have an IRB.

Source: Code of Federal Regulations, Protection of Human Subjects.

Three basic ethical principles seek to protect human subjects in biomedical and behavioral research:

1 **Respect for persons:** This recognizes the importance of personal dignity and autonomy of people, as well as the need for special protection of certain populations, such as children or prisoners.

2 **Beneficence:** This highlights the obligation to protect people from harm by maximizing benefits and minimizing risks.

3 **Justice:** This principle stands for fairness in the distribution of the benefits and burdens of research.

Source: NIH Office of Human Subjects Research.

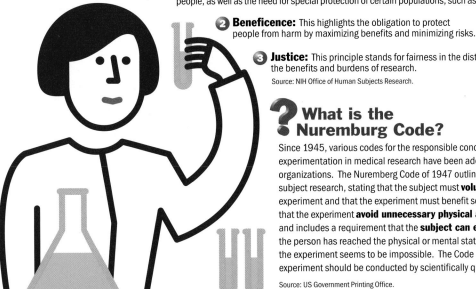

What is the Nuremburg Code?

Since 1945, various codes for the responsible conduct of human experimentation in medical research have been adopted by different organizations. The Nuremberg Code of 1947 outlines conduct of human subject research, stating that the subject must **voluntarily consent** to the experiment and that the experiment must benefit society. It also requires that the experiment **avoid unnecessary physical and mental suffering,** and includes a requirement that the **subject can end the experiment** if the person has reached the physical or mental state where continuation of the experiment seems to be impossible. The Code also states that the experiment should be conducted by scientifically qualified people.

Source: US Government Printing Office.

ACTION ITEMS

Resources

- **CLINICALTRIALS.COM™** An Internet resource for finding clinical trials in the United States and Canada. The site also provides thousands of local and national organizations that are associated with specific illnesses.
  www.clinicaltrials.com

- **NIH Office of Human Subjects Research (OHSR)**
  www.206.102.88.10/ohsrsite/about.html

- **The Food and Drug Administration**
  www.thebody.org/fda/fdapage.html

- **FDA Center for Drug Evaluation and Research**
  www.fda.gov/cder

- **National Library of Medicine**
  www.nlm.nih.gov

- **The Scripps Research Institute Molecular and Experimental Medicine**
  www.scripps.edu/mem

- **The Journal of Experimental Medicine**
  www.jem.org

? Can I participate in a clinical trial? [255]

There are opportunities for patients interested in cutting-edge treatments and drug therapies to participate in clinical trials. But not everyone who wants to participate in a clinical trial can due to limits on the number of participants and specific eligibility criteria.

Source: FDA Consumer Magazine.

? Why should I participate?

It's critical that people from diverse backgrounds participate in clinical trials. That way we'll make progress. Also, a clinical trial can get you access to a new treatment. You may benefit greatly—your health may improve and symptoms may subside. And even if you receive a placebo, you will be contributing to the long-term improvement of medicine.

Source: *Understanding Clinical Trials from the Patient's Perspective*, Delaney; US Food and drug Administration; *Why volunteer? Clinical Trials of Medical Treatments*, FDA.

? What are the risks?

Before participating in a clinical trial, consider carefully the risks and benefits. While **the benefits can be great, the risks can be significant.** For example, in 1992, tests of a promising hepatitis B drug severely damaged the liver in 10 patients participating in a clinical trial. Some died and others required liver transplants.

Also, don't forget—you are participating in an experiment on the safety and effectiveness of a new treatment or drug—there is no guarantee the treatment will work for you. There may be some risks that are not yet known. Also, if you are participating in a clinical trial with control groups, you may get an older treatment or a placebo. In these types of experiments, patients either receive the current therapy for the disease or a placebo—"sugar pills" that produce no therapeutic benefit. **Because patients are randomly assigned to either the group treated with the experimental drug or to a group receiving the standard therapy or placebo, there's no guarantee you'll get the experimental treatment.** Source: FDA .

? Can I be experimented on without my consent?

No. Anyone participating in a clinical trial must sign a consent form. The form will tell you what treatment will be given, what kind of problems might occur, and other treatments that might work for your condition. The informed consent form also indicates which costs are covered by the study and which must be paid by you or your insurance plan. If the participating subject is a child, a parent or guardian must sign the form. Be sure you understand the clinical trial, the protocol and the risks and the benefits before you sign a consent form.

? Do I have to pay to participate?

Studies funded by the federal government are free for the patient. Many studies funded by drug companies also do not cost anything. Some costs, however, may be paid by a patient's health insurance or managed-care plan.

What should I know about experimental medicine?

Experimental medicine is the avenue for progress in medicine.

! CONSUMER ALERT

Most online pharmacies are legitimate businesses, but you should not buy drugs on web sites that
- are not registered on a search engine
- offer to prescribe a prescription drug without a physical exam
- sell drugs not approved by the FDA
- do not offer you the opportunity to ask questions of a registered pharmacist
- do not provide a US phone number and address.

Before buying, check with the National Association of Boards of Pharmacy to see if the pharmacy possesses a valid pharmacy license and has met state practice standards.

Source: *Questions About CDER*, www.fda.gov/cder/about/faq/.

- **NIH Program on Clinical Trials.** A joint FDA/National Institutes of Health resource, it currently contains only NIH studies, but plans eventually to include all federally and privately financed clinical studies.
  www.lhncbc.nlm.nih.gov/clin

- **CancerNet.** Run by the National Institute of Health's NIH's National Cancer Institute (NCI) it provides information on clinical trials. You also can call NCI's Cancer Information Service at 800.4.CANCER.
  www.cancernet.nci.nih.gov

For information about clinical trials for rare diseases, see:
www.rarediseases.info.nih.gov/ord/researchct.html

- **ACTIS, the AIDS Clinical Trials Information Service** provides a range of information about AIDS research, including drug trials and vaccine trials. Call: 800.TRIALS.A.
  www.actis.org

- **CenterWatch Clinical Trials Listing Service** This site provides information on over 5,000 active clinical trials.
  www.centerwatch.com

THE THREE MAIN CATEGORIES OF PRIVATE HEALTHCARE RESEARCH:

BIOTHERAPY AND BIOTECHNOLOGY

Research to develop products, cures, treatments and vaccinations for various diseases and conditions. Done by private companies, universities and the federal government.
Example: Medtronic, which tests, develops and sells medical devices such as pacemakers.

Source: medtronic.com.

HEALTHCARE

Research to ensure that the available medical treatments reach the appropriate people. Many private foundations support research that educates researchers, policymakers, health care providers and the public about particular diseases, their treatment and prevention strategies. Private foundations also fund research to evaluate existing health services for effectiveness and to provide the underserved better access and health care.
Example: The Robert Wood Johnson Foundation, through its research funding, seeks to improve the health and healthcare of all Americans.

POLICY

Research to design policy that governs the way health care is provided in the US. Funders of this type of research support work that informs Congress about issues such as prescription drug costs, caring for the uninsured and Medicare. This work often is political and ideological. While funders' goals may sound similar, the means to achieving their aims often differ significantly.
Examples: The Heritage Foundation, a conservative organization, conducts and funds research to support more patient choice and free-market competition. The Commonwealth Fund, a more liberal foundation, supports research focused on expanding insurance coverage and improving care for vulnerable populations.

Sources: heritage.org, cmwf.org.

How does the private sector fund medical research?

1 Private foundations: These organizations are not-for-profit. Their funding usually comes from the philanthropic contributions of wealthy individuals. A board of directors, with assistance from foundation staff, decides which research projects are funded. Private foundations fund health research by giving grants to independent research organizations that compete for these grants by submitting proposals. This process is highly selective. **Example:** The Robert Wood Johnson Foundation provided $560 million worth of grants in 2001.

Source: rwjf.org.

2 Private corporations: These companies are for-profit, which means that their first priority is to conduct research that will lead to new or improved products and increase industry profits. Both pharmaceutical and biotech companies devote billions of dollars to private medical and health care research.

Companies conduct most of their research within their internal research and development (R&D) departments. However, sometimes companies contract with outside research organizations to help them with their projects, such as scientists working for universities or in private labs .
Example: in 2001, Bristol-Myers Squibb spent $2.2 billion on research (out of revenues of $19.4 billion).

3 Disease groups: Non-profit organizations such as the American Heart Association and the Juvenile Diabetes Research Foundation raise money for research. Their missions are to find cures for specific diseases or conditions by using donations to fund research projects or educate the public about the benefits of medical research. **Example:** in 2003, the Juvenile Diabetes Research Foundation will spend $100 million on research.

Source: jdrf.org.

How do drugs move through the development & approval process?

It's a complicated and intensive process. On average it takes about **$800 million** over the course of 10 to 15 years to develop a new prescription medicine that is approved by the Food and Drug Administration (FDA). Drug companies attribute high drug costs to the cost of research and development. Critics challenge these assertions, arguing that drug companies are profitable and spend less on R&D than they do on marketing, advertising and administration.

Despite the disagreement, it is clear that the drug approval process is costly and takes a significant amount of time. The clinical trials take up most of the time in the approval process — generally several years.

Sources: Tufts Center for the Study of Drug Development; FDA.

CONTROVERSIES

Major issues include:

1 How much money pharmaceutical companies spend on research and development as compared to marketi

2 Whether corporate funding of universi research influences the review proces and reporting of findings.

3 Whether research on health policy is shaped to support a particular ideological or political agenda.

ACTION ITEMS
If you would like to contribute

Research! America This national non-profit organization's mission is to make medical and health research a much higher national priority.

1101 King Street, Suite 520
Alexandria, VA 22314
800.366.CURE
www.researchamerica.org

If you are concerned about a particular illness, you might consider one of these:

American Diabetes Association
800.342.2383
www.diabetes.org

American Heart Association
800.AHA.USA.1
www.americanheart.org

American Cancer Society
800.ACS.2345
www.cancer.org

American Foundation for the Blind
800.232.5463
www.afb.org

The FDA is responsible for the drug approval process, which has numerous steps:

1 Sponsor (usually a drug company) **tests the drug on animals** to discover how the drug works and if it is potentially safe and effective for humans.

2 Sponsor prepares an **investigational new drug application (IND)** which outlines the proposal for human testing in clinical trials.

3 Phase 1 studies typically involve 20 to 80 people. Designed to assess the safety of the drug with a small number of patients.

4 Phase 2 studies involve anywhere from a few dozen to 300 people. Tests the effectiveness of the treatment. Looks for side-effects and determines best dosage.

5 Phase 3 studies involve several hundred to 3,000 people to verify that the drug is effective. Usually randomized trials.

6 The pre-NDA (new drug application) period is commonly when FDA and drug sponsors meet to discuss the possible NDA.

7 Submission of the NDA marks the formal request to the FDA to consider a drug for approval.

8 After the FDA receives an NDA, the agency has 60 days to decide whether to file it. The FDA can refuse to file an application that it deems incomplete.

9 If the FDA decides to file the NDA, the agency assigns a review team to evaluate the sponsor's research on the drug's safety and effectiveness.

10 The FDA reviews the information that's on the drug's label, including guidance on how to use the drug.

11 The FDA inspects the facility where the drug will be manufactured.

12 If the FDA reviewers find that the benefits of a drug outweigh the risks, the agency will approve the medication. If the agency has concerns, it will find the drug either "approvable" or "not approvable." "Approvable" means the drug can most likely be approved if certain issues are resolved. "Nor approvable" means there are significant deficiencies and that it is not clear that the FDA will approve the drug in the future without significant additional data.

Sources: From Test Tube to Patient: Improving Health Through Human Drugs, US FDA, Center for Drug Evaluation and Research, 1999; The FDA's Drug Review Process: Ensuring Drugs are Safe and Effective, FDA Consumer Magazine; Experimental Treatments Unapproved but Not Always Available, FDA Consumer Magazine.

There are 3 main areas of healthcare research done by the private sector:

Biotherapy and biotechnology

Healthcare

Policy

American Liver Foundation
800.GO.Liver or 888.4HEP.USA
www.liverfoundation.org

American Lung Association
212.315.8700
www.lungusa.org

Arthritis Foundation
800.283.7800
www.arthritis.org

Asthma and Allergy Foundation of America
202.466.7643
www.aafa.org

Cystic Fibrosis Association
800.FIGHT CF
www.cff.org

Juvenile Diabetes Research Foundation
800.533.CURE
www.jdrf.org

Lupus Foundation of America
301.670.9292
www.lupus.org

March of Dimes
www.modimes.org

National Kidney Foundation
800.622.9010
www.kidney.org

The National Parkinson Foundation
800.327.4545
www.parkinson.org

? How much does the federal government spend on medical research?

Department of Health and Human Services (HHS), the government's main healthcare agency, has a budget of

$460 billion

of which **$375 billion** is for **Medicare and Medicaid,** the programs that pay for healthcare for nearly 74 million Americans.

Within the HHS, the **National Institutes of Health** has a budget of

$20 billion

The NIH supports 35,000 research projects nationwide. It also conducts over 1,200 projects in its own facilities and has 27 institutes and centers under its jurisdiction.

Source: National Institutes of Health.

Other government agencies that fund health research:

The Centers for Disease Control has a budget of

$3.7 billion

The CDC is the lead federal agency for protecting the health and safety of Americans. Its mission is to promote health and quality of life by preventing and controlling disease, injury and disability.

The Agency for Health Care Research and Quality has a budget of

$301 million

The AHRQ funds research to improve the quality of healthcare, promote patient safety and reduce medical errors, advance the use of information technology in healthcare.

The Department of Defense

has a healthcare system that spans the globe. Among the many topics studied are patient safety, patient satisfaction and the development of vaccines in the case of a bioterrorist attack. The DOD also funds research in identifying epidemics caused by germ warfare.

The Veterans Health Administration

has its own office of research and development, which oversees more than 100 Veteran Affairs medical centers. Funded with taxpayer dollars, the VHA invested

$350 million

in health research in 2001.

Sources: hhs.gov.

ACTION ITEMS Get more information

For general information on the world's premier medical research organization, contact:

National Institutes of Health
301.496.4000
nih.gov

Or, visit the NIH institute that interests you:

National Cancer Institute
nci.nih.gov

National Eye Institute
nei.nhi.gov

National Heart, Lung, and Blood Institute
nhlbi.nih.gov

National Human Genome Research Institute
nhgri.nih.gov

National Institute on Aging
nia.nih.gov

National Institute on Alcohol Abuse and Alcoholism
niaaa.nih.gov

National Institute of Allergy and Infectious Diseases
niaid.nih.gov

National Institute of Arthritis and Musculoskeletal and Skin Diseases
niams.nih.gov

National Institute of Biomedical Imaging and Bioengineering
nibib.nih.gov

❓ What are the goals of NIH research?

1. Foster creative discoveries, innovative research strategies and their applications to advance the nation's ability to protect and improve health.

2. Develop and improve the nation's ability to prevent disease.

3. Improve medical and associated sciences with an eye on the nation's economic well-being and to ensure a high return on the public's investment in research.

4. Serve as a leader and promoter of the highest level of scientific integrity, public accountability and social responsibility.

Source: National Institutes of Health.

❓ How does the NIH set research priorities?

Given the importance of protecting the nation's health and thousands of requests for funding, setting priorities is a complicated task for NIH. A booklet, *Setting Research Priorities*, is available online at **www.nih.gov/about/ researchpriorities.htm.** This booklet details the principles and mechanisms that guide the NIH's decision-making process.

❓ Which research initiatives or programs receive the most money from the NIH?

(billions of dollars)

- CARDIOVASCULAR $2.1
- BEHAVIORAL/SOCIAL $2.6
- AIDS $2.8
- PEDIATRICS $3.1
- WOMEN'S HEALTH $4.1
- NEUROSCIENCES $4.7
- BRAIN DISORDERS $4.8
- CANCER $5.8
- PREVENTION $6.9
- CLINICAL RESEARCH $8.0

Though not in the top 10, **bioterrorism** funding increased over 500% ($1.7 billion) from 2002 to 2003. Funding for emerging infectious diseases increased by nearly 300% ($1.5 billion). Vaccine development funding increased by 70 % ($1.2 billion).
Source: National Institutes of Health.

❓ What is the federal government's role in medical research?

The federal government plays an incredibly significant role in American healthcare.

It funds programs that provide care and conducts and supports medical research.

National Institute of Child Health and Human Development
nichd.nih.gov

National Institute on Drug Abuse
nida.nih.gov

National Institute on Deafness and Other Communication Disorders
nidcd.nih.gov

National Institute of Dental and Craniofacial Research
nidr.nih.gov

National Institute of Diabetes and Digestive and Kidney Diseases
niddk.nih.gov

National Institute of Mental Health
nimh.nih.gov

National Institute of Environmental Health Sciences
niehs.nih.gov

National Institute of General Medical Sciences
nigms.nih.gov

National Institute of Neurological Disorders and Stroke
ninds.nih.gov

National Institute of Nursing Research
nih.gov/ninr

National Library of Medicine
nlm.nih.gov

10 of the most advanced medical technologies

1 GENETIC ENGINEERING (designing our children)

Newborn children with genetic defects from missing genes, such as Von Wildebrand's Disease, can have that gene "replaced" so they will not have the bleeding disorder. Soon we will be able to control and change or replace any genetic birth defect and eventually any genetic characteristic.

2 TISSUE ENGINEERING (growing synthetic organs)

Bio-resorbable materials are allowing blood vessel stem cells to grow on a "scaffold" that dissolves leaving a living blood vessel tree, on which specific organ stem cells are then "seeded," resulting in synthetically grown organs from a person's own tissues. Soon we will be able to replace injured or diseased organs with "new" ones—indefinitely.

3 ROBOTIC SURGERY (operating rooms without people)

The success of the current robot surgery systems will move to replacing all the people in the operating room, with the surgeon operating from outside a "clean room" operating room. Surgeons will rehearse and "edit" their procedures on virtual reality images of their patients, then the robot will execute the surgery under the surgeon's supervisory control.

4 TOTAL BODY IMAGING (the virtual human) 195

The total body scans of today will lead to highly sophisticated full 3D representation of each individual—a personal holographic medical electronic representation or Holomer—with all the information about the person so that it actually behaves as the person. It will be used for surgical planning and rehearsal, prediction of the effects of a medicine or diet or health plan, or be able to simulate "aging" like Dorian Gray.

5 BIOSURGERY (operating on individual cells, mitochondria or DNA)

New scientific imaging and therapy tools are working at the cellular level. Doctors will operate on parts of the cell, such as the mitochondria, nucleus or even directly on the DNA to change the biology and chemistry of a person.

6 BRAIN MACHINE INTERFACE (direct brain connection)

Monkeys with computer chips implanted in their brains are being taught to think to make a robotic arm feed themselves —"thoughts into action." Severely handicapped persons will be receiving these chips and be given a chance to take care of themselves or begin to interact with their environment, gaining new level of independence.

7 CONTROLLED CELLULAR METABOLISM (suspended animation)

Discoveries that hibernating animals do so because a molecule from their brain "turns off" the drive for oxygen at the cellular level is leading to the search for a signaling molecule or environmental factor that is responsible. Using profound hypothermia, dogs have had their hearts stopped for up to two hours, and successfully resuscitated without apparent injury. Short term "suspended animation" will be used for injured persons until they can be transported to a hospital. Anesthesia may soon be replaced.

8 INTELLIGENT PROSTHESES (cyborg)

Microelectro-mechanical systems (MEMS) have changed simple mechanical parts such as pacemakers, hearts, limbs or hip replacements into sophisticated, "intelligent" engineered prostheses that can replace human organs or tissues. There will continue to be more opportunities to replace nearly every system in the body with even more sophisticated systems.

9 NANOTECHNOLOGIES (nanobots)

More than 1000 times smaller than a single cell, nanotechnology is building materials and "machines" atom-by-atom. Entire "engines" that function like the flagella of a bacterium or materials ten times the strength of titanium have been created. Initially, this technology will be used to deliver drugs or chemicals to a precise spot, to attack or repair a specific spot on a cell membrane. It will be decades before there are little "nano-bots" traveling in the blood stream.

10 LONGEVITY (extending lifespan) 9

The oldest known living human was only 125 years old; however there is a strain of mice which have been engineered (using anti-telomerase and various apoptosis factors) to extend their life span to 3 times normal. These discoveries may extend the average human lifespan to greater than 125 or 150 years.

Moral and ethical issues raised by the technologies

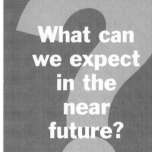
What can we expect in the near future?

① GENETIC ENGINEERING

Is it ethical to interfere with the natural process of creating our children? Who will be allowed to receive the genes that provide greater intelligence, strength, etc? What happens to those whose engineering goes wrong?

② TISSUE ENGINEERING

Should we grow only organs that humans have, or should we engineer new organs that can give properties humans do not have, such as hearing in the ultrasound (like bats), seeing in the infra-red (like hummingbirds)? Will an unlimited supply of organs allow humans to live beyond their natural lifespan?

③ ROBOTIC SURGERY

Initially optimizing surgical precision will be possible, but then will we be able to operate in seconds and minutes rather than hours? What happens if the robotic system malfunctions? Who is to blame?

④ TOTAL BODY IMAGING 195

Will we be able to predict our probable natural life span and aging? Will we download our holomer into cyberspace and become even more powerful in the information world than the real world?

⑤ BIOSURGERY

If we begin operating on individual cells, will we change what it means to be human? Will we create totally unexpected variations?

⑥ BRAIN MACHINE INTERFACE

Along with intelligent prostheses, artificial organs and the Internet will humans "create" their own evolution? Will we download into the Internet and become a single node on the massive global intelligence?

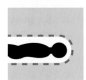
⑦ CONTROLLED CELLULAR METABOLISM

Short-term hibernation can be beneficial, but will the science fiction of decades or longer of hibernation arrive, with all the questions of what happens when you awaken a hundred years later? Will no one be allowed to die, but put into hibernation until a cure is found?

⑧ INTELLIGENT PROSTHESES

If I totally replace all my body parts with synthetic replacements, am I still human—should I just "download" myself? Will some devices directly attach us to the Internet, and loose our own identity of self?

⑨ NANOTECHNOLOGIES

The head of a pin has billions of atoms, so we will not be able to assemble large structures from nanotechnology—they will be "self-assembled". What happens if they are out of control—the gray goo?

⑩ LONGEVITY 9

There are more than enough people on the planet, what happens when people don't die for centuries? Will this be the way the human species can make the journey to outer planets and the stars?

By **Richard M. Satava, MD FACS**
Professor of Surgery, University of Washington Medical Center (Seattle) and Program Manager, Advanced Biomedical Technologies Defense Advanced Research Projects Agency (DARPA)

The future: one view of the

According to William Haseltine, CEO and Founder of Human Genome Sciences, genome science has added a new dimension to the traditional physician's black bag. He calls this new set of tools

regenerative medicine.

Haseltine lists four separate approaches, each one occurring at a higher level of biological organization:

LEVEL	POTENTIAL
1 Cell	The ability to use the innate capacity of human body to **build** itself, maintain **and repair** itself.
2 Tissue	The power to **create replacement parts** for parts that no longer work.
3 Organ	The use of micro-structures to create **neuromechanical prostheses**.
4 Organism	The capability to go beyond mere replacement to **revivification** of body parts—that are younger and better than the ones they are replacing.

1 Build and repair

This is the key attribute of regenerative medicine, putting the body's innate talent for restoring itself to work. We always knew that a wound could close and heal. But the talent goes much deeper than that. When surgery is performed on a baby in utero, the surgical scars are gone by the time the baby is born.

Mind-blowing thought: We change utterly. The atoms we are made of today are not the atoms we were made of 10 years ago, or will be made of 10 years from now. We are continually recreating ourselves—the same selves—out of fresh matter.

Genome science takes this insight, and seeks to extend the healing process to the highest degree.

This insight is implicit in insulin, a drug developed from a single gene of an actual individual's body that controls the metabolism of millions of people. But insulin is generalized medicine, the same from person to person. The new drugs will be individualized to match the patient's unique requirements.

Our knowledge of how cells work has advanced tremendously in recent years. We know cells operate according to signals—they rest, they go to work, they even commit suicide on command. In a sense, the challenge for regenerative medicine is a simple one: It is to learn what these signals are, where they can be found, and what specific responses they can trigger.

We know that, as we get older, our ability to heal and restore ourselves diminishes. The signals become confused, or they are not issued. The challenge may be simply to remind the body of its capabilities, to extend life far beyond its current accepted range. Match the signal to the protein, and we can remind the body how to fight cancers and other diseases.

2 Create replacement parts

In the past, if a heart or kidney went bad, that was the end for you. In the present, we have developed advanced but traumatic organ transplantation methodologies. In the future, we may simply grow our own new organs.

If there is a nick in an organ, the first kind of regenerative medicine will restore it to function. But if it is damaged beyond repair, the second kind, called tissue engineering, is required.

Animal research has seen advances. A "cookbook" of tissue engineering procedures is in its second edition. Blood, bone and cartilege are grown as callus and folded, origami-style, into functional units. Already, surgeons are fashioning new blood vessels from sheets of lab-grown muscle. "You just roll it around a straw."

3 Neuromechanical prostheses

Beyond "tissue-bending" lies the challenge of creating intricate new anatomical structures. Using the tissue generating techniques described above, functioning new heart valves have been built. Penile tissue regeneration has already seen major advances.

The key technology to creating neuromechanical prostheses is developing processes that occur at the microscopic level. Artificial bone and cartilage are being reengineered from the atomic level up. Researchers have created a replacement thymus gland. A German group has already fitted a couple dozen people with titanium ear implants. Electrode implants are allowing paralyzed

ACTION ITEMS

Interesting reading

- **The Double Helix: A Personal Account of the Discovery of the Structure of DNA**
  James D. Watson

- **Understanding Cloning**
  compiled by Sandy Fritz, edited by Scientific American; Foreword by William Haseltine

- **Stem Cells and the Future of Regenerative Medicine**
  edited by The Committee on Biological and Biomedical Application of Stem Cell Research Material

- **Life Script: How the Human Genome Discoveries Will Transform Medicine and Enhance your Health**
  Nicholas Wade

- **The New Genetics: Medicine and the Human Genome. Molecular Concepts, Applications and Ramifications**
  Sara L. Tobin and Ann Boughton

- **Genetics and Public Health in the 21st Century: Using Genetic Information to Improve Health and Prevent Disease**
  edited by Muin J. Khoury, Wylie Burke and Elizabeth Thomson

biotech revolution

people to move their limbs again. Experiments with retinal replacements are allowing people with macular degeneration to make out visual signals again.

The possibilities for nano-based genomic prostheses are vast. Imagine unobtrusive counterparts that are based on the body itself, and capitalize on the body's natural chemistry and functionality.

4 Revivification of body parts

The final level of regenerative medicine goes beyond replacement of cells tissue, and organs with something just as good. It replaces them with something better. It reverses aging. It makes the organism younger.

Stem cells are building blocks that may be coaxed into becoming any other cell type. They therefore hold the key to endless mysteries of human biology. Someday they may provide a cure for diabetes, Parkinson's, spinal-cord degeneration and Alzheimer's.

In stem cell biology, scientists replace tired proteins with vital, versatile, unaged proteins. The evidence so far suggests that the embryonic clock can actually be turned back—that the signals to deteriorate and age can be reversed.

This process, and not making endless replicant sheep and cows, may be the great use of cloning.

Using cloning techniques, however, it appears to be possible to implant a kidney that is younger than the kidney that went bad, even before it went bad. We already see this happening with bone marrow transplants —the new cells reproduce blood cells that are younger than the body "should" be capable of producing.

The implications of this fourth category are awesome. For openers, the brain turns out to be eminently suitable for this kind of cellular refreshment. In time, this biochemical fountain of youth may push human longevity beyond its current accepted absolute limit of 125 years.

There is hardly a way to get one's arms around the implications of Haseltine's future. A society whose citizens live to be 125 and older needs to reexamine many assumptions—family size, healthcare, insurance, retirement, education. Currently we know only what to do with people until they're 65.

This is an exerpt from an essay about William Haseltine's lectures to the Masters Forum, in April 2001. It was written by Michael Finley.

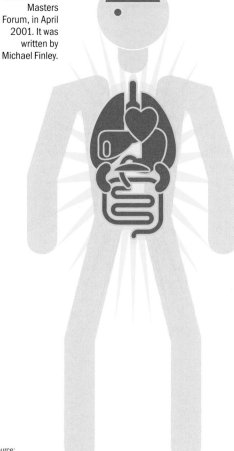

Source: www.mastersforum.com.

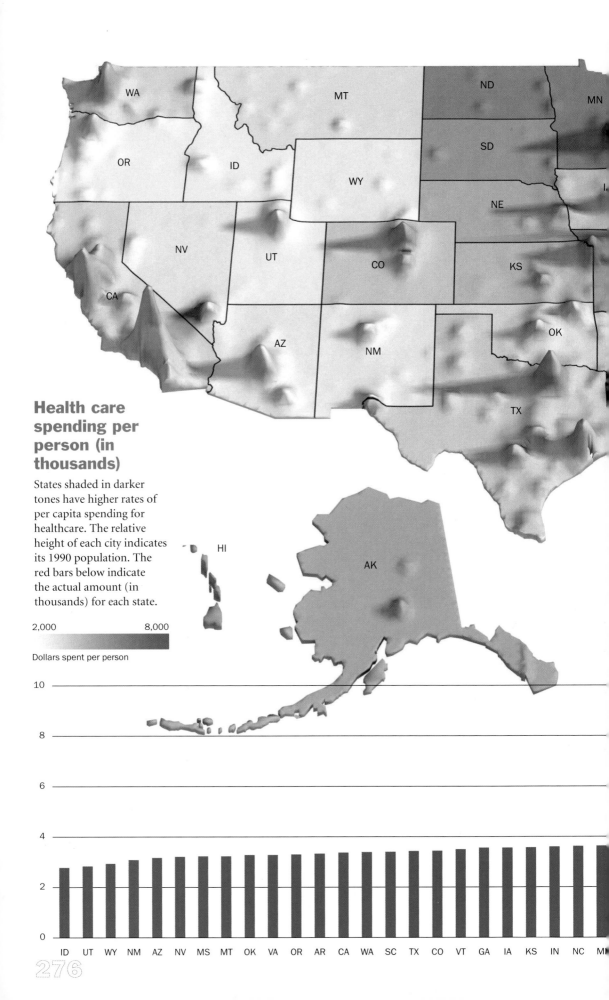

Health care spending per person (in thousands)

States shaded in darker tones have higher rates of per capita spending for healthcare. The relative height of each city indicates its 1990 population. The red bars below indicate the actual amount (in thousands) for each state.

2,000   8,000

Dollars spent per person

Elderly Americans spend 19% of their income on healthcare, those in poorest health spend 29%.

Source: iog.wayne.edu.

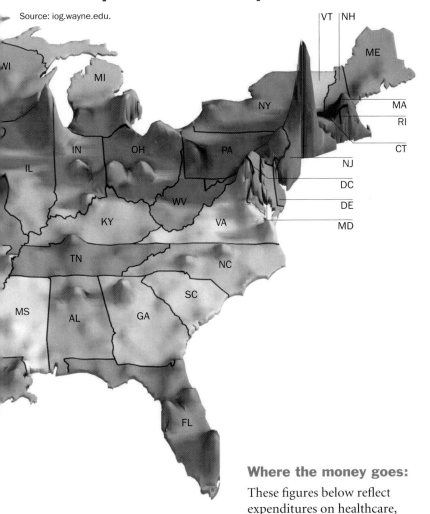

VT NH
ME
MA
RI
CT
NJ
DC
DE
MD

MI
NY
WI
IN
OH
PA
IL
WV
KY
VA
TN
NC
SC
MS
AL
GA
FL

Which states spend the most on health care?

In general, people in states with older populations spend more on healthcare.

Florida, which has the highest median age (38.7, compared to the national median of 37.5) is close to the top, spending almost $60,000 per capita in 1998. Utah, with the youngest population (median age 26.7) ranks second lowest in spending.

Source: US Census Bureau, Statistical Abstract of the United States.

Where the money goes:

These figures below reflect expenditures on healthcare, which include: hospital care, the services of physicians and other professionals, prescription drugs and nursing home care.

Graying and spending: both on the rise.

One reason that age-related spending is likely to increase: we're living longer. In 1950, the over-65 population totalled 7% of all Americans, or 9 million people.

By 2000, we had 35 million people over 65.

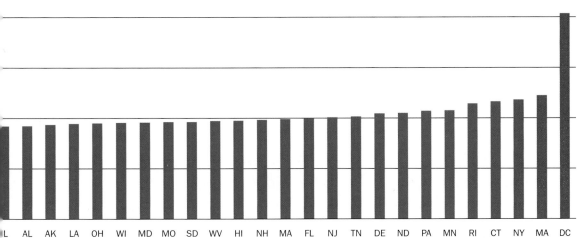

L AL AK LA OH WI MD MO SD WV HI NH MA FL NJ TN DE ND PA MN RI CT NY MA DC

What makes healthcare costs go up?

Insurance premiums cost more

An aging and longer-living population, reduction of managed care programs, increases in inpatient hospital care, and increases in use of all healthcare resources all contribute to higher costs.

Diagnosis and treatment cost more

Healthcare providers have access to increasingly advanced medical technologies, but at higher costs. For example, physicians have rapidly adopted MRI scans over older CT scan technology; MRIs allow physicians to view up to **15%** more detail than CT scans but at a cost that's over **150%** higher.

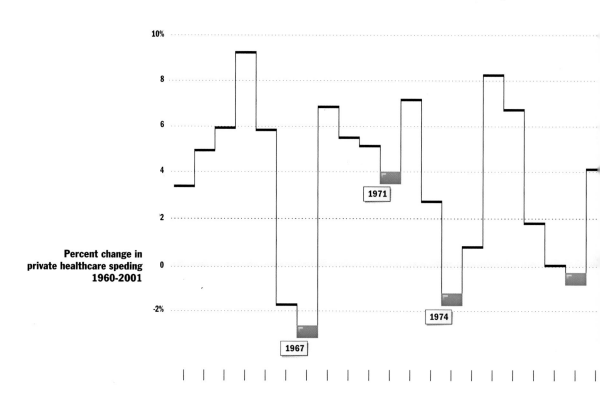

Percent change in private healthcare speding 1960-2001

When has government action pushed costs down?

1967

Originally envisioned by FDR in 1939 as "healthcare for all," **Medicare was signed into law by President Johnson.** As a result, the average person paid **1.4 percent** less than in 1967.

1971

With inflation rising to 4.5 percent **President Nixon issued an executive order freezing healthcare costs** and wages. The average person paid **1.5 percent** less than in 1971.

1974

The **Kassebaum-Kennedy Act regulated costs** by limiting what healthcare providers and pharmaceutical companies could charge. The average person paid **4.5 percent** less than in 1973.

ACTION ITEMS Minimize your costs

Compare costs for drugs: prescription, name brand and generic

Medscape Drug Information
www.medscape.com/druginfo

Destination RX
www.destinationrx.com

RX List
www.rxlist.com

Know where to find low-cost community resources for healthcare services

State-by-state list of toll-free Medicaid help lines
www.cms.hhs.gov/medicaid/tollfree.asp

Society for Healthcare Consumer Advocacy
www.shca-aha.org

People's Medical Society
www.peoplesmed.org

Government requirements push costs up

The number of government mandates has increased **25-fold** over the last decade. Costs associated with Federal government regulations were **$78.2 billion** in 1997, and mandates passed by State legislatures comprise from **8 percent** in Oregon to **22 percent** in Maryland of total healthcare costs.

Prescription drugs cost more

There are more new drugs introduced every year, and they're increasingly expensive. For example, in 1990 there were **4** prescription drugs for allergy relief, costing an average **.98¢ per dose**; today there are more than **17** such drugs, averaging **$3.41 per dose**.

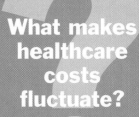

What makes healthcare costs fluctuate?

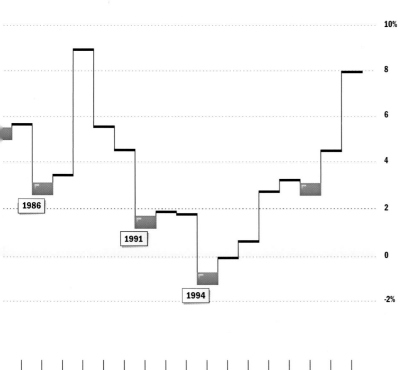

Public demand for more and better care drives costs up.

Public demand for cost containment incites government action, which drives costs down—at least temporarily.

Since 1961 there have been nine major contractions in the cost of healthcare; six of these were the direct result of government intervention. But the factors pushing expenses up are unrelenting: in each of the six government-initiated contraction healthcare **costs began to rise steadily within 8 months** of reaching their lowest point.

Source: Kaiser Family Foundation
May 2002 Chartbook.

1986
President Reagan imposed economic controls on health-care spending in response to public outcry over soaring costs. The average person paid **3 percent** less than in 1985.

1991
With the economy stagnating, **a federal task force was formed to investigate universal healthcare.** The average person paid **3.4 percent** less than in 1990.

1994
Universal healthcare legislation ultimately died in Congress. However, government and other health-care purchasers used managed care and other changes to reduce costs by **3 percent** from the previous year.

Research common diagnoses, treatments and associated costs

MedlinePlus Health Information
www.medlineplus.gov

Food and Drug Administration
www.fda.gov

The Mayo Clinic
www.mayoclinic.com

Know what to do if you can't afford a doctor

Medicaid and Medicare
cms.hhs.gov/medicaid/

Volunteers in Healthcare
www.volunteersinhealthcare.org

Source: Agency for Healthcare Research and Quality.

? Does all this mean people in the US live longer?

No. As an average American, **your life expectancy is among the lowest in the industrialized world:** 76.2 years (compared to 81.2 years in Japan). And at 6.4 per thousand births, the US has one of the highest infant mortality rates among industrialized nations.

Why? Life expectancy seems to be influenced more by lifestyle factors (eating, smoking and exercise habits) than by the availability of medical care. And heroic measures to save sick and premature infants are used here more extensively than elsewhere, contributing to a higher infant mortality rate but also to a higher rate of live births.

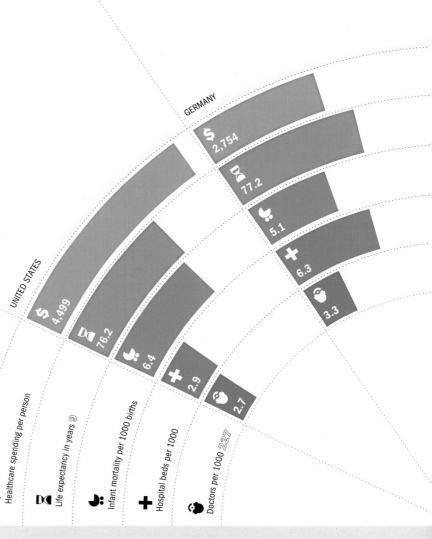

GERMANY

$ 2,754

DC 77.2

5.1

+ 6.3

3.3

UNITED STATES

$ 4,499

DC 76.2

6.4

+ 2.9

2.7

$ Healthcare spending per person

DC Life expectancy in years

Infant mortality per 1000 births

+ Hospital beds per 1000

Doctors per 1000 227

ACTION ITEMS — Understanding healthcare economics

Compare fees, specialties and backgrounds for physicians in your area

American Medical Association

www.ama-assn.org

Physician Reports

www.physicianreports.com

Compare insurance costs in your state to those in other states

Centers for Medicare and Medicaid Services

cms.hhs.gov

Bureau of Labor Statistics

www.bls.gov

Know when to perform routine preventative checkups, and which ones are recommended for you

Healthfinder

cms.hhs.gov

National Guideline Clearinghouse

www.guideline.gov

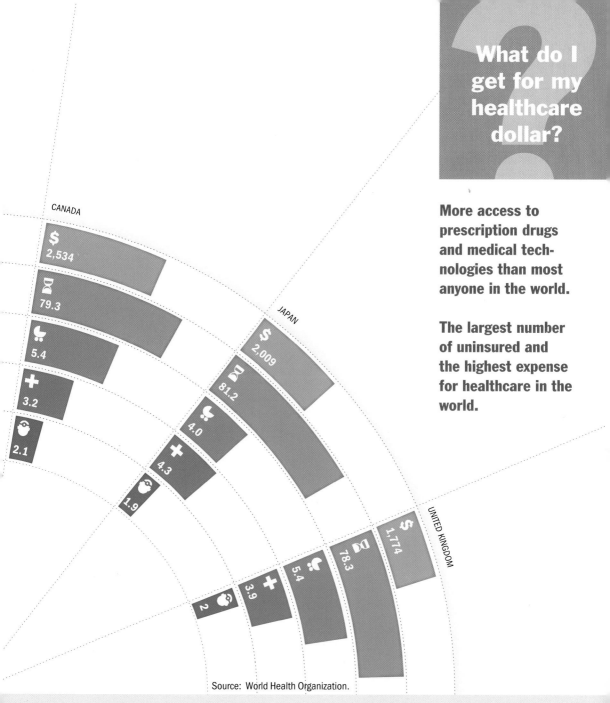

What do I get for my healthcare dollar?

More access to prescription drugs and medical technologies than most anyone in the world.

The largest number of uninsured and the highest expense for healthcare in the world.

CANADA
$ 2,534
79.3
5.4
+ 3.2
2.1

JAPAN
$ 2,009
81.2
4.0
+ 4.3
1.9

UNITED KINGDOM
$ 1,774
78.3
5.4
+ 3.9
2

Source: World Health Organization.

Research cost projections for hospital care and doctors' services

Centers for Medicare and Medicaid Services

cms.hhs.gov

Bureau of Labor Statistics

www.bls.gov

Health Research and Educational Trust

www.hospitalconnect.com/aha/hret/

Research healthcare procedures, issues, and insurance plans

Kaiser Family Foundation

www.kff.org

Agency for Healthcare Research and Quality

www.ahcpr.gov

Georgetown University Health Policy Institude

www.healthinsuranceinfo.net

? Why do a few people spend most of the money?

One theory is that **our healthcare system isn't used very efficiently,** with the "nervous well" spending vast, question-ably necessary dollars. Another is that new **medical technologies can result in significantly higher spending** often without corre-spondingly higher benefits to patients.

The situation has left policymakers in an ongoing debate about our healthcare priorities, and how much a society should spend taking care of a small number of ill people. And it has given insurers strong incentives to practice "favorable risk selection" to avoid insuring the small percentage of high-cost individuals.

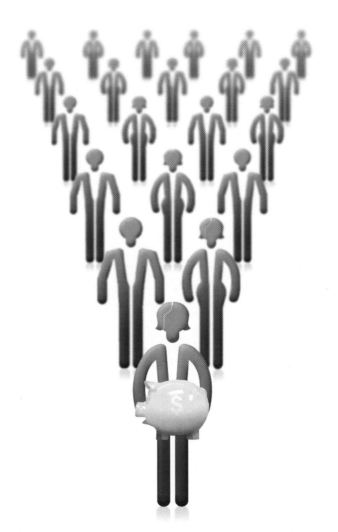

Three percent of all US healthcare dollars buys care for half our population...

ACTION ITEMS   Be your own advocate

Find the primary care doctor that's right for you

Many physicians make information available on the internet about their training, background, views about healthcare and which services they provide. You'll need to find out if the practice is taking new patients and whether it accepts your insurance plan. It's always a good idea to set up an appointment to visit with the doctor about his approach to your care before you make your decision.

Know what to ask your doctor when getting medical tests or prepar-ing for surgery

The most important questions to ask about any surgery is why the procedure is necessary for you and whether there are alternatives to surgery. Patients who are well informed about their treat-ment tend to be more satisfied with the outcome, so be sure you understand the answers your doc-tor offers.

For "Quick Tips: Talking with Your Doctor" and "Quick Tips: Getting Medical Tests" visit:
www.ahcpr.gov/consumer/

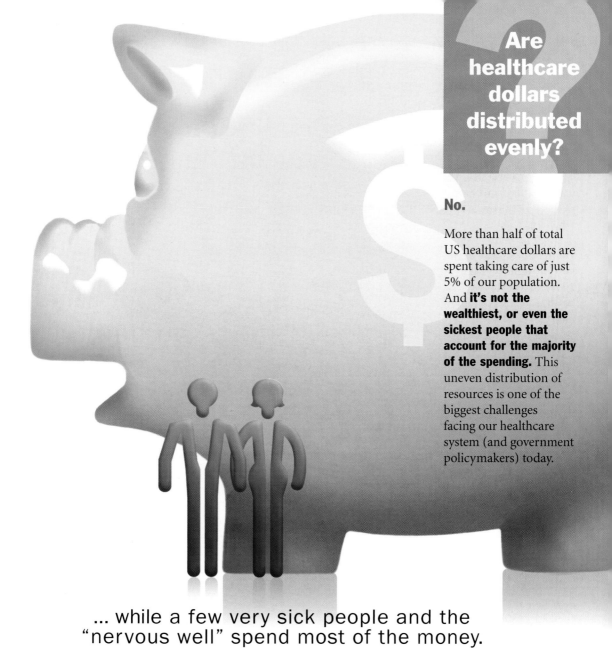

Are healthcare dollars distributed evenly?

No.

More than half of total US healthcare dollars are spent taking care of just 5% of our population. And **it's not the wealthiest, or even the sickest people that account for the majority of the spending.** This uneven distribution of resources is one of the biggest challenges facing our healthcare system (and government policymakers) today.

... while a few very sick people and the "nervous well" spend most of the money.

Source: HealthAffairs.org.

Get a second opinion

Getting a second opinion from another doctor is a good way to make sure having a given procedure is the best alternative for you. Many health insurance plans require patients to get two opinions before having non-emergency operations (and Medicare pays for second opinions). If your plan doesn't require a second opinion, you may still ask to have one. Check with your insurance company or your employee benefits office to verify your coverage.

Help prevent medical errors

Medical errors are one of the nation's leading causes of death and injury. Here are four quick tips to minimize your risks:

- Speak up if you have questions or concerns.
- Make sure that someone, such as your personal doctor, is in charge of your care.
- If you have a test, don't assume that no news is good news. Ask about the results.
- If you're hospitalized, consider having an advocate present to act on your behalf or help you make decisions in the event your capacity is diminished.

283

❓ Terminal care: what's the myth, what's reality?

In 1984, a flawed study reported that 77 percent of healthcare expenditures happen in the last six months of life—a statistic that has been widely quoted (and refuted) in the twenty years since.

The reality is that current terminal care spending runs closer to 15 percent of our national healthcare bill—still a number that many feel is disproportionately high.

The question of how high is *too high* is one that number-crunching will never answer. It is a question of human values, and we should expect many complex and potentially disturbing policy implications as decision makers try to balance our desire for unlimited healthcare with what has been termed "the high cost of dying".

Source: The Milbank Quarterly; Journal of the American Medical Association

❝ 77 cents of

spend on healthcare

last **6 months**

☐ TRUE

ACTION ITEMS Investigate end-of-life controversies

❶ What is meant by the term "medical futility"?

Roughly one-third of Medicare spending goes to those who live less than a year after treatment, leading many to believe that aggressively prolonging lives is "futile" and serves only to drive costs up. Most studies, though, suggest otherwise: that costs are high because patients are usually the sickest right before they die, but that many who are severely ill and/or elderly do recover. The dilemma becomes how to predict for whom help will be "futile"...and who makes the call.

Source: Century Foundation.

❷ How do advance directives 317 **affect costs?**

As a result of medicine's ability to save and prolong lives with technology-intensive care, many patients are turning to living wills and such to guide their care in the event they're incapacitated. But researchers are finding that these "advance directives" have little affect on patients' experiences—or on our national healthcare bill.

Source: The SUPPORT Principal Investigators.

In the United States, the majority of our healthcare dollars are spent maintaining life—or at least the quality of life— in the face of impending death.

At least that's what most folks think.

every dollar you will be spent during the of your life. "

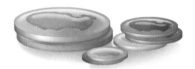

☑ FALSE

3 **Will healthcare ultimately be rationed in the United States?**
Many healthcare economists believe that rationing care—withholding at least some medical services from those who might potentially benefit from them—has become an economic necessity in the United States. Some believe, in fact, that our current system encourages covert rationing by placing financial limits on healthcare. Should such rationing become an accepted practice, with universal rules for its administration?
Source: Your Doctor in the Family.

4 **Oregon is currently the only state to legalize physician-assisted suicide.**
The state's Health Division reports that no patients suggested concern over the cost of treating illness as a motivator for seeking life-ending help. The primary reasons patients cited for choosing physician-assisted suicide were losing autonomy (85%), a decreasing ablity to participate in activities that made life enjoyable (79%) and losing control of bodily functions (58%).
Source: Oregon Department of Human Services.

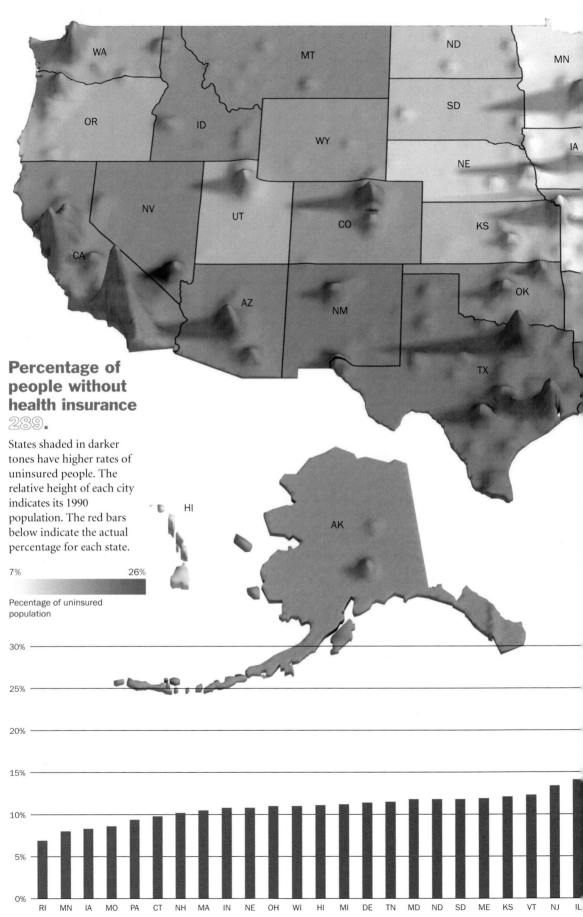

Percentage of people without health insurance
289.

States shaded in darker tones have higher rates of uninsured people. The relative height of each city indicates its 1990 population. The red bars below indicate the actual percentage for each state.

7%   26%

Pecentage of uninsured population

18,000 adults die every year
in the US because a lack of insurance keeps them from getting proper care.

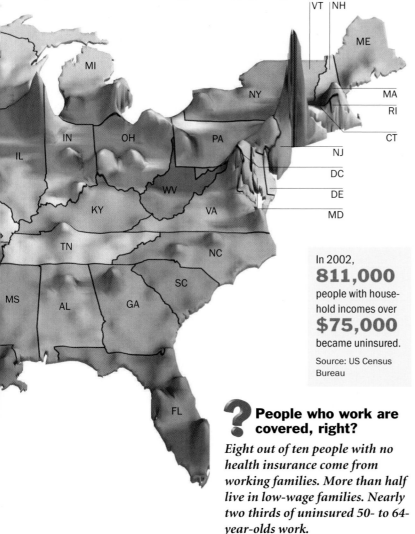

VT NH

ME

MI

NY

MA

RI

CT

IN   OH   PA

NJ

IL

DC

WV

DE

KY   VA

MD

TN

NC

SC

MS   AL   GA

FL

Quite a few. Nearly 44 million people lacked health coverage for all of 2002.

This was 14.2% of the total US population of 282 million—an increase of 2.4 million from the previous year.

Source: coveringtheuninsured.org.

In 2002,
811,000
people with house-hold incomes over
$75,000
became uninsured.

Source: US Census Bureau

? People who work are covered, right?

Eight out of ten people with no health insurance come from working families. More than half live in low-wage families. Nearly two thirds of uninsured 50- to 64-year-olds work.

Consequences

Not surprisingly, people who go without health insurance tend to get sicker and die earlier. Research from The American College of Physicians and The American Society of Internal Medicine shows that the uninsured tend to be sicker when admitted to hospitals and are more likely to die there. In a Florida study, those without insurance were more likely to be diagnosed with skin, colorectal, breast and prostate cancers at later, more dangerous stages.

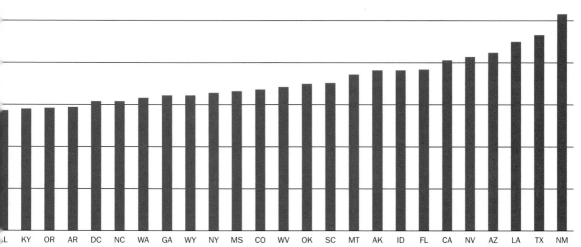

L KY OR AR DC NC WA GA WY NY MS CO WV OK SC MT AK ID FL CA NV AZ LA TX NM

? How does medical insurance work?

Private, independent insurance companies collect a premium from each individual purchasing medical insurance. Each company puts this money into a fund to pay for medical care to policyholders who need it (that includes you, of course, when you need it) after claims are submitted to the companies. The kind of coverage you receive (and the cost of it) differs from company to company.

The system usually works because insurance companies spread their risk over a wide range of people. healthy people pay more in premiums than they withdraw. This difference subsidizes sicker people with large claims. (Healthy people are in fact usually paying lower premiums than higher-risk payers. Besides, they might become ill themselves one day.)

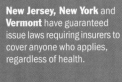

Find out more about the companies you are interested in by getting the company's **AM Best** rating. This is an independent rating company that grades insurance companies on their financial stability, and their ability to pay claims.

? When does medical insurance *not* work?

New Jersey, New York and **Vermont** have guaranteed issue laws requiring insurers to cover anyone who applies, regardless of health.

States **with NO guaranteed issue** laws are:

Alabama	Maryland
Alaska	Mississippi
Arizona	Missouri
Arkansas	Montana
California	Nebraska
Colorado	Nevada
Connecticut	N. Carolina
Delaware	Oklahoma
Florida	S. Carolina
Georgia	Tennessee
Illinois	Texas
Kansas	

Affordable prices are easier to find in these states.

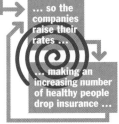

When states pass "guaranteed-issue" laws ...

... it forces insurance companies to accept everyone, without adjusting premiums based on risk ...

... so the companies raise their rates ...

... making an increasing number of healthy people drop insurance ...

As the spiral continues with risk pools getting worse, companies find it is no longer profitable to do business, so they may decide to get out of the state altogether, leaving people to search for alternatives.
Source: Kiplinger.com.

There is no sure way of finding affordable health insurance for yourself. If you live in Kentucky, Maine or Washington, you will have few choices of any kind. In rural areas of the country you might not save money by joining an HMO because there may not be enough patients or doctors to make running one economical. Association plans (which can offer good deals) are unavailable in some states. And your state may limit your options for raising deductibles or cutting back on your coverage to lower the price.

ACTION ITEMS

Know these terms

Benefit
Amount payable by the insurance company to a claimant, assignee or beneficiary.

Capitation
Capitation represents a set dollar limit that you or your employer pay to an HMO, regardless of how much you use (or don't use) their services.

Co-Insurance
Co-insurance refers to money that an individual pays for services, after a deductible has been paid.

Co-Payment
Co-payment is a predetermined (flat) fee that an individual pays for healthcare services, in addition to what the insurance covers.

Deductible
The amount an individual must pay for healthcare expenses before insurance covers the costs.

Exclusions
Medical services that are not covered by insurance.

LOS
LOS refers to the length of stay in a hospital.

Maximum Dollar Limit
The maximum amount of money that an insurance company (or self-insured company) will pay for claims within a specific time period.

Out-of-Plan
Refers to physicians, hospitals or other health care providers who are considered nonparticipants in an insurance plan (usually an HMO or PPO).

? What are different types of health insurance?

Type of insurance	What it's for	Typical costs covered
Major Medical (sometimes called *catastrophic insurance*)	Injury or sickness	Charges by doctors and hospitals for medically necessary services
Medicare 297	Injury or sickness	Charges by doctors and hospitals for medically necessary services
Long-Term Care 305	Unable to perform certain activities of daily living (ADLs)	Fixed payment for each day spent in a nursing home
Accidental Death and Dismemberment (AD&D)	Accidental death or loss of one or more limbs or eyes	Fixed payment for accidental death or loss of up to two limbs (usually half of death benefit for each).
Dental	Dental problems or prevention	Charges by dentists for necessary services
Disability 135	Loss of income due to injury or sickness	Fixed payments while unable to work

? What should I know about health insurance?

A health insurance plan protects you by promising to pay for medical care or to provide medical care.

> Americans insure themselves against dying but not against disability. (Only about four million people in the US have disability insurance.) Yet one in seven people becomes disabled for at least five years before age 65. Between ages 35 and 65, one in five will become disabled.
>
> Source: MSN Money Central Insurance.

? What's a viatical settlement?

Patients with terminal illnesses may consider selling their life insurance policies to a viatical settlement company for a lump sum cash payment. This company becomes the beneficiary of the policy, pays the premiums, and collects the face value of the policy when the original holder dies.

Source: WebMD Health.

? What's a flexible spending account?

Some employers offer FSAs to their employees to help them save money. Set aside an amount of dollars in an FSA, and pay no tax on it, putting the amount towrad medical expanses that insurance companies don't cover. The account must be established for 12 months, and the money can only be used for medical expenses during that time.

Source: Cliffs Notes *Understanding Health Insurance*.

Out-of-Pocket Maximum
A predetermined, limited amount of money that an individual must pay before an insurance company or (self-insured employer) will pay 100%.

Outpatient
A patient receiving health care services (such as surgery) when they do not stay overnight in a hospital or inpatient facility. Many insurance companies specify tests and procedures (including surgery) that will not be covered unless they are performed on an outpatient basis.

Pre-Admission Certification
Prior approval by a case manager or insurance company representative (usually a nurse) for a person to be admitted to a hospital.

Primary Care Provider (PCP)
A healthcare professional (usually a physician) who is responsible for monitoring an individual's overall healthcare needs.

Provider
A healthcare professional (usually a physician) who provides healthcare services.

Usual, Customary and Reasonable (UCR) or Covered Expenses
An amount customarily charged for similar services and supplies required for treatment.

Waiting Period
A period of time when you are not covered by insurance for a particular problem.

Source: Health Insurance Resource Center: healthinsurance.org.

*S*usan and her husband Ben used to joke that their 6-year-old son Michael was the family athlete—"A T-ball prodigy," said Ben.

"It seemed like he got sick overnight," said Susan, shaking a head of red curls. "One minute he was a normal kid, and the next he could hardly walk."

Their pediatrician confirmed the bad news: Michael had a brain tumor. In less than 12 hours he was in the operating room.

At her son's bedside, Susan, her face creased with worry, was struck by how small and helpless her little boy looked. Thank goodness they had health insurance. She couldn't imagine having to face enormous hospital bills while her son's life was in danger.

"The day I filled out the paperwork for my family's health insurance was crazy," Susan remembered with a frown. "It was so busy. I just picked the first option and signed the papers."

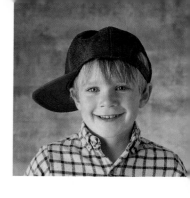

Michael's parents were unfamiliar with their family's health coverage.

What if he needed a bone marrow transplant? Would her plan cover it? Susan sobbed.

As Ben comforted his wife, Dr. Bellows entered the room and bent over her young patient. "Looking better," she smiled. "Let's talk about what happens next."

Over the next hour, Susan and Ben huddled with the doctor learning about possible future treatments, side-effects and more than they thought they'd ever need to know about health plans. With relief, they discovered Dr. Bellows could help navigate their health plan's referral system if Michael needed specialty care.

"Look over your health plan information," she advised. "Your plan's web site probably has most of the information you need."

"We have a lot to learn," Susan said taking Ben's hand in hers. "We need to make sure Michael gets the care he needs. And, we'll do whatever it takes."

Some policies require your primary care doctor to make referrals only to other doctors in the same medical group. If the specialist you need isn't in your plan's network of doctors, you may have to pay more to see that specialist. Check out your options before you need to.
Source: National Health Law Program.

The Consumers Guide to Health Insurance is available from the Health Insurance Association of America.
202.824.1600
www.hiaa.org/consumer/guidehi.cfm

Healthcare in America is changing rapidly. 25 years ago, most people in the US had fee-for-service insurance coverage. That meant you could go to any doctor, hospital or other provider, and you and your insurance would each pay part of the bills.

Today, **more than half of all Americans who have insurance are enrolled in a managed-care plan**—a way of providing services and paying for them. There are three different types of managed-care plan: **PPOs, HMOs and POS plans.**

What are my health plan choices?

Choosing between health plans is not as easy as it once was. Although there is no one best plan, there are some plans that will be better than others for you and your family's health needs. Plans differ, both in how much you have to pay and how easy it is to get the services you need. Although no plan will pay for all the costs associated with your medical care, some plans will cover more than others.

Health insurance plans are usually described as either **fee-for-service** or **managed care.**

With any health plan, there is a basic **premium,** which is how much you or your employer pay, usually monthly, to buy health insurance coverage. In addition, there are often other payments you must make, which will vary by plan. In considering any plan, you should try to figure out its total cost to you and your family, especially if someone in the family has a chronic or serious health condition.

Source: The Agency for Healthcare Research and Quality, ahcpr.gov.

Fee-for-service plans

With fee-for-service plans (sometimes called indemnity plans), you can use any medical provider (doctor, hospital). You or they send the bill to the insurance company, which pays part of it. Usually, you have a deductible—such as $200—to pay each year before the insurer starts paying.

Once you meet the deductible, most fee-for-service plans pay a percentage of what they consider the "usual and customary" charge for covered services. The insurer generally pays 80% of the usual and customary costs and you pay the other 20%, which is known as coinsurance. If the provider charges more than the usual and customary rates, you will have to pay both the coinsurance and the difference.

The plan will pay for charges for medical tests and prescriptions as well as from doctors and hospitals. It may not pay for some preventive care, like check-ups.

Managed care plans 295

PPOs (Preferred Provider Organizations) are a form of managed care closest to fee-for-service plans. A PPO has arrangements with doctors, hospitals and other providers of care who have agreed to accept lower fees from the insurer for their services. As a result, your cost sharing should be lower than if you go outside the network. In addition to the PPO doctors making referrals, plan members can refer themselves to other doctors, including ones outside the plan.

If you go to a doctor within the PPO network, you will pay a copayment (a set amount you pay for certain services—say $10 for a doctor or $5 for a prescription). Your coinsurance will be based on lower charges for PPO members.

If you choose to go outside the network, you will have to meet the deductible and pay coinsurance based on higher charges. In addition, you may have to pay the difference between what the provider charges and what the plan will pay.

ACTION ITEMS

Choosing a health plan

Whether you choose a fee-for-service plan or a form of managed care, you must examine a benefits summary or an outline of coverage—the description of policy benefits, exclusions and provisions that makes it easier to understand a particular policy and compare it with others.

Look at this information closely. Think about your personal situation. You may not mind that pregnancy is not covered, but you may want coverage for psychological counseling. Is the coverage for your whole family or just yourself? Are you concerned with preventive care and checkups? Or, would you be comfortable in a managed-care setting that might restrict your choice somewhat but give you broad coverage and convenience?

Here are some of the things you should look at when comparing health insurance plans:

Coverage

What medical services are covered?
- Inpatient hospital services
- Outpatient surgery
- Physician visits (in the hospital)
- Office visits
- Skilled nursing care
- Medical tests and x-rays
- Prescription drugs
- Mental health care
- Drug and alcohol abuse treatment
- Home health care visits
- Rehabilitation facility care

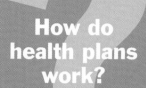

HMOs

HMOs (Health Maintenance Organizations) are the oldest form of managed-care plan. HMOs offer members a range of health benefits, including preventive care, for a set monthly fee. There are many kinds of HMOs. If doctors are employees of the health plan and you visit them at central medical offices or clinics, it is a staff or group model HMO. Other HMOs contract with physician groups or individual doctors who have private offices. These are called individual practice associations (IPAs) or networks.

HMOs will give you a list of doctors from which to choose a primary care doctor. This doctor coordinates your care, which means that generally you must contact him or her to be referred to a specialist.

With some HMOs, you will pay nothing when you visit doctors. With other HMOs there may be a copayment, like $5 or $10, for various services.

If you belong to an HMO, the plan only covers the cost of charges for doctors in that HMO. If you go outside the HMO, you will pay the bill. This is not the case with point-of-service plans.

POS

POS (Point-of-Service) Plans. Many HMOs offer an indemnity-type option known as a POS plan. The primary care doctors in a POS plan usually make referrals to other providers in the plan. But in a POS plan, members can refer themselves outside the plan and still get some coverage.

If the doctor makes a referral out of the network, the plan pays all or most of the bill. If you refer yourself to a provider outside the network and the service is covered by the plan, you will have to pay coinsurance.

Source: The Agency for Healthcare Research and Quality, ahcpr.gov.

Where do I get these plans?

Group Policies

You may be able to get group health coverage—either indemnity or managed care—through your job or the job of a family member. Many employers allow you to join or change health plans once a year during open enrollment. But once you choose a plan, you must keep it for a year. Discuss choices and limits with your employee benefits office.

Individual Policies

If you are self-employed, or if your company does not offer group policies, you may need to buy individual health insurance. Individual policies often cost more than group policies. Some organizations—such as unions, professional associations or social or civic groups—offer health plans for members. You may want to talk to an insurance broker who can tell you more about the fee-for-service and managed-care plans that are available for individuals. Some states also provide insurance for very small groups or the self-employed.

Medicare 297

Americans age 65 or older and people with certain disabilities can be covered under Medicare, a Federal health insurance program. In many parts of the country, people covered under Medicare now have a choice between managed care and fee-for-service plans. They also can switch their plans for any reason.

Medicaid 303

Medicaid covers some low-income people (especially children and pregnant women) and disabled people. Medicaid is a joint federal-state health insurance program that is run by the states. In some cases, states require people covered under Medicaid to join managed-care plans. Insurance plans and state regulations differ, so check with your state Medicaid office to learn more.

Health plans have gone through enormous changes and finding the one that's right one for you takes careful planning.

- Physical therapy
- Speech therapy
- Hospice care
- Maternity care
- Chiropractic treatment
- Preventive care and checkups
- Well-baby care
- Dental care
- Other covered services

What conditions are covered or excluded?
Are pre-existing conditions covered?

Benefit procedures

- What types of utilization review, pre-authorization or certification procedures are required?

Costs

- How much is the premium?
- Are there any discounts available for good health or healthy behaviors (e.g., non-smoker)?
- How much is the annual deductible?
- What coinsurance or co-payments apply?
- What is the maximum out-of-pocket expense?

Source: Health Insurance Association of America, hiaa.org.

DEFINITIONS

Capitation represents a set dollar limit that your health maintanence organization (HMO) pays to your primary care physician for providing medical treatment to you and your dependents. This fee is usually paid to the physician on a monthly basis. The physician gets no more nor no less than this set fee no matter how much you use his or her services.

Health Maintenance Organizations (HMOs) represent "pre-paid" or "capitated" healthcare plans in which individuals pay small fees or copayments for specified healthcare services over and above the monthly premiums paid to be a member of the HMO. Services are provided by physicians and allied healthcare personnel who are employed by, or under contract with the HMO. HMOs vary in design. Depending on the type of HMO, services may be provided in a central facility, or in an individual physicians office. HMO's are available on both an individual and employer group basis.

Preferred Provider Organizations (PPOs) are a group of healthcare providers who have agreed by contract to furnish medical services to members of a health plan at discounted rates.

Point-of-Service Plan (POS) allows a choice of whether to receive services from a participating or nonparticipating provider.

Exclusive Provider Organization (EPO) ia a type of preferred provider organization where individual members use particular preferred providers rather than having a choice of a variety of preferred providers. EPOs are characterized by a primary physician who monitors care and makes referrals to a network of providers.

Indemnity health insurance plans are also called **"fee-for-service."** These are the types of plans that primarily existed before the rise of HMOs, IPAs and PPOs. With indemnity plans, the individual pays a predetermined percentage of the cost of healthcare services, and the insurance company pays the additional percentage ultimately adding up to 100% of charges. For example, an individual might pay 20% for services and the insurance company pays 80%. The fees for services are defined by the providers and vary from physician to physician. Indemnity health plans offer individuals the freedom to choose any physician or hospital.

Fee-for-Service is a healthcare system where physicians and other providers receive payment based on their billed charge for each service provided.

❓ What's the difference between managed and non-managed care?

Available plans

Philosophy

Coverage

Providers

Costs

Payment to providers

ACTION ITEMS

How to handle your disputes

1 **Talk to your doctor about the situation.** This is an important first step because you'll need your doctor's help and advice.

2 **Call your state insurance or health department** to find out the appeals processes that are required in your state.

3 **Look up your plan's grievance procedures** and follow them.

4 **Keep good records:** keep your paperwork in order and maintain a log of every call you make to your plan. Record the date of the call and the name of the person with whom you spoke. Take careful notes about what you asked and

the answer you received. If you send a letter, always keep a copy

5 **Complete your plan's internal appeal process.** Most require written documentation of the issue you're appealing. Follow the instructions carefully. Answer all questions thoroughly, supply crucial information, including the service or procedure you believe should be covered, support from your doctor and any information from your insurance benefit booklet you believe is helpful to your cause.

6 If your internal appeal isn't successful, **find out if external reviews are required in your state.**

Managed Care	Non-Managed Care
● HMO ● POS ● EPO ● PPO (in-network)*	● Indemnity ● PPD (out-of-network)* ● POS (out-of-network)*
● Wellness, proactive care, disease management efficiency and cost effectiveness	● Freedom of choice ● Open access
● Physician visits ● Hospitalization ● More preventative medicine	● Physician visits ● Hospitalization
● Except in emergencies, network providers give maximum benefits	● Any provider ● No referrals necessary
● Lower premiums and co-pays	● Higher premiums ● Co-pays ● Deductibles ● Coinsurance
● Capitation, salary, case rate, discounted fee-for-service or combination	● Fee-for-service ● Balanced billing ● Usual, customary and reasonable

Know your plan's review process and what avenues are open to you to raise grievances.

* If you are enrolled in a PPO or PSO and you have chosen to be "out-of-network," your coverage works like non-managed care. If you have chosen to be "in-network," your coverage works like managed care.

Ask the plan for the procedures about external reviews. Again, follow instructions.

7 If your external appeal isn't successful and you still believe the procedure you are seeking should be covered, explore other avenues: **consider contacting an attorney.**

Where to go for help

A Consumer Guide to Handling Disputes with your Private or Employer Health Plan, *Kaiser Family Foundation*
www.kff.org/consumerguide

HealthCareCoach
www.healthcarecoach.com

Fact Sheets: Getting the Best Out of Managed Care
www.healthlaw.org/pubs/FS/managedcarefacts.shtml

Georgetown University Health Policy Institute
www.healthinsuranceinfo.net

Health Assistance Partnership
www.healthassistancepartnership.org

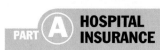

HOSPITAL INSURANCE

PART **A**

$0

Most people get Part A automatically when they turn age 65 at no cost, because they or a spouse paid Medicare taxes while they were working.

❓ What does Medicare Part A help to cover?

In a hospital: semiprivate room, meals, general nursing and other hospital services and supplies. Includes inpatient care you get in critical access hospitals and mental health care. **Does not include:** private duty nursing or a TV or telephone in your room.

In a skilled nursing care facility: semiprivate room, meals, skilled nursing and rehabilitative services.

At home: part-time skilled nursing care, physical therapy, occupational therapy, speech-language therapy, home health

aide services, medical social services, durable medical equipment (wheelchairs, etc.) and medical supplies.

Hospice care: drugs for symptom control and pain relief (for people with a terminal illness). Hospice care is usually given in your home, but short-term hospital care is covered when needed so the usual caregiver can rest.

Blood: pints of blood you get at a hospital or skilled nursing facility during a covered stay.

MEDICAL INSURANCE

PART **B**

$58.70

per month, in 2003

In some cases this amount may be higher if you did not choose Part B when you first became eligible at age 65.

❓ What does Medicare Part B help to cover?

Medical services include: doctor's services (not routine exams), outpatient medical and surgical services and supplies, diagnostic tests. Second surgical opinions, outpatient mental health care, outpatient physical and occupational therapy.

Clinical laboratory services: blood tests, urinalysis and more.

At home: same as part A.

Outpatient hospital services: services and supplies received as an outpatient as part of a doctor's care.

Blood: pints of blood you get as an outpatient or as part of a Part B covered service.

Preventive services:
bone mass measurements
once every 24 months

colorectal cancer screening
fecal occult blood test once every 12 months
fexible sigmoidoscopy once every 48 months
colonoscopy once every 24 months (if you are at risk for colon cancer)

pap test and pelvic examination
once every 12 months (includes a breast exam)

diabetes services and supplies
glucose monitors, test strips, lancets, diabetes self-management training

shots (vaccinations)
flu shot once a year in fall or winter
pneumonia shot (one may be all you need)
hepatitis B shot

prostate cancer screening
digital rectal exam once every 12 months
PSA test once every 12 months

glaucoma screening
once every 12 months

mammogram screening
once every 12 months

Source: Centers for Medicare and Medical Services.

ACTION ITEMS Enrolling for Medicare

Don't wait until you're 65 to sign up!

Pay close attention to enrollment dates because applying late can delay your coverage. Call or visit your local Social Security office to enroll 800.772.1213 or go to www.ssa.gov.

- Enrollment starts three months before the month you turn 65.
- Enrollment ends three months after the month you turn 65.

For example, if Bill turns 65 on May 2, he is allowed to enroll in Medicare any time between February 1 through August 31.

What if I'm already receiving benefits from Social Security?

If you're already receiving benefits, you are automatically entitled to Medicare Part A (Hospital Insurance) and Part B (Medical Insurance) starting the first day of the month you turn age 65. You'll receive your Medicare card in the mail about three months before your 65th birthday.

What if I'm not getting Social Security benefits?

You can apply for both Social Security benefits and Medicare online. Call the Social Security Administration at 800.772.1213 or go online at www.ssa.gov for more information.

NEW DRUG BENEFIT

PRESCRIPTION DRUG COVERAGE

$35.00

per month, available in 2006

New $400 billion legislation, endorsed by the AARP and AMA and signed into law in November 2003, will offer a Medicare prescription drug benefit, promote competition and assist rural healthcare providers. Until the drug benefit is available in 2006, seniors will be able to purchase discount drug cards beginning mid-2004. Low income seniors will also get a $600 annual subsidy.

? What will the new drug benefit cover?

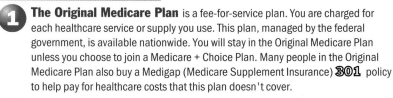

	your costs with	your costs without	
premium	$420	$0	**Should I sign up?**
deductible	$250	$250	
75% coverage from $250 to $2,250	$500	$2,000	◀ $810 If you spend more than $810 per year ($67.50 per month) on prescription drugs, the new Medicare drug benefit will save you money.
no coverage from $2,250 to $5,100	$2,850	$2,850	
95% after $5,100	5%	100%	**Who pays?** You / Medicare

HEALTH PLAN CHOICES

Medicare health coverage comes in two forms:

1 **The Original Medicare Plan** is a fee-for-service plan. You are charged for each healthcare service or supply you use. This plan, managed by the federal government, is available nationwide. You will stay in the Original Medicare Plan unless you choose to join a Medicare + Choice Plan. Many people in the Original Medicare Plan also buy a Medigap (Medicare Supplement Insurance) **301** policy to help pay for healthcare costs that this plan doesn't cover.

2 **Medicare + Choice Plans** provide care under contract to Medicare. There are two types of Medicare + Choice Plans. (These are not available everywhere.)

- Medicare Managed Care Plans (like HMOs and PPOs)
- Medicare Private Fee-for-Service Plans

If you belong to a Medicare + Choice Plan, the plan must cover at least the same benefits as Medicare Part A and Part B. However, your costs may be different, and you may have extra benefits, like coverage for prescription drugs or additional days in the hospital.

? What is Medicare?

Medicare is government health insurance.

These people are eligible:

People age **65** or older

Some people with **disabilities** under age 65

People with end-stage **renal** disease

In the US... **96.4%**

of people age 65 and older have Medicare.

What if I'm turning 65 or am older?

You can delay taking your Part B medical insurance if: (1) you or your spouse (of any age) continue to work and (2) you are covered under a group health plan from that current employment.

What if I'm under age 65 and disabled?

You can delay your Part B if (1) you or any member of your family is currently working, and (2) you have group health plan coverage from that current employment. Ask your employer or health benefits representative for .

What if I need a new card?

If you need to order a new card or want additional information contact the Social Security Administration.

800.633.4227

www.medicare.gov

Source: Medicare.

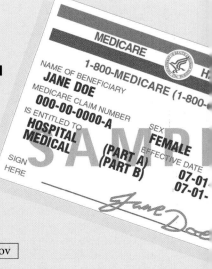

An HMO (Health Maintenance Organization) **is a health plan that is also involved in how your healthcare is delivered.** Managed care refers to health plans coordinating your healthcare with you and the providers that participate in the plan. HMOs are the most common type of coordinated care.

A Medicare HMO is an HMO that has contracted with the federal government under the Medicare + Choice program to provide health benefits to persons eligible for Medicare that choose to enroll in the HMO, instead of receiving their benefits and care through the traditional fee-for-service Medicare program.

Source: medicarehmo.com.

How do Medicare HMOs work?

How you get care varies across plans. Make sure you know the rules before you need care.

Keep your Medicare card but don't present it for payment purposes.

To receive covered care in an HMO, you **must get prior approval** from your primary care doctor.

If you don't get prior approval, neither Medicare nor the HMO will pay for the services. (They also will not pay for any services outside the HMO network.)

The only exceptions to this are for emergency or urgently needed service you receive outside the plan's service area. To guarantee payment in these cases, you must follow any rules your HMO has.

How do I enroll?

To be eligible, you must:

- be a Medicare beneficiary
- reside in an area served by a Medicare HMO
- not have end-stage renal disease
- not be receiving Medicare hospice benefits

HMOs must have at least one **open enrollment period** each year. You may enroll in a Medicare HMO without health screening during one of these advertised 30-day open enrollment periods.

When you enroll, you must choose a primary care doctor or one will be assigned to you. Usually you can change your doctor for any reason, but you must pick another from the plan's network.

What are the possible advantages of a Medicare HMO?

- Preventive healthcare
- Improved care coordination
- Extra benefits, reduced costs
- Less paperwork, simpler pay system
- Avoids the need for Medigap

What are the possible dis-advantages of a Medicare HMO?

- Limits choice of doctors, specialists, hospitals, nursing homes and other service providers
- May not be able to receive care from those you've been using for years
- Limited coverage when you are traveling outside the service area of the HMO
- May make getting Medigap more difficult

ACTION ITEMS
Questions you should ask

Yourself...

1. Do you have a trusted physician you don't want to leave? Does he or she participate in a Medicare managed care plan? If not, are you willing to change your primary care doctor?

2. Do you need to see a specialist regularly? If so, are you willing to change providers if your regular specialist is not part of an HMO you're considering?

3. Do you live in a continuing care retirement community (CCRC) whose skilled nursing facility is not part of the HMO? Do you live in an area where the long-term-care facilities are not part of the HMO? If so, are you willing to go out of the area for needed, covered services?

4. Do you travel or spend time in a second home? If so, does the HMO have arrangements with other plans in those areas to provide healthcare services while you're there?

The HMO...

1. How much does the plan cost? What is the premium? Are there any co-payments? What services are covered? What services aren't?

2. Can you choose your primary care physician? Can you change physicians within the plan? If so, how long must you wait? Are participating

❓How much does an HMO plan cost?

Your out-of-pocket expenses depend on:

Whether the plan charges a monthly premium in addition to your monthly Part B premium.

How much the plan decides you must pay for each visit.

The type of care you need and how often you receive it.

The average out-of-pocket expenses for **prescription drugs** for unhealthy people enrolled in Medicare HMOs in 2001 was **$2,088** (a 56% increase from 1999.) Those who were in good health spent an average of **$158** on prescription drugs (a 47% increase from 1999.)

Source: *USA Today.*

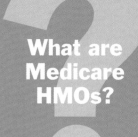
Medicare HMOs are healthcare plans under contract with the government to offer an alternative to direct Medicare services.

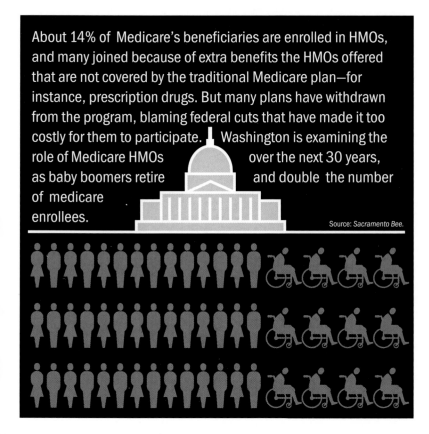

About 14% of Medicare's beneficiaries are enrolled in HMOs, and many joined because of extra benefits the HMOs offered that are not covered by the traditional Medicare plan—for instance, prescription drugs. But many plans have withdrawn from the program, blaming federal cuts that have made it too costly for them to participate. Washington is examining the role of Medicare HMOs over the next 30 years, as baby boomers retire and double the number of medicare enrollees.

Source: *Sacramento Bee.*

primary care doctors accepting new patients?

❸ Where do you go for care? To a central facility or individual doctor's office? Are the locations convenient? How long do you have to wait for a routine appointment?

❹ Which hospitals does the plan use? Do you have a choice? Where do you go for emergencies? How are "emergency" and "urgently needed" care defined? Do you need prior approval? Who do you call and how long does it take? How soon must you notify the HMO after receiving emergency care?

❺ What additional services, (e.g., ambulances) are available to you? What about services for any medical condition for which you are being treated? Remember, you can't be denied coverage because of a preexisting condition.

❻ What percentage of the HMO's patients receive preventive health services and screenings?

❼ What is the HMO's record in providing skilled nursing care, physical therapy or home health care? What are the rules on these types of care? You may want to ask nearby nursing homes, therapists and other caregivers about how the HMO treats its elderly and disabled members.

❽ Can the HMO cancel your membership? For what reason(s)?

Source: Pennsylvania Association of Non-Profit Homes for the Aging.

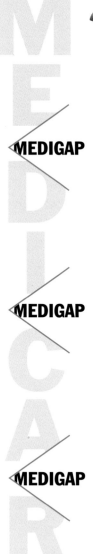

? What is a Medigap policy?

A Medigap policy is a health insurance policy sold by private insurance companies to **fill the "gaps" in Original Medicare Plan coverage.** There are ten standardized Medigap plans called "A" through "J."

When you buy a Medigap policy, you pay a premium to the insurance company. This premium is different than the Medicare Part B premium you must also pay. **As long as you pay your premium, your policy is automatically renewed each year.**

If you buy a Medigap policy, it only covers *your* healthcare costs. It doesn't cover any healthcare costs for your spouse. In some states, insurance companies may refuse to renew a Medigap policy bought before 1990. At the time these policies were sold, state law was not required to say the Medigap policies had to be renewed automatically each year. **Medigap policies only help pay healthcare costs if you have the Original Medicare Plan. You don't need to buy a Medigap policy if you are in a Medicare + Choice Plan.**

Source: Centers for Medicare and Medical Services, medicare.gov.

? Why would I want to buy a Medigap policy?

You may want to buy a Medigap policy because Medicare doesn't pay for all of your healthcare. There are "gaps" or costs that you must pay in the Original Medicare Plan. **Remember, no Medigap policy will cover all the gaps in the Original Medicare Plan.**
If you are in the Original Medicare Plan, a Medigap policy may help you:

- lower your out-of-pocket costs
- get more health insurance coverage

What you pay out-of-pocket in the Original Medicare Plan will depend on the following:

- whether your doctor or supplier accepts "assignment" (which means takes Medicare's approved amount as payment in full)
- how often you need healthcare
- what type of healthcare you need
- whether you buy a Medigap policy
- which Medigap policy you buy
- whether you have other health insurance

If you live in Massachusetts, Minnesota or Wisconsin, different types of standardized Medigap plans are sold in your state.

? Who can buy a Medigap policy?

To buy a Medigap policy, you generally must have Medicare Part A and Part B. If you are under age 65 and you are disabled or have End-Stage Renal Disease (ESRD), you may not be able to buy a Medigap policy until you turn 65.

? What is Medigap select?

It's a type of Medigap policy available in some states. If you buy this policy, you are buying one of the ten standardized Medigap plans A through J. With a Medicare Select policy, you must use specific hospitals and, in some cases, specific doctors to get full insurance benefits (except in an emergency). For this reason, Medicare Select policies generally cost less than other Medigap policies.

ACTION ITEMS

Shop carefully if you buy Medigap

1 Review your yearly healthcare expenses.
Write down your yearly expenses for healthcare. This will help you shop for the Medigap policy that is right for you.

2 Think about your future needs.
Consider benefits you may need in the future. Think about your medical history, your family's history and your health risks when considering future healthcare needs and costs.

3 Find out who sells Medigap policies near you.
Call 800.MEDICARE (800.633.4227). Select option "0" for customer service to get information on Medigap policies in your area.

Or, go on-line to www.medicare.gov and select "Medicare Personal Plan Finder."

4 Call the insurance companies
You should plan to call more than one insurance company that sells Medigap policies in your state. Make sure the ones you choose to call are honest and reliable. Call several and ask questions:
- Is this company licensed in this state?
- Which Medigap policies do you sell?
- What is the cost of the policy?
- What has been the cost of this Medigap policy for the past few years?
- How is the price decided?

❓ Can I keep seeing the same doctor?

In most cases, yes. If you are in the Original Medicare Plan and you have a Medigap policy, you can go to any doctor, hospital or other healthcare provider who accepts Medicare. However, if you have Medicare Select T, you must use specific hospitals and, in some cases, specific doctors to get your full benefits.

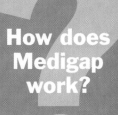
❓ What do Medigap policies cover?

Each standardized Medigap policy covers basic (core) benefits. Medigap policies pay most, if not all, of the Original Medicare Plan coinsurance and outpatient copayment amounts. Policies may also cover Original Medicare Plan deductibles. Some policies cover extra benefits to help pay for things Medicare doesn't cover.

Medigap plans A through J basic (core) benefits include:

- the Medicare Part A coinsurance amount for **days 61-90 ($210 per day in 2003)**, and days **91-150 ($420 per day in 2003)** of a hospital stay

- Coverage of up to **365 more days of a hospital stay during your lifetime** after you use up all Medicare hospital benefits

- **the coinsurance or copayment amount** for Medicare Part B services after you meet the $100 yearly deductible (in 2003)

- **the first three pints of blood** or equal amounts of packed red blood cells per calendar year, unless this blood is replaced

❓ What do Medigap policies *not* cover?

- long-term care
- vision or dental care
- hearing aids
- private-duty nursing
- unlimited prescription drugs

Medigap is additional insurance for those who have an original Medicare plan. 297

FACTORS THAT MAY AFFECT THE COST OF YOUR MEDIGAP POLICY

 Whether you are male or female.
Some companies offer discounts for females.

 Whether you smoke.
Some companies offer discounts for non-smokers.

 Whether you are married.
Some companies offer discounts for married couples.

 Whether the insurance company uses medical underwriting.
This is a process that an insurance company uses to review your health and medical history, and decide whether to accept your application for insurance, how much to charge you and whether to make you wait for some benefits.

There are huge rate differences for similar policies: rates range from $352 to $6,659 for all types of Medigap coverage, but even among plans with identical benefits, consumers' costs vary widely, according to an analysis by Weiss Ratings.
Source: CBS Marketwatch.

If you aren't in the open enrollment period, ask:
- Will you accept my application?
- Will I have to wait for pre-existing conditions to be covered?

5 **Choose the best policy for you.**
Carefully review the Medigap policy benefits, costs and company reputations. If you're still unsure, talk with someone you trust or an impartial insurance agent about your choice.

6 **Get it in writing.**
Once you have decided on the policy you want, the insurance company must give you a clearly worded summary of your policy. Read it carefully.

 Buy the policy.
Don't pay cash. Pay for your policy by check, money order or bank draft. And, make it payable to the insurance company, not the agent. Get a receipt.

 Follow up.
Make sure you get a copy of your policy within 30 days. If you don't, call your insurance company. If you don't get your policy in 60 days, call your state's insurance department.

❓ What is Medicaid?

Medicaid is a federal-state entitlement program that pays for medical assistance for certain people and families with low incomes and resources.

Eligibility, services and payment are complex and vary considerably from state to state. A person may be eligible for Medicaid in one state but not in the neighboring state. Within broad national guidelines established by federal statutes, **each state:**

 establishes its own eligibility standards

 determines the type, amount, duration and scope of the services

 sets the rate of payment

 administers its own programs

❓ Who pays for Medicaid?

Medicaid operates as a vendor payment program. States either pay health care providers directly on a fee-for-service basis, or they may pay through various prepayment arrangements, such as HMOs. States may impose nominal deductibles, coinsurance or copayments on some Medicaid recipients for certain services, However, **these recipients are always excluded from cost sharing:**

- pregnant women
- children under 18
- hospital and nursing home patients

In addition, all Medicaid recipients are exempt from copayments for emergency services and family planning services.

❓ What is the basis for eligibility?

Medicaid does not provide medical assistance for all poor persons unless they are living in certain circumstances, which include:

 individuals who meet the requirements of the Aid to Families with Dependent Children (AFDC) program that were in effect in their state on July 16, 1996.

 children under age 6 whose family income is at or below 133% of the federal poverty level (FPL)

 pregnant women whose family income is at or below 133% of the FPL (services to these women are limited to their pregnancy and aftercare)

 supplemental security income (SSI) recipients in most states

 people who get adoption or foster care assistance from Social Security

 children under age 19, in families with incomes at or below the FPL

In order to receive federal matching funds, states must cover the groups listed above. But states also have the option of providing Medicaid coverage for other groups (called "categorically related") including **certain aged, blind or disabled adults**.

 States can also cover **medically needy** people who would be eligible for Medicaid except that their income/resources are above the level set by their state. They can become immediately eligible for Medicaid by "spending down"—incurring medical expenses that reduce their income to the state's "medically needy" level.

ACTION ITEMS
Applying for Medicaid

To obtain Medicaid coverage, you need to apply in the state in which you live. Depending on your state, your options for applying may include:

- filling out an application at your local Medicaid office
- submitting an application at another location in your community, like a specific health center
- completing an electronic form on the Internet
- answering application questions by telephone

To find out how your state takes applications, you'll need to contact your local office. Here are some suggestions for getting the proper contact information.

① Look in the phone book
The phone number for your local office can probably be found in the blue pages of your phone book. Frequently, the office listing is under "medical assistance."

❓ What does Medicaid cover?

To be eligible for federal matching funds, states must provide medical assistance for certain basic needs, including:

- inpatient hospital services
- outpatient hospital services
- prenatal care
- vaccines for children
- physician services
- nursing facility services for people 21 or over
- family planning services and supplies
- rural health clinic services
- home health care for people eligible for skilled nursing services
- laboratory and x-ray services
- pediatric and family nurse practitioner services
- nurse-midwife services
- early and periodic screening , diagnostic and treatment services for children under 21
- federally qualified health center and ambulatory services

States may also receive federal matching funds to provide an additional 34 optional services, including prescribed drugs, transportation services, rehabilitation and physical therapy services, and home and community-based care to certain people with chronic impairments.

❓ How does Medicaid work?

Medicaid provides healthcare assistance for people with low incomes.

❓ Who gets Medicaid? | Percent of each population group

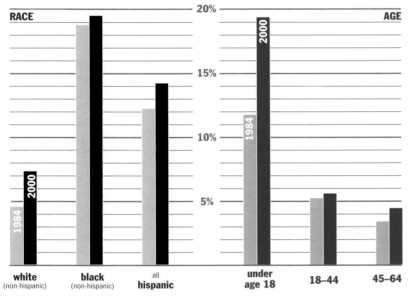

RACE

- white (non-hispanic)
- black (non-hispanic)
- all hispanic

AGE

- under age 18
- 18–44
- 45–64

20%
15%
10%
5%

1984 / 2000

Sources: Centers for Medicare and Medical Services, *World Almanac.*

2 **Call your local Social Security office**
If you have trouble finding the local office phone number in your phone book, call your local Social Security office. They can give you the phone number and address of your local Medicaid office.

3 **Call toll-free information**
Most states have a toll-free number to help answer your questions. Most toll-free operators can provide you information on how and where to apply.

4 **Go on-line**
You can find the state contact information at http by visiting www.cms.hhs.gov/medicaid/statemap.asp and select your state program from the map.

77% of American adults have planned and saved for their retirement but only 3% have saved any money to cover their expected long-term care costs.

Source: The American Society on Aging

? What is long-term care insurance?

Long-term care insurance covers your care if you have a disease such as **Alzheimer's,** or other cognitive impairments, or if you have trouble with two of these six **ADLs (activities of daily living):**

BATHING

CONTINENCE

USING THE TOILET

EATING

DRESSING

"TRANSFERRING" (i.e., moving from bed to chair)

Long-term care insurance can include three benefit triggers:

1 physical impairment benefit trigger

2 cognitive impairment benefit trigger

3 medical necessity benefit trigger

? What is a benefit trigger?

It's a term that an insurance company uses to describe the ways an evaluator will decide when to pay you benefits. Different companies use different triggers for home care coverage and nursing home care.

Source: mrtlc.com.

Physical impairment is the most common trigger. Some policies pay benefits when you cannot perform more than two of the six ADLs. Some policies specify whether you need **substantial assistance** with the ADLs. For other, more consumer-friendly policies, **standby assistance** with ADLs will qualify you for benefits.

Your policy usually pays benefits for **mental incapacity**, when you cannot pass certain tests of mental function. This is obviously an important part of coverage if you have symptoms of Alzheimer's or other dementia.

Some long-term policies will pay benefits if your **doctor certifies that medical care is necessary,** even though your case may not be related to either of the first two triggers, but fewer and fewer companies are selling policies with this trigger because they are not tax-qualified (TQ).

ACTION ITEMS Evaluating policies

Make sure your policy includes the right features and options.

1 **Guaranteed renewable**—ensures that the insurance company can't cancel your policy if it finds out you're in poor health.

2 **Benefit period**—the number of years of coverage you're buying. These come in three-year, five-year or lifetime varieties. Statistically, fewer than 15% of nursing home residents remained for more than five years. Still, your best bet is to purchase a policy with the longest benefit period you can afford.

3 **Daily benefit**—the number of dollars available per day, usually ranging from $30 to $200. The

higher the coverage, the greater the cost. Ask your state insurance office how much care costs in your area. Then factor in your Social Security and pension benefits, which you can use to help pay for care. Finally, balance what you think you'll need with what you can afford. Most people try to cover 80 to 100% of the daily cost of long-term care.

4 **Elimination period**—the number of days you'll pay for care out-of-pocket before your coverage kicks in. Policies range from zero to 100 days. The shorter the waiting period, the higher the premiums. Most planners suggest a waiting period of 30 days. And make sure you only have to meet the waiting period once.

42% of Americans 65 and older will enter a nursing home during their lifetimes. The current annual cost of a one-year stay is $57,700. Women have a 50% greater likelihood of needing nursing home care than men.

What are the insurance premiums for this kind of care?

They are not cheap, but if you can afford it and you want to preserve some assets for your children, you probably need the insurance. Of course premiums vary based on age, sex, where you live and what kind of policy you get, but an annual premium for a 40-year old male might be $400, going up to $3,000 for a man or woman aged 70 or over.

You can keep premiums down by choosing a longer waiting period (the time between qualifying for benefits and actually taking them), taking lower benefits or coverage that ends after a certain time. Also, many employers offer long-term care insurance as an employee benefit.

Source: insbuyer.com.

Remember, long-term care is not just for when you are older, possibly needing help in your own home, or a stay in a nursing home. If you have a bad car accident at any age you could be in bed for months. 40% of those getting long-term care today are under 65.

Will Medicare, Medigap or my private medical insurance pay for long-term care?

Medicare will not cover all long-term care needs. Medicare provides some coverage for skilled nursing care, but it is limited to 100 days in each benefit period, and only following a hospital stay.

A high percentage of people will need long-term care. It is worth evaluating your probable needs and planning ahead for them.

---

5 **Benefit triggers**—the conditions that activate benefits. Your benefits should be triggered if you become mentally or physically impaired or need assistance with at least two activities of daily living (ADLs). These include bathing, dressing and eating. Get a policy that gives you maximum coverage—and that allows you, not the insurance company, to pick the advocate who will make those calls.

6 **Inflation rider**—increases the benefit amount by a simple or compound inflation rate each year. If you purchase the policy before you're 75, get an inflation rider. If you buy at 55 or 60, get the most generous rider you can afford. Can't afford it? Reduce the starting daily benefit. It's more important to have inflation coverage than a big daily benefit.

7 **Home care coverage**—benefits for care at home as well as in an institution. You want the option of staying home to receive care.

8 **Definition of nursing home care**—facility classifications. You want to be covered for skilled, intermediate, respite or custodial care.

What else do you look for?

Make sure the company you buy from has been in the LTC coverage business for more than 10 years and has A or higher ratings from more than one rating service, such as AM Best.

Complex molecules
Big proteins from biotech

Many of our most promising new drugs are developed through biotechnology. Broadly defined, biotechnology is the use of living organisms (usually cells) to manufacture products. Most biotech drugs are proteins—large molecules that dwarf traditional drugs not only in size but also in complexity.

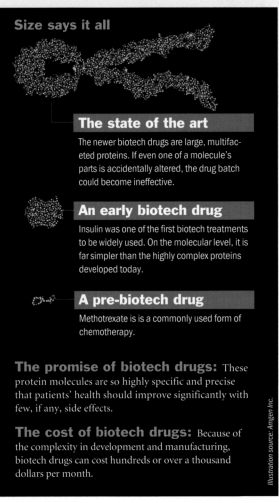

Size says it all

The state of the art
The newer biotech drugs are large, multifaceted proteins. If even one of a molecule's parts is accidentally altered, the drug batch could become ineffective.

An early biotech drug
Insulin was one of the first biotech treatments to be widely used. On the molecular level, it is far simpler than the highly complex proteins developed today.

A pre-biotech drug
Methotrexate is is a commonly used form of chemotherapy.

The promise of biotech drugs: These protein molecules are so highly specific and precise that patients' health should improve significantly with few, if any, side effects.

The cost of biotech drugs: Because of the complexity in development and manufacturing, biotech drugs can cost hundreds or over a thousand dollars per month.

Illustration source: Amgen Inc.

Complex manufacturing
Sustaining cell life

To produce a biotech drug, scientists usually insert an isolated gene into living "host" cells, which will, under the right conditions, make copies of the desired protein molecule. The key to mass production, then, is to keep high numbers of these host cells alive and flourishing in a tightly controlled liquid environment. The process is delicate and labor-intensive, as even minor shifts in temperature, oxygen supply or acidity could kill the cells. ■ The cost and materials for biotech manufacturing can be 20 to 100 times higher than for synthetic drug manufacturing. Some biotech companies spend over $250 million in facility costs before their product even begins the earliest clinical trials.

Complex markets
The push to sell before time runs out

■ **Drug development is expensive.** It takes a drug company an average of **14 years** and as much as **$800 million** to get a drug from pre-clinical trials through FDA approval. 255 ■ Only 3 of 10 marketed drugs produce revenues that match or exceed average research and development costs.
■ **Patent life may be short.** Companies are often pressed to recoup their investment before their patent expires. Companies typically patent drug compounds during the research phase, long before the drug makes it to market. This leaves drugs with an average effective patent life of 11 to 12 years; products in non-drug markets enjoy an average of 18.5 years on patent. ■ **Generics may lurk on the horizon.** A generic drug has the same active ingredients as its corresponding brand-name drug. If a generic is made, sales of the brand original can plummet by 50% or more.

ACTION ITEMS
How to reduce your drug expenses

Ask for a generic.

About half of brand-name drugs have generic equivalents. Ask your pharmacist to fill your prescription with a generic drug if one is available. Your savings can be 50% or more.

Although generic drugs are required to have the same active ingredients as the brand original, your doctor may, in some instances, consider a brand-name drug medically preferable for you. If your doctor has written "Brand Necessary" on your prescription, ask for the reason and discuss whether a generic is an option.

Consider purchasing online— but exercise caution.

Buying prescription drugs online can save you money—as well as the hassle of waiting in line at the pharmacy. However, not all sources are reliable or even ethical. You could be at risk for receiving the wrong drug or dose, counterfeit or contaminated medicine, or no drug at all.

- Make sure the pharmacy website is licensed by the National Association of Boards of Pharmacy. Visit www.nabp.net.
- Do not order from a site that does not offer access to a registered pharmacist who will answer your questions.
- Beware of sites that allow you to get a prescription by filling out a questionnaire instead of seeing a doctor.

We use more drugs...

National health expenditures for prescription drugs totaled $91 billion in 1991 and are projected to reach about $243 billion in 2008. A driving factor in this increase: the growing number of older Americans, the population that uses more Rx drugs than any other age group.

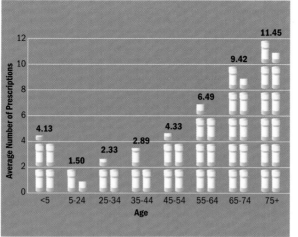

Average Number of Prescriptions by Age, 1997

Source: NWDA, 1998 Industry Profile & Healthcare Factbook.

...And our drugs do more

It's true that scientific improvements can lead to higher drug prices. But in many cases, drug advances provide cost-effective alternatives to more invasive, less successful treatments in other realms of patient care. **Examples:** ■ Increased use of asthma drugs that reduces emergency room visits ■ Cholesterol-lowering drugs that decrease risks of needing bypass surgery ■ A breast-cancer drug that reduces incidence and the need for surgery and hospitalization ■ Drugs for depression that decrease absenteeism and lost productivity in the workplace

Why do drugs cost so much?

In a word: complexity. Today's drugs are extremely complicated to develop and mass produce. Market conditions are also complex, with drug companies forced to recoup their investments within a compressed time frame. These complexities often translate into higher drug costs.

Drugs around the globe

Why are drugs cheaper in some other countries?

Most developed countries control drug prices directly or indirectly by limiting reimbursement or profits. In developing countries, drug companies are often forced to slash prices to realize any sales at all.

Are there laws against importing prescription drugs?

Although the US has banned the importation of drugs, there are certain circumstances under which illegal importation is overlooked—for example, when domestic treatment is not available or if the product has no foreseen risk.

Where research dollars come from

Americans' higher drug prices cover 50% of the drug industry's research costs. US tax dollars support about 80% of government-funded biomedical research worldwide, only a small fraction of which is involved directly in drug discovery. *Source: Business Week*

Buy a larger supply.

Some mail order programs and pharmacies offer discounts if you buy in bulk—for example, a 90-day supply instead of a 30-day supply. If you have insurance prescription coverage, make sure you'll be covered for quantities that exceed a 30-day supply.

Or buy a smaller supply.

By law, prescription drugs cannot be returned after purchase. So if you're trying a drug for the first time and you don't have prescription coverage, ask your pharmacist for a one-week supply. This way, if you have side effects you can't tolerate, you don't risk losing the money you've spent on the remaining 3 weeks.

Resources

● **Cost Containment Research Institute**
News and guidelines on getting drugs at lower prices

www.institutedc.org

202.478.0481

● **Rxaminer**
Searchable database of generic drugs

www.rxaminer.com

TIP

At every medical visit, ask your doctor if there are free samples of the drugs you use.

Source: institutedc.org.

?Which countries have the best overall health systems?

Using five performance indicators, the World Health Organization ranked 191 countries' health systems.

THE FIVE INDICATORS ARE:

● the overall level of **population health**

● **health inequalities** within the population

● the overall level of **heath system responsiveness** (patients' satisfaction and how well the system works)

● **distribution of responsiveness** within the population (how well people of varying economic status find that they are served by the health system)

● distribution of the **health system's financial burden** within the population (who pays the costs)

THE RESULTS: (numbers are out of a possible 1.000)

1 France 0.994 **2 Italy** 0.991 **3 San Marino** 0.988 **4 Andorra** 0.982 **5 Malta** 0.978 **6 Singapore** 0.973 **7 Spain** 0.972 **8 Oman** 0.961 **9 Austria** 0.959 **10 Japan** 0.957 **11 Norway** 0.955 **12 Portugal** 0.945 **13 Monaco** 0.943 **14 Greece** 0.933 **15 Iceland** 0.932 **16 Luxembourg** 0.928 **17 Netherlands** 0.928 **18 United Kingdom** 0.925 **19 Ireland** 0.924 **20 Switzerland** 0.916 **21 Belgium** 0.915 **22 Colombia** 0.910 **23 Sweden** 0.908 **24 Cyprus** 0.906 **25 Germany** 0.902 **26 Saudi Arabia** 0.894 **27 United Arab Emirates** 0.886 **28 Israel** 0.884 **29 Morocco** 0.882 **30 Canada** 0.881 **31 Finland** 0.881 **32 Australia** 0.876 **33 Chile** 0.870 **34 Denmark** 0.862 **35 Dominica** 0.854 **36 Costa Rica** 0.849 **37 United States** 0.838 **38 Slovenia...** 0.838

...17 of the last 30 countries in this World Health Organization ranking are in Africa. The very last country, with a score of 0.000, is Sierra Leone.

ACTION ITEMS

Get the full report

The 206-page World Health Report 2000 summarized above can be obtained online at www.who.int or by calling the WHO Publications Center USA at 202.974.3000.

Dr. Gro Harlem Brundtland, Director General of WHO, describes this report as "a wake up call to the global community." The ultimate goal is to help governments of all countries to lower major risks to health, and thereby raise the healthy life expectancy of their populations. The report makes the following recommendations:

1 Governments, especially health ministries, should play a stronger role in formulating

risk prevention policies, including more support for scientific research, improved surveillance systems and better access to global information.

2 Countries should give top priority to developing effective, committed policies for the prevention of globally increasing high risks to health, such as tobacco consumption, unsafe sex in connection with HIV/AIDS and, in some populations, unhealthy diet and obesity.

3 Cost-effectiveness analyses should be used to identify high, medium and low priority

Healthcare spending in four high-income countries

In this chart, the highest amount spent in each category (1.0 on the outer rings) is used as an index to compare with the other countries' numbers in that category .

Of the four countries, the chart shows that Denmark and Sweden each had the highest expenditures on drugs; Sweden was also the highest spender on health employment, physicians, and hospital beds; while the US spent more than the other three on national health as a % of GDP, on healthcare in general, and on magnetic resonance imaging and computerized tomography scanners.

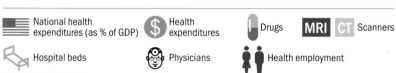

National health expenditures (as % of GDP) • $ Health expenditures • Drugs • MRI CT Scanners

Hospital beds • Physicians • Health employment

The United States rates 37 out of 191 in the World Health Organization's World Health Report.

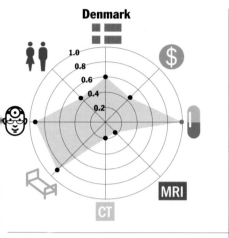

Denmark

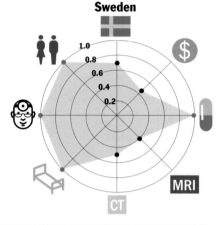

Sweden

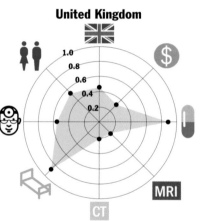

United Kingdom

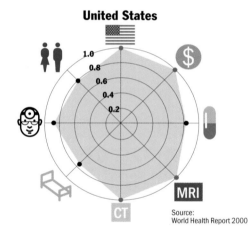

United States

Source:
World Health Report 2000

---

interventions to prevent or reduce risks, with highest priority given to those interventions that are cost-effective and affordable.

4 Intersectoral and international collaboration to reduce major extraneous risk to health, such as unsafe water and sanitation or a lack of education, is likely to have large health benefits and should be increased, especially in poorer countries.

5 Similarly, international and interesectoral collaboration should be strengthened to improve risk management and increase public awareness and understanding of risks to health.

6 A balance between government, community and individual action is necessary. For example, community action should be supported by nongovernmental organizations, local groups, the media and others. At the same time, individuals should be empowered and encouraged to make positive, life-enhancing health decisions for themselves on matters such as tobacco use, excessive alcohol consumption, unhealthy diet and unsafe sex.

Source: World Health Organization.

❓ What is medical malpractice?

Medical malpractice applies to situations when negligent actions by a healthcare provider results in harm to the patient. Negligence in the malpractice world is when a healthcare provider fails to meet standards of skill and care generally exercised by other providers in the community. A claim of malpractice can arise out of an error in diagnosis, treatment or illness management.

Source: Black's Law Dictionary, Sixth Edition.

❓ Does malpractice law work?

There is disagreement about whether our malpractice system functions well. Some say that there are too many malpractice suits, that awards are too high and that doctors are suffering as a result of high medical malpractice insurance. You will hear this group talking about **"tort reform"** and the importance of putting a limit on the dollar amount a plaintiff can receive in a malpractice lawsuit. Others find the system a just way to compensate victims of medical negligence and believe that caps on awards unfairly penalize victims of malpractice.

❓ What should I do if I think I have a malpractice claim?

If you believe you have been harmed by a healthcare provider and are considering pursuing a medical malpractice claim, consult an attorney. Ask friends and family for the names of reputable lawyers and be sure to check references of any attorney you contact. **Carefully consider whether you want to pursue a claim.** Cases are time consuming and can be exhausting. Also, most people who file malpractice claims and go to court lose their cases. In 2000, only 38 percent of jury verdicts went in favor of the claimant. **Each state has laws**—known as statutes of limitations—that specify a certain amount of time within which a malpractice claim may be filed. If you believe you are the victim of malpractice, don't wait too long before contacting an attorney.

Source: FindLaw for the Public, public.findlaw.com.

ACTION ITEMS — Getting information on malpractice

In a number of states, you can get information about your doctor's malpractice history.

For example, in Massachusetts, consumers can view malpractice about doctors online. Call your state insurance division or medical board to find out what malpractice information is available and how you can get it.

Empower yourself with information about your doctor, but use caution when interpreting medical malpractice information. A record of malpractice does not mean your doctor has been sued and found guilty. If a doctor has settled a claim, it is not necessarily an admission of wrongdoing, but may be an effort to avoid an expensive lawsuit. Also, keep in mind that malpractice histories tend to vary by specialty. Some doctors work primarily with high-risk patients, and these doctors may have

❓ What is an arbitration agreement?

Some doctors ask patients to sign arbitration agreements before they will see them. Agreeing to arbitration with your doctor generally means that you are giving up your right to go to court. Instead, any disputes will be decided by an outside arbitrator. Before signing an arbitration agreement, think about it and weigh the pros and the cons. **Make sure you understand the rights you are giving up.** For example, if you give up the right to sue the doctor, you may be giving up the right to gather evidence from the provider or from independent witnesses. On the other hand, arbitration can allow a decision to be reached faster and less expensively than a full-fledged law suit and can reduce the amount of money you have to pay a lawyer.

No matter what you decide, don't make the decision without careful deliberation. Before you go to an appointment, call and ask office staff about the doctor's arbitration policy. Does he require all patients to sign these agreements? Find out if your state has laws about arbitration (see below). If you're uncomfortable signing an arbitration agreement and the doctor insists, look for a new doctor.

A number of states have passed laws regulating arbitration agreements. 313 To find out if your state has such protections, call or visit the web site of your local or state bar association. Another source of information is the American Arbitration Association at www.adr.org or 800.778.7879.

Source: webmd.com.

Medical malpractice laws are designed to protect patients' rights to pursue a lawsuit if they are injured as a result of negligence.

Source: FindLaw for the Public, public.findlaw.com.

> EIGHT TIMES AS MANY PATIENTS ARE INJURED BY MEDICAL MALPRACTICE AS EVER FILE A CLAIM.

> SIXTEEN TIMES AS MANY PATIENTS ARE INJURED AS RECEIVE ANY COMPENSATION.

malpractice histories that are higher than average because they specialize in cases or patients who are at very high risk for problems.

No matter what you find out, consider discussing your concerns with your doctor. Be careful about choosing a doctor solely based on malpractice information. 229

Sources: www.massmedboard.org; webmd.com.

Insurance companies are paying victims of medical negligence on average approximately **$30,000.** Average payouts have stayed virtually flat for the last decade.
Total national costs of negligence in hospitals are estimated to be between
$17 billion
and
$129 billion
each year.

Source: Center for Justice & Democracy.

YOU pay for malpractice law suits.

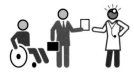
Doctor is sued for malpractice.

Doctor contacts his insurance provider.

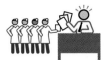
Insurance provider needs more money to cover the growing number of lawsuits.

Doctor's malpractice insurance premiums skyrocket.

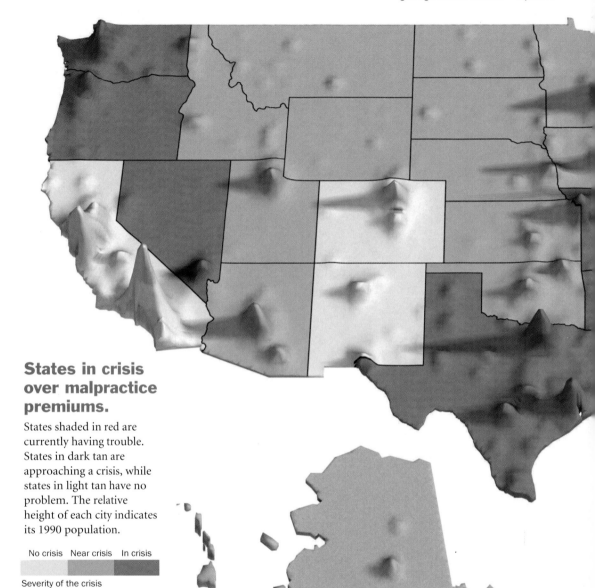

States in crisis over malpractice premiums.

States shaded in red are currently having trouble. States in dark tan are approaching a crisis, while states in light tan have no problem. The relative height of each city indicates its 1990 population.

No crisis   Near crisis   In crisis

Severity of the crisis

Premium Increases in Non-reform States

State	Premium Increase in 2002	State	Premium Increase in 2002
Arkansas	112%	North Carolina	50%
Connecticut	40%	Ohio	60%
Florida	75%	Oregon	80%
Georgia	40%	Pennsylvania	40%
Maryland	37%	South Carolina	42%
Missippi	99%	Tennessee	65%
Nebraska	36%	Texas	40%
Nevada	50%	Virginia	113%
New Hampshire	50%	Wyoming	38%

Source: Medical Liability Monitor, 2002.
*Highest increase among specialty physicians as reported in MLM Survey, 2002

Doctor passes the costs onto the next patient, either directly or through the HMO, which must increase it's premiums.

OR

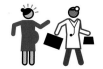

Doctor moves to another state where costs are more stable, sometimes leaving patients with no care.

OR

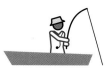

Doctor retires early, which also can leave an area without a doctor.

In 2003, 62% of final-year medical school residents ranked medical liability as their top concern— a 59% increase since 1995.

Source: ama-assn.org.

Medical Malpractice Liability Average Premium Increases by Specialty

Specialty	Summer 2001	Winter 2001	Summer 2002
Internists	10%	22%	26.3%
General Surgeons	10%	21%	23.7%
Ob/Gyns	9%	19%	19.4%

Source: Medical Liability Monitor

To put it mildly, we're in a full-blown crisis.

The current system for handling medical liability 311 is failing. Catapulting insurance premiums are forcing more and more physicians to compromise patient care or seek refuge in states that have better liability reform. Some have even closed their practices.

So far, 18 states are in medical liability crisis— roughly 40% of the country. And America is responding. Organizations such as the American Medical Association have designated medical liability reform as a top priority. Congress is attempting to pass legislation that will help stabilize the medical liability system.

Source: ama-assn.org.

How are states dealing with high malpractice premiums?

The General Accounting Office (GAO) supports the Congress in meeting its Constitutional responsibilities. On the topic of the dramatic rise in malpractice premiums for physicians, GAO points to multiple factors. The most important being the rapid increase of high awards. However, among other factors is the decrease in investment income caused by under-pricing premiums to compete for business during the 1990's.

Premiums vary by medical specialty and by state, and even by cities within a state. For example, a Florida insurer increased rates to general surgeons by 75% from 1999 to 2002. A Minnesota insurer raised rates by 2% for the same group.

States are trying different approaches to medical liability reform. California enacted the Medical Injury Compensation Reform ACT (MICRA) in 1975. Many current proposals for state or national medical liability reform use it as a model. Since enactment, average costs for medical malpractice premiums have increased three times faster nationally than in California. Savings are estimated at more than $1 billion per year.

Minnesota has also experienced lower than national growth in premium rates. This is primarily due to mandatory prescreening that prevents cases without merit going to trial.

Sources: General Accounting Office, American Medical Association, California Medical Association.

*H*ealthy her entire life until, at age 84, she got severe food poisoning, Heidi was admitted to the hospital where she stayed for a week. When she returned home, she was weaker than she'd been her entire life, and very unhappy about her deteriorating health. Her prognosis for a full recovery was good, yet she felt terrible. Accustomed to living independently, she hated that she couldn't sleep in her own bedroom upstairs, that she needed a nurse almost around the clock and that her children and grandchildren had to take care of her until she got better.

Several years before she got sick, Heidi had written advance directives—a living will and a medical power of attorney. Her wishes were crystal clear— she wanted to die in her home, not in a hospital or other care facility, she did not want any "extraordinary measures" taken and she did not want to be hooked up to any machines for artificial breathing

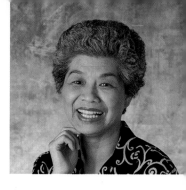

Heidi's advance directives allowed her to die at home as she wished.

or nutrition. She appointed her granddaughter as her healthcare proxy. She wanted to die a peaceful death in her own home.

One afternoon, Heidi became gravely ill. The visiting nurse said that if she wasn't taken to the hospital, she would die soon. Her granddaughter was with her and asked Heidi if she wanted to go to the hospital. Again, Heidi emphasized her desire to avoid the hospital. She then became delirious. Her family wondered whether Heidi should be taken to the hospital, but they decided that, to stay true to the living will and Heidi's wishes, she should stay in her own home.

Heidi slowly stopped eating. Hospice workers provided medication to ease Heidi's pain and let the family know what to expect in the next few weeks. Two weeks later, Heidi died. She was in her living room, with her family close by.

Advance directives clarify your wishes about medical care when you are unconscious or too ill to communicate. As long as you can express your own decisions, your advance directives will not be used and you can accept or refuse any medical treatment.

It is essential that you have honest and open discussions with your proxy, family members and physicians about their willingness to support and, if necessary, advocate to ensure that your wishes are carried out. If you learn they are not willing to support your choices, you may wish to consider appointing a non-family member who will honor your wishes or change your physician before a conflict arises.

❓ What are advance directives?

They are oral and written instructions about your future medical care, in case you become unable to speak for yourself.

There are two types of advance directives:

LIVING WILL

MEDICAL POWER OF ATTORNEY

Both documents require families to talk together about the issues surrounding serious illnesses and death. This discussion is hopefully well before any medical emergency. You also should ask your doctor any questions you may have about the kind of care you want at the end of life. All states have laws authorizing the use of some type of advance directive, but the laws they are regulated by differ from state to state.

❓ Who should have them?

Any adult over the age of 18 should have advance directives.

❓ What's a living will?

A living will is a document in which you communicate your wishes about medical treatment should you be unable to communicate at the end of life. A living will also is called a directive to physician, declaration or medical directive. The living will outlines the kind of treatment you want if you are in a terminal condition.

❓ What's a medical power of attorney?

A medical power of attorney is a written document where you appoint someone you trust to make decisions about your medical care if you can't make such decisions yourself. This type of advance directive, also called a **health care proxy, is the** appointment of a healthcare agent or a durable power of attorney for healthcare. The person you appoint through a medical power of attorney can speak for you any time you are unable to make your own medical decisions, not only at the end of life.

❓ Why do I need advance directives?

Advance directives **clarify your wishes about medical care when you are unconscious** or too ill to communicate. As long as you can express your own decisions, your advance directives will not be used and you can accept or refuse any medical treatment.

❓ Do I need both documents?

Yes, you can best protect your treatment wishes by having both documents. The appointment of a healthcare proxy ensures a more flexible form of decision making, since the agent can respond to unanticipated changes and base decisions not only on written or verbal expressions of treatment wishes, but also on general knowledge of the patient. **A living will is also important.** If your agent becomes unavailable or unwilling to serve, the living will serves as a guide to medical decision making. The living will also can reassure your proxy that he or she is following your wishes and ease the burden of decision making. If the agent's decisions are challenged, the living will can provide evidence that the agent is acting in good faith.

❓ Will my advance directives be honored in an emergency?

No. Generally, advance directives such as living wills and medical powers of attorney are not effective in medical emergencies. There generally isn't time to consult the directions in an advance directive or determine a person's underlying medical condition. **Once the person comes under the care of a physician, the living will can be evaluated** and the instructions of a health care agent determined in light of that person's overall prognosis.

ACTION ITEMS

Resources

Aging with Dignity
- Five Wishes® and Five Wishes Video. This advance directive document and 25-minute video highlight the importance of advance care planning.

  888.5.WISHES
  www.agingwithdignity.org.

Gundersen (WI) Lutheran Medical Foundation
- Making Choices: Planning in Advance for Future Healthcare Choices
- Making Choices: Planning Guide and/or Video

  800.362.9567 ext. 6748

National Hospice & Palliative Care Organization (NHPCO)
- Advance medical directives

  703.837.1500
  www.nhpco.org and www.kitslegacy.org

Partnership for Caring (PFC)
- Advance Directives
- Talking About Your Choices
- Q & A (a selection of titles on relevant topics)
- Whose Death Is It, Anyway?

  800.989.9455
  www.partnershipforcaring.org

❓ Where do I get the documents?

Your local hospital or long-term care facility may distribute them. Some physicians make them available to their patients. You can also get them for a nominal charge through Partnership for Caring by calling 800.989.9455. You can download them at no charge from www.partnershipforcaring.org .

❓ What do I do with the signed documents?

Make photocopies of the completed documents. Keep the original in an accessible but safe location (not a safe deposit box). **Give copies to your proxy,** an alternate proxy if you have one, your doctor and anyone else who might be involved with your healthcare.

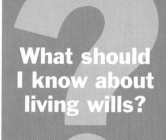

What should I know about living wills?

It is well worth taking the time to make your wishes known about what you want done if you become terminally ill and unable to communicate.

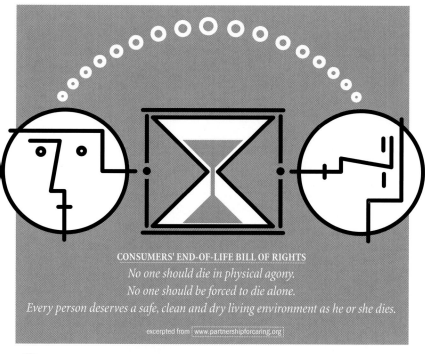

CONSUMERS' END-OF-LIFE BILL OF RIGHTS
No one should die in physical agony.
No one should be forced to die alone.
Every person deserves a safe, clean and dry living environment as he or she dies.

excerpted from www.partnershipforcaring.org

❓ What happens if my doctor (or family) won't honor my wishes?

There is no simple answer to this question. For this reason it is essential that you have honest and open discussions with your proxy, family members and physician about their willingness to support and, if necessary, advocate to ensure that your wishes are carried out. If you learn they are not willing to support your choices, you may wish to consider appointing a non-family member who will honor your wishes or change your physician before a conflict arises.

Hospice Net
- What questions should I ask about Hospice Care?
- Frequently Asked Questions about Hospice

www.hospicenet.org/html/questions-pr.html

National Hospice Foundation (NHF)
- Hospice Care: A Consumer's Guide to Selecting a Hospice Program
- Hospice Care and the Medicare Hospice Benefit

800.338.8619
www.hospiceinfo.org

Americans For Better Care of the Dying
www.abcd-caring.org

Growth House—Guide To Death, Dying, Grief, Bereavement and End Of Life Resources
www.growthhouse.org

Last Acts
www.lastacts.org

Handbook for Mortals. Oxford University Press 1999.
Joanne Lynn and Joan Harrold

A Good Death: Challenges, Choices and Care Options
Charles Meyer

Dying Well
Riverhead Books, 1997

A will is perhaps the most important legal document the average American will ever sign.

But, over

70%

of adults in America do not have a will.

Key words

Probate is the process of legally passing ownership of property from a dead person to his heirs or beneficiaries. Probate courts administer the process.

Beneficiaries are family members, friends or charitable organizations who will receive your assets as your will directs. Your will includes specific gifts (such as jewelry or a specified amount of money) to named beneficiaries.

The executor is a person or institution named in your will and appointed by the probate court, who collects and manages your assets, pays your debts and expenses and any taxes that might be due, and then distributes your assets to the beneficiaries.

? What makes a will legal?

In all states except Louisiana, these are the requirements for a will to be legal:

- **The testator** (that is, the person whose will is being made) **must be an adult.**

- The testator **must be of sound mind.**

- The will must specifically **state that it is your will.**

- The will must do what wills are supposed to do, such as: **appoint beneficiaries of your "worldly goods;" appoint a guardian for your minor children; appoint an executor.**

- The will must be **signed and dated by the testator, in front of the required number of witnesses.**

? Can my will be contested?

Usually a challenge to have a will invalidated comes from people who believe that they are potential heirs or beneficiaries, but to whom you left nothing. Their objections might be:

- **The will was not properly drawn up, signed or witnessed, according to the requirements of the particular state.**

- **You lacked mental capacity when the will was made.**

- **There was fraud, force or undue influence on you when you made the will.**

- **The will is a forgery.**

If the will is held to be invalid, the probate court may invalidate all provisions or just the ones that are challenged. If the entire will is invalidated, the proceeds are usually distributed as though you had died intestate (with no will). The distribution is according to the laws of the state that has the probate court.

? How do I find a lawyer to write a will for me?

The best way is to get a referral from someone whose judgement you trust—friends, associates or your employer. In addition, your local bar association maintains a list of State Bar-certified lawyer referral services in your area.

ACTION ITEMS

You should review your will:

1 every five years

2 if you have lost the one you had

3 when you get married

4 when you have your first child

5 if you decide to change the provisions of your will

6 if you move to another state

7 if your executor(s), guardian(s) or trustee(s) move to another state

Keep in touch with them. You should think about making a new will when they move.

How can my will provide for my minor children?

Children who are minors (under 18 in most states) cannot legally own anything except for small amounts—under $5,000, in most states. However there are three ways to leave property to your minor children:

● **Appoint a property guardian** to manage your child's inheritance. The role is different from that of the **personal guardian** whom you will be naming in other parts of your will. (The personal guardian raises the child, if necessary, and may or may not be the same person as the property guardian.)

● **Create a custodian account.** This is usually better than appointing a property guardian. Your will states that you are making a bequest to the Uniform Transfer to Minors Act. This act permits your named custodian to manage the property as she sees fit for the benefit of your child, without having a court review her actions annually, as is the case with property guardians.

● **Establish a trust for your child.** Unlike your will, which is public, the content of a trust is private. There are no limits to the length of time that a trust is in effect, although most trusts distribute money until the recipient is about 35. A trust can be made before you die or as part of your will. **A trust is generally considered to be the best way to provide for minors.**

What is not included in a will?

Life insurance
Because cash proceeds from an insurance policy on your life are paid to the person you named as the beneficiary of the policy, it is very important to keep this information current. Monies to deceased beneficiaries will be left to your estate if you die.

Retirement plans
Assets held in retirement plans (401(k), or an IRA) are transferred to the person you named as beneficiaries in the plan documents.

Jointly owned assets
Real estate, cars, bank accounts and other property jointly held passes to the joint tenant on your death, not in accordance with any directions in your will.

Laws vary from state to state, and you should check with your State Bar (the Estate Planning, Trust and Probate Law Section) about what laws are currently on the books.

What happens if I die without making a will?

Without a will, the state, and not you, will decide who is entitled to your personal items. A court will appoint a guardian for your child if she is under 18. Most likely, the court will appoint your spouse as the guardian, but a bond may have to be posted. The court will also, among other regulations, require an annual accounting of income and expenses, and any investment of the money from your estate by the guardian may be limited.

Do I need a will?

Yes. Having a will allows you—and not the state—to determine how your estate will be distributed and how your family will be protected.

If you die without a will and have minor children, the court will have to appoint a guardian to manage your child's share of your estate. This can cause major problems and expense.

Source: Understanding Children, understandingchildren.com, TOP and Civitas; pcwills.com; legal-zoom.com; New York State Bar Association; State Bar of California.

8 if you get divorced

9 if you've had a significant increase in wealth

10 if there has been a change in estate tax laws

For more information:

National Association of Financial Estate Planning

www.nafep.com

TIP
If the value of your estate is around the $700,000 mark or higher, you should consider finding a good estate planner to minimize estate taxes.

Bring a family member or friend with you to check-ups so that they can support you, help you ask questions and make you feel more comfortable.

*A*t was just a routine x-ray, but there it was, a spot on my mother's lung," said Kate, a young wife and mother. "She's only 67, but she really relies on me to help her make decisions. Dad's much older and in a nursing home, so it's really left to me."

Thinking the spot could be cancer, Betty's doctor suggested she see a surgeon.

Tapping the x-ray with his pen, the surgeon said, "The location of this tumor makes a biopsy impossible." Assuming the tumor was malignant, he recommended surgery the next week to remove a part of Betty's lung (a lobectomy).

"Everything felt so rushed," Kate said. "I told Mom that we should get more information before the surgery, but she was so anxious that she went ahead and scheduled it.

Borrowing her son's computer, Kate went online to learn more about lung cancer.

Make treatment decisions based on as much information as possible. Talk to your doctor about all your options. Always ask the pros and cons of every procedure. If your doctor visit is for a specific reason, consider doing research before you see the doctor.

Almost all users found the health information they got online useful and 80% learned something new.
Source: Pew.

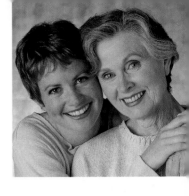

A positron emission tomography (PET) scan shows tissue and organs as well as the body's structure. Doctors can actually see increased metabolic activity in an area of the body that could indicate cancer, allowing for earlier diagnosis for some cancers. These scans are usually available only at larger hospitals or medical centers.
Source: MayoClinic.com.

Betty and her daughter Kate used the Internet to research her medical condition and avoid unneccessary surgery.

"I found a ton of stuff," she said with excitement. She learned about something called a PET scan 257 that could determine whether Betty's tumor was benign without surgery.

"I showed Mom what I found and once she saw that the PET meant no surgery, at least for now, she was really excited" Kate said. "So now we had information we could take back to the doctor."

Unfortunately they learned that the hospital where the doctor wanted to perform the surgery didn't have PET scans available. "We weren't giving up," Kate said with her mother nodding in agreement. "I went back online and started looking up hospitals. There was one 100 miles away that had one."

The PET scan showed no cancer and the surgery was cancelled. "We're so relieved," Kate said. "I'm thrilled that I could find all this information and not even leave my house. It made the difference."

Be an active healthcare consumer. Ask questions. Do research.

Choose your hospital carefully. Check with The Leapfrog Group to see if your hospital's safety records are listed.
www.leapfroggroup.org

? What's my best source for finding information fast?

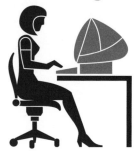

The **Internet** 325 gives you immediate access to information. It's also your gateway to other resources: people, doctors, tools, medical literature, etc. Use it like a "yellow-pages" for your health.

You can begin with a search engine like **Google.com** or **Yahoo.com**. Type some key words in the search box and you're off and running. Or, go directly to a trusted web site that provides consumer health information, such as **MayoClinic.com** or **WebMD.com**. You'll find medical literature at **bmj.com**. This site also gives you access to PubMed, an online database where you can find the most recent research information.

Look for information before your next doctor visit. Your doctor can explain anything you don't understand or verify what applies to your situation. 325

? Where do I begin?

Define your topic and what you want to learn about it. If the topic is asthma, do you want information for adults or children? Are you looking for causes or treatment? **First, locate your resources:**

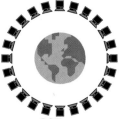

Internet 325
You may have access at work, home or at a library. Use search engines to find legitimate sources of information. What is a "legitimate" source? Look for the source of the information, the author's professional background, when the information was last updated and review the site's publication policy. Online support groups are often available, giving you support 24-hours a day!

People
Find experts or people who have information—doctors, nurses, pharmacists, dietitians. Each of these can offer a unique perspective. Check patient organizations to connect with people with the same illness.

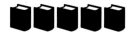

Libraries
Make a list of libraries in your area. Many hospitals and universities have libraries you may access, in addition to your local public library.

Community
Check the newspaper for listings of local support group meetings. A community senior center may provide access to the Internet or other resources. Your local hospital has resources through its patient education and social work departments. Look in the yellow pages for local chapters of national organizations.

Source: Wisconsin Library Services.

? How can I find information at a medical library?

Medical libraries are located at medical, nursing and dental schools, large medical centers and some community hospitals. Look in your telephone book under "hospitals," "schools" or "universities." Or call the National Network of Libraries of Medicine at **800.338.7657.**

These libraries contain medical and nursing textbooks, health-related journals, computer databases, drug reference books, medical and diagnostic laboratory testing manuals, as well as medical dictionaries and encyclopedias. Librarians can help you locate what you need. If you can't take materials home, most libraries have photocopiers available.

Source: National Institutes of Health.

? What information does the government provide?

The federal government operates many clearinghouses and information centers that offer free information and resources. The Health Information Resource Database includes 1,800 organizations and government offices that provide health information upon request.

For a free list, go to **www.health.gov/nhic**

or contact: Health Information Resource Database
PO Box 1133, Washington, DC 20013-1133
800.336.4797

Source: National Institutes of Health.

ACTION ITEMS   Don't believe everything you read

Not sure what to believe? It's easy to feel overwhelmed by health information. It's everywhere you look—magazine articles, television news, billboards, the Internet. You're bombarded, but how do you know these stories are accurate? Ask yourself these questions:

1 **Who's the source?** Does the author or company providing the information benefit from positive publicity? This, in itself, isn't an indication that the information isn't true, but it's something to take into consideration.

2 **How does it compare with other evidence?** Look at other sources for corroboration of the findings.

3 **Are there two sides to the story?** Is the information balanced? Does the story tell the pluses and the minuses? If it sounds too good to be true, it probably is.

4 **Do you understand the numbers?** 153 Statistics are great, if you understand them. Researchers often report findings within a range. Are these numbers on the high side? Or the low side? Do you understand what they mean to you?

5 **Where'd they get that?** Does the story or report identify the original source of the information so that you can verify it?

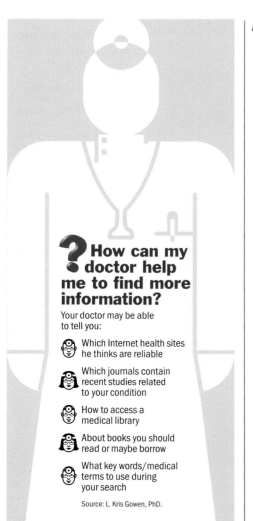

? How can my doctor help me to find more information?

Your doctor may be able to tell you:

- Which Internet health sites he thinks are reliable
- Which journals contain recent studies related to your condition
- How to access a medical library
- About books you should read or maybe borrow
- What key words/medical terms to use during your search

Source: L. Kris Gowen, PhD.

? How can I find information at my local library?

Ask the librarian to explain what resources are available in the library. Public libraries can provide basic information and resources to get you started.

Library computers are available for a variety of purposes. Use them to:

- Search the library's collection of books and other resources
- Search databases for magazine, newspaper and medical journal articles
- Search the Internet for online information
- Use software programs to create documents, spreadsheets and slideshows

Most libraries offer free computer classes on basic computer skills, email, effective web searching, word processing and basic research skills.

BEYOND THE LIBRARY WALLS

If you can't get to a library, then a library can come to you. You can receive materials by mail and some even deliver right to your front door.

Services for People with Disabilities

Need special assistance? Most libraries have resources for people with hearing, sight and mobility impairments.

Don't be shy! Ask for help. Librarians are your best resource. They're there to help you find what you need!

Sources: National Institutes of Health; D. Kemper. *Healthwise Handbook: A self-care guide for you.*

? Can I find good healthcare information?

Define your topic and what you want to know about it.

The Internet gives you immediate access to information and is the gateway to other resources, as well.

Sources: Wisconsin Library Services and Using the Internet.

According to the Wall Street Journal, some of the best medical information can be found right in your mailbox in health newsletters like those published by Harvard, Johns Hopkins, Tufts and the Mayo Clinic.

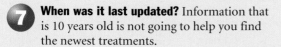

6 **Who paid for the study?** Some studies are funded by entities that benefit from the results. Look for independent studies that support reported findings.

7 **When was it last updated?** Information that is 10 years old is not going to help you find the newest treatments.

8 Add up your evidence and decide if it's truth or fiction.

Source: Fairness & Accuracy in Reporting.

TIP
The US Department of Health and Human Services can refer you to reliable online information.

healthfinder.gov

CONSUMER ALERT

When your doctor says, "Something's not right," whether it's a diagnosis of cancer or pneumonia, you're bound to feel alarmed or even panicked. Take heart. Health information is increasingly consumer friendly, making it easier for you to understand and interpret. And, if you don't understand it, ask your doctor. There are no stupid questions! It's well worth the effort for your peace of mind and your health!

Source: National Institutes of Health.

It's called e-health and millions are doing it— going online to research health topics.

According to a 2002 Harris Poll, 80% of all online adults look for healthcare information on the Internet.

In 2002, **110 million people** went online for health information. That's 13 million more than 2001.

% of adults looking for health information online

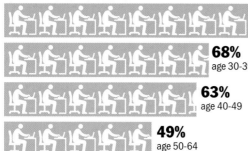

82% age 18-29

68% age 30-39

63% age 40-49

49% age 50-64

26% age 65+

Source: Harris Interactive.

? What is healthfinder.gov and how can it help me?

Healthfinder®, developed by the US Department of Health and Human Services and other federal agencies, is a resource for finding the best health information on the Internet. You'll find information and links to Web sites from over 1,800 organizations in English and Spanish. Sections include:

Help for healthcare choices
Information to help you on a wide range of topics —from finding background on healthcare providers, to hospitals and nursing homes ratings, to guides for selecting health insurance.

Health news
Updated daily on new studies and treatments.

Online tools
Check your diabetes or cancer risks, estimate your risk of a heart attack, learn whether you need professional help for depression symptoms.

Health library
Health information from A to Z — prevention and wellness, diseases and conditions, and alternative medicine—plus medical dictionaries, an encyclopedia and journals .

Directory
Selected health information web sites from government agencies, clearinghouses, non-profits and universities.

Children's area
Kids 8-12 can play games that teach about fire safety, nutrition and healthy habits, enter art contests and research several health-related topics, including smoking, alcohol, feelings and exercise.

Source: Healthfinder®.

? What kind of support can I find?

If you want face-to-face support, such as ongoing support group meetings, the Internet can help you find local and national non-profit organizations that provide education and support. If you prefer something more anonymous, many web sites offer "communities" that you can access online. Communities are online discussions about specific topics. When accessing these communities, you can choose to keep your name and other identifying information private.

The American Diabetes Association, for example, conducts online community forums on topics like eating right and healthy living. Or, you can choose a topic for people who are newly diagnosed with diabetes or who have either Type 1 or Type 2 diabetes. Read what other people have to say and ask your own questions.

General health web sites also have communities or forums on a variety of health topics. You can write (post) a question to these communities. People can read your question and respond if they wish.The best thing about online communities is that they're open 24 hours a day—whenever you need a little help.

Another source of support you can find on the Internet is centered around special online events. Often doctors or other healthcare professionals are online at specific times to answer questions for group members.

Source: American Diabetes Association.

ACTION ITEMS   Evaluating web sites

Look critically at the content of a web site before you decide if it is a good source of information. In other words, consider the source! Below are suggestions on what to look for. If you're still not sure about something you found, ask your doctor.

Be wary of web sites that:
- Offer "cures" for incurable diseases
- Sell drugs without a doctor's prescription
- Sell subscribers' lists

Source: AARP.

Check the quality of web health information by asking yourself questions about:

Content

Is the content factual, current, comprehensive and referenced? Does the site provide an editorial review process?

Author

Is the author qualified to write about this subject? What are the author's credentials and training? Are there any conflicts of interest?

?What are some reliable sites I can use?

American Academy of Family Physicians
`www.familydoctor.org`
Questions and answers about common health concerns and medicines, herbal remedies and dietary supplements, advice about self care and a listing of family physicians and practices.

Centers for Disease Control and Prevention
`www.cdc.gov`
Information about various health issues including traveler's health, data and statistics and publications.

HIV InSite
`www.hivinsite.com`
Information on HIV/AIDS treatment, prevention and policy.103

Health Care Choices
`www.healthcarechoices.org`
Health Care Choices is a non-profit corporation that seeks to educate the public about the health care system. The site contains information about hospitals, physicians and health insurance.

Health Care Coach
`www.healthcarecoach.org`
Run by the National Health Law Program, a nonprofit legal organization, this site contains popular articles, a question and answer section, action steps for advocating for yourself and your family, and other topics including lowering costs and women's health.

KidsHealth
`www.kidshealth.org`
Provides families with health care information with separate areas for children, teens and parents. The site features articles, animations, games and resources.

Mayo Clinic
`www.mayoclinic.com`
Contains information about specific diseases and medications. It includes guides to assist consumers in making health care decisions and an "ask the specialist" service.

Medline plus
`www.medlineplus.gov`
Sponsored by the National Library of Medicine and the National Institutes of Health, this site covers many topics and includes a medical encyclopedia. It also offers current health news and interactive tutorials. The site has links to numerous sites from around the world, including a link to the regular Medline site, a database of references to over 11 million articles published in more than 4,000 biomedical journals.

National Cancer Institute
`www.cancer.gov`
Information about various types of cancer, research programs and funding, clinical trials and cancer-related statistics.87

NOAH: New York Online Access to Health
`www.noah-health.org`
Sponsored by a consortium of libraries in New York, NOAH seeks to provide access to consumer health information in English and Spanish that is accurate, timely, relevant and unbiased. The site contains information and resources on a variety of health topics.

Source: Medical Library Association.

Frequently used Internet terms

Browser The software application used to display the Internet. The most popular are Microsoft Internet Explorer and Netscape Navigator.

Cookie A software program that contains a user's personal information, such as passwords or web sites they have visited. Web sites use "cookies" to make it easier for users to get back onto a site. It also builds a profile of the user, which many people find objectionable for privacy reasons.

Discussion board These areas of web sites allow people to read and write messages about a particular topic. Also called newsgroups, forums, discussion groups and bulletin boards.

E-newsletter Many organizations and businesses produce newsletters that are sent through the Internet to people's email addresses.

Internet Service Provider (ISP) A company that provides access to the Internet.

Link Also called hyperlink, links are usually underlined in blue on a web page and when a cursor is placed over it and clicked, it will take you to a new page, web site or document.

Portable Document Format (PDF) An Adobe Systems software application that displays documents to readers. When a document is "PDF'd" it retains the formatting and graphics that might be lost in another program.

Search engine A program that searches for keywords in documents or web sites. Google (google.com) and AltaVista (altavista.com) are examples of search engines.

Source: The Web Content Style Guide, G. McGovern, R. Norton and C. O'Dowd.

?How can I use the Internet to get healthcare information?

The Internet is an incredibly powerful source of information.

?Are my online activities private?

There are no absolutes when it comes to privacy on the Internet. Reputable web sites have privacy policies that are usually easy to find. These policies state how your information will be used. Read them. However, you have little recourse if the web site violates its own policy. According to the Federal Electronic Communications Privacy Act (ECPA), it is not illegal to read or disclose an electronic communication if the communication is "readily accessible" to the public.

Your posts to newsgroups and listserves are considered public messages that can be viewed by anyone at anytime. Some Internet service providers (ISPs) publicly list all their subscribers, including personal information. Ask your ISP about its policy. You can request your information be removed. Some ISP's sell their lists to marketing companies. Again, ask about your ISP's policy.

Purpose

Is the information written to inform you? Or explain something to you? Or is it trying to persuade you to do something? Is it balanced in terms of pros and cons?

Disclosure

Is the purpose of the site adequately explained? How the content was developed? Who owns the site? And, who pays for content development? Is it clear if the site is selling a product or services?

Sources: Gerald Tucker Memorial Medical Library, Health Summit Working Group.

CONSUMER ALERT

Look past the fluff! Most Internet users rate a web site's credibility by how attractive they find the site rather than any documented criteria, such as privacy and security policies, source information or how often information is updated. Read this information before you review the site's content. It should be easy to find. If it isn't, keep looking—it may be that the source of the information has buried its identity. There are plenty of credible web sites. Don't settle for less.

Source: Consumers Union, How Do People Evaluate a Web Site's Credibility?

YOUR CONTACT INFORMATION:

Name

Phone

Address

Date of birth

City/State/Zip

❏ Living will ❏ Organ donor

PRIMARY CARE PHYSICIAN:

Name

Phone

Address

Fax

City/State/Zip

Email

PRIMARY EMERGENCY CONTACT:

Name

Phone

Address

Phone

City/State/Zip

Email

SECONDARY EMERGENCY CONTACT:

Name

Phone

Address

Phone

City/State/Zip

Email

PRIMARY INSURANCE COMPANY:

Name

Phone

Address

Policy number

City/State/Zip

Subscriber number

SECONDARY INSURANCE COMPANY:

Name

Phone

Address

Policy number

City/State/Zip

Subscriber number

ADVOCATE/HEALTHCARE PROXY:

Name

Phone

Address

Phone

City/State/Zip

Relationship

MEDICATIONS:

1 _____
Dose _____ times per day _____ Begin _____ End _____

Reason _____

2 _____
Dose _____ times per day _____ Begin _____ End _____

Reason _____

3 _____
Dose _____ times per day _____ Begin _____ End _____

Reason _____

4 _____
Dose _____ times per day _____ Begin _____ End _____

Reason _____

5 _____
Dose _____ times per day _____ Begin _____ End _____

Reason _____

6 _____
Dose _____ times per day _____ Begin _____ End _____

Reason _____

7 _____
Dose _____ times per day _____ Begin _____ End _____

Reason _____

8 _____
Dose _____ times per day _____ Begin _____ End _____

Reason _____

9 _____
Dose _____ times per day _____ Begin _____ End _____

Reason _____

ALLERGIES:

_____   _____
Allergen   Reaction

_____   _____
Allergen   Reaction

_____   _____
Allergen   Reaction

FAMILY MEDICAL HISTORY (MOTHER, FATHER, GRANDPARENTS, CHILDREN):

_____   _____
Relationship   Condition

_____   _____
Relationship   Condition

_____   _____
Relationship   Condition

_____   _____
Relationship   Condition

EMERGENCY NUMBERS:

Rescue _____   Poison control _____

Fire _____   Other _____

Police _____   Other _____

CONTACTS (SPECIALISTS, DENTISTS, HOSPITALS, REHAB CENTERS, TESTING FACILITIES, ETC.):

Health care Provider/Facility _____   Phone _____

Address _____   Fax _____

City/State/Zip _____   Email _____

Health care Provider/Facility _____   Phone _____

Address _____   Fax _____

City/State/Zip _____   Email _____

Health care Provider/Facility _____   Phone _____

Address _____   Fax _____

City/State/Zip _____   Email _____

Health care Provider/Facility _____   Phone _____

Address _____   Fax _____

City/State/Zip _____   Email _____

Health care Provider/Facility _____   Phone _____

Address _____   Fax _____

City/State/Zip _____   Email _____

Health care Provider/Facility _____   Phone _____

Address _____   Fax _____

City/State/Zip _____   Email _____

Health care Provider/Facility

Phone

Address

Fax

City/State/Zip

Email

Health care Provider/Facility

Phone

Address

Fax

City/State/Zip

Email

Health care Provider/Facility

Phone

Address

Fax

City/State/Zip

Email

Health care Provider/Facility

Phone

Address

Fax

City/State/Zip

Email

Health care Provider/Facility

Phone

Address

Fax

City/State/Zip

Email

Health care Provider/Facility

Phone

Address

Fax

City/State/Zip

Email

Health care Provider/Facility

Phone

Address

Fax

City/State/Zip

Email

IMPORTANT HEALTHCARE EVENTS (SYMPTOMS, DIAGNOSES, SURGERIES, TREATMENTS, ETC.):

Date (M/D/Y)

Date (M/D/Y)

Date	Height/ Weight	Blood Pressure	LDL/HDL	Triglycerides

GLUCOSE	PSA (M)	PAP (W)	MAMMOGRAM (W)	OTHER TESTS
GLUCOSE	PSA	PAP	MAMMOGRAM	OTHER TESTS

REVIEWERS

The following experts read and reviewed various sections of this book under the direction of FACCT. We deeply thank them for their time, direction, diligence and knowledge.

Understanding Yourself
Elizabeth Hays, MD; Greenfield Health
Sam W. Ho, MD; PacifiCare Health Systems
Sunil Khanna, PhD; Department of Anthropology, Oregon State University
Gabrielle Meyers, MD; Utah Health Sciences Center

Staying Healthy
L. Kris Gowen, PhD, EdM, FACCT/Portland State University
Sam W. Ho, MD; PacifiCare Health Systems
Kathleen Weaver, MD, FACP; State of Oregon Health Policy and Research

Diseases & Conditions
Diana Bianco, JD; FACCT
Peter Block, MD; Emory Health Care
Py Driscoll, MD; Highland General Hospital
Cynthia Ferrier, MD; Greenfield Health
L. Kris Gowen, PhD, EdM, FACCT/Portland State University
David Hays, MD; Greenfield Health
Elizabeth Hays, MD; Greenfield Health
Chuck Kilo, MD, MPH; Greenfield Health
Sam W. Ho, MD; PacifiCare Health Systems
Katie Maslow; Alzheimer's Association
Susan Prows, PhD MPH; FACCT
Ellen Stovall; National Coalition for Cancer Survivorship
Daniel H. Solomon, MD, MPH; Brigham and Women's Hospital

Diagnosis
William A. Barnett, OD; South River Eye Care; Bowie Optometric Group
Py Driscoll, MD; Highland General Hospital
Cynthia Ferrier, MD; Greenfield Health
Sam W. Ho, MD; PacifiCare Health Systems
Lisa D. Kelly, MD; Kelly Eye Care
Chuck Kilo, MD, MPH; Greenfield Health

Treatment
Cynthia Ferrier, MD; Greenfield Health
Scott Hurlbert, MD
Lisa D. Kelly, MD; Kelly Eye Care
Chuck Kilo, MD, MPH; Greenfield Health
Molly C. McKenna, PhD; clinical psychologist
Gabrielle Meyers, MD; Utah Health Sciences Center
John C. Meyers, PharmD; Oregon Health & Science University
Susan Prows, PhD, MPH; FACCT
Michael D. Skokan, MD; The Oregon Clinic P.C.

People
William A. Barnett, OD; South River Eye Care; Bowie Optometric Group
David Hays, MD; Greenfield Health
Lisa D. Kelly, MD; Kelly Eye Care
Connie Leben, PMHNP; Sundstrom & Associates, PC
Molly C. McKenna, PhD; clinical psychologist
Jeffrey A. Poland, OD; Lifetime Eyecare Center; president, Maryland Optometric Association

Places
James D. McMahan, MD; Advanced Aesthetic & Reconstructive Surgery, Inc.

Technology
Cynthia Ferrier, MD; Greenfield Health
John C. Meyers, PharmD; Oregon Health & Science University
Lee Michels, MD; Radiology Associates, PC
Blackford Middleton, MD, MPH, MSc; Partners Healthcare
Karen Williams; National Pharmaceutical Council

Money
Robert Berenson, MD; AcademyHealth
Jack A. Friedman; Regence Blue Cross Blue Shield of Oregon
Susan Prows, PhD, MPH; FACCT
Shelley Rouillard; Health Rights Hotline

Legal
Diana Bianco, JD; FACCT

FACCT–Foundation for Accountability is a non-profit organization with a mission to improve healthcare for Americans. FACCT advocates for a healthcare system where consumers are partners in their care and help shape the delivery of care. FACCT accomplishes its mission through monitoring health policy and informing healthcare leaders and consumers on the impact of these policies.

www.facct.org

FACCT Staff
Nancy Bateman, FACCT's Editor & Communications Program Manager, has been writing about healthcare for two decades. As a healthcare journalist her writing has appeared nationwide in print publications and on the Internet for Websites such as WebMD and HealthAnswers. She was one of the many health writers involved with A.D.A.M. Inc.'s award-winning health illustrated encyclopedia.

Diana Bianco, JD
Aryne Blumklotz, MPH
Michelle DuBarry
L. Kris Gowen, PhD, EdM
Kim Meyers, MPH
Barbara Porter
Susan Prows, PhD, MPH

Our appreciation to Greenfield Health System for their major contributions and their collaboration with FACCT on this book.

www.greenfieldhealth.com

INFORMATION ARCHITECTS

Explanation Graphics

Nigel Holmes

A fellow information architect whose work & contributions to the field cannot be overestimated from his ground-breaking 16 years at TIME to being a key team member of many of RSW's recent publications including, *Understanding USA*, *Diagnostic Tests for Men and Women* & *Understanding Children*. This is his seventh book project with RSW.

    staff: Sharon Stea

www.nigelholmes.com

Pentagram

Kit Hinrichs, partner

Pentagram is an international design consultancy, specializing in graphic design, product design, architecture & interactive design. Powerful contributions to *Understanding USA*.

    staff: Belle Howe
              Takayo Muroga

www.pentagram.com

Medical Broadcasting Company

Linda Holliday, president

MBC is a provider of marketing strategies and solutions for the healthcare & pharmaceutical industries. Contributed in a seminal manner to *Understanding Children*.

    staff: Alex vonPlato
              Anne Wren
              Maryann Porch
              Jamie Cohen
              Rob Macoviak
              Tom Mullins

www.mbcnet.com

Agnew Moyer Smith Inc.

John Sotirakis, principal designer

AMS is a nationally recognized design firm helping businesses untangle complex communication problems & explain important ideas by making their messages visible, understandable & accessible. Important contributions to *Understanding USA*, *Understanding Children* & *Wills, Trusts & Estate Planning*.

    staff: Kurt Hess, principal illustrator
              Mary Beth Baniecki
               Bill DeRose
              Mike Duda
              Jack Kelley
              Don Moyer
              Amy Oriss
              Christina Papp
              Mimi Wlodek
              Cat Zaccardi

www.amsite.com

Ingo Fast

Ingo Fast's whimsical drawings convey the explorative spirit of a child's playful character. They can be seen in newspapers, magazines & books.

www.ingofast.com

Rigsby Design

Lana Rigsby, principal

For over a decade they have been focused on helping companies and institutions communicate in ways that are clear at all scales.

    staff: Thomas Hull
              Travis Rimel
              Sara Gray

www.rigsbydesign.com

SPONSORS

Understanding Healthcare owes its publication to the vision and commitment of Johnson & Johnson. As the world's most comprehensive and broadly based healthcare company, whose operations span the entire healthcare universe, from consumer and pharmaceutical to medical devices and diagnostics, Johnson & Johnson is dedicated to improving the quality of life for people around the world. Through its support of this book, Johnson & Johnson is helping to raise awareness of essential information about accessing medical care today.

www.jnj.com

This book would not have been possible without the generous support of UnitedHealth Group. UnitedHealth Group, through its family of companies, is a leader in advancing, promoting and facilitating health. It is their belief that consumers should have access to trustworthy information as they make decisions to improve their health, that of their families and the communities in which they live.

Special thanks to Steve Hemsley, President and Chief Operating Officer of UnitedHealth Group, for his early recognition of the potential of this project.

www.unitedhealthgroup.com

As a part of its commitment to improving people's lives in the information age, the Markle Foundation focuses on using information and communications technologies to address critical public needs, particularly in the areas of healthcare and national security. The Markle Foundation's overarching goal in the health area is to accelerate the rate at which information technology enables consumers and the health system that supports them to improve health and healthcare.

www.markle.org

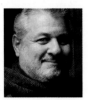

Richard Saul Wurman, with the publication of his first book at the age of 26, began the singular passion of his life: making information understandable. In his best-selling book, *Information Anxiety*, in 1989 (& then again in 2000 with *Information Anxiety2*), RSW developed an overview of the motivating principles found in his previous works. Each of his 80-some books focuses on some subject or idea that he personally had difficulty understanding. They all stem from his desire to know rather than from already knowing; from his ignorance rather than his intelligence; from his inability rather than his ability.

RSW has received both M. Arch. & B. Arch. degrees from the University of Pennsylvania, in 1959 graduating with highest honors & the Arthur Spayd Brookes Gold Medal. He established a deep personal & professional relationship with the architect Louis I. Kahn. He is a fellow of the American Institute of Architects (FAIA). He has been awarded several grants from the National Endowment for the Arts, a Guggenheim Fellowship, two Graham Fellowships & two Chandler Fellowships. In 1991, RSW received the Kevin Lynch Award from MIT for his creation of the ACCESS travel guides & was honored by a retrospective exhibition of his work at the AXIS Design Gallery in Tokyo, Japan on the occasion of their 10th Anniversary. He received the Chrysler Design Award, a Doctorate of Fine Arts by the University of the Arts in Philadelphia, an Honorary Doctorate of Letters from Art Center College of Design & an Honorary Doctorate of Fine Arts from the Art Institute of Boston. In 2003, he was inducted into the Art Director's Hall of Fame.

He chaired the International Design in Aspen in 1972, the first Federal Design Assembly in 1973 & the National AIA Convention in 1976 before creating & chairing TED (Technology, Entertainment & Design) Conferences from 1984-2002. He continues chairing TEDMED Conferences.

RSW & his wife, novelist & lyricist Gloria Nagy, have four children & five grandchildren. They live in Newport, RI with Max & Abraham (their dogs).

David Lansky is the President of FACCT– Foundation for Accountability, a non-profit group that provided collaboration & fact checking for this book.

For more than 20 years, Dr. Lansky has advocated for a more responsive & accountable healthcare system. As an expert in quality measurement & healthcare accountability, he is a sought after speaker nationally & internationally. His inspirational vision of what healthcare can be for consumers inspires national leaders & policymakers to look at new methods of improving the US healthcare system.

Lansky has served as a board member or advisor to numerous healthcare projects & programs, including the National Quality Forum, the Joint Commission on Accreditation of Healthcare Organizations, the National Patient Safety Foundation, The Leapfrog Group & President Bush's 2002 Economic Summit.

Prior to FACCT, Lansky was a senior policy analyst for the Jackson Hole Group during the national healthcare reform debate of 1993-94. He also led the Center for Outcomes Research & Education at Oregon-based Providence Health System.

Loren Barnett Appel has assisted RSW on 11 of his last publications including four focusing on healthcare, two on financial issues, the critically acclaimed *Understanding USA* & *Understanding Children*.

Loren has served as director for TOP contributing as production manager, researcher, writer & information architect. Her unique skills have meshed with the method of producing TOP books using a virtual office to manage the activities of many of the best information architects in the US.

Loren has lived & worked in Newport, RI & now resides in Annapolis, MD with her husband James & daughter Helen.

A selection of books authored, co-authored, published & designed by Richard Saul Wurman:

1960s
Cities: A Comparison of
  Form and Scale
The Notebook and
  Drawings of Louis I.
  Kahn
Urban Atlas: 20 American
  Cities (with Joseph
  Passonneau)
Various Dwellings
  Described in a
  Comparative Manner
1970s
Aspen Visible
Guidebook to Guidebooks
Making the City
  Observable
Man Made Philadelphia
  (with J.A. Gallery)
The Nature of Recreation
  (with Alan Levy &
  Joel Katz)

Our Man Made
  Environment Book 7
  (with Alan Levy)
What-If, Could-Be: An
  Historic Fable of the
  Future
Yellow Pages Career
  Library (12 volumes)
Yellow Pages of Learning
  Resources
1980s
Baseball Access
Dog Access
Football Access
Hawaii Access
Las Vegas Access
London Access
Los Angeles Access
Medical Access
New Orleans Access
New York City Access
Olympic Access

Paris Access
Polaroid Access
Rome Access
San Francisco Access
Summer Games Access
Tokyo Access
Hats
Information Anxiety
Wall Street Journal Guide
  to Understanding
  Money & Markets
Washington, DC Access
What Will Be Has Always
  Been, The Words of
  Louis I. Kahn
Winter Games Access
1990s
Barcelona Access
Boston Access
C, The Charleston Guide
California Wine Country
  Access

Chicago Access
Danny Goodman's
  Macintosh
  Handbook
  (with Danny
  Goodman)
Florence/Venice/Milan
  Access
Follow the Yellow Brick
  Road
  (with Loring Leifer)
Fortune Guide to Investing
  in the 90's
Information Architects
N, The Newport Guide
On Time, Airline Guide to
  North America
Office Access
San Diego Access
Twin Peaks Access
  (with David Lynch)
USAtlas

2000s
Understanding USA
Can I Afford To Retire?
Information Anxiety2
Drugs: Prescription,
  Non-prescription &
  Herbal
Heart Disease &
  Cardiovascular Health
Wills, Trusts & Estate
  Planning
Diagnostic Tests for
  Men
Diagnostic Tests for
  Women
Understanding Children
  (with Civitas)
1000 - Richard Saul
  Wurman's Who's
  Really Who
Understanding
  Healthcare